A GLOBAL SCIENTIFIC VISION - PREVENTION, DIAGNOSIS, AND TREATMENT OF LUNG CANCER

Edited by **Marta Adonis**

A Global Scientific Vision - Prevention, Diagnosis, and Treatment of Lung Cancer
http://dx.doi.org/10.5772/63687
Edited by Marta Adonis

Contributors
John Anthony Alvan Nichols, Petr Starostik, Stephan Jahn, Trevor Rogers, Tao Sun, Yuan Qin, Wei-Long Zhong, Shuang Chen, Guanghu Wang, Cheng Zule, Hongju Mao, Peter Lee, Karen Zeman, Corey Carter, Christina Brzezniak, Li Zhang, Keely FitzGerald, Chantal Vidal, Purna Chaitanya Konduri, Hyuntae Yoo, Chuan-Mu Chen, Romeo Ioan Chira, Alexandra Chira, Petru Adrian Mircea, Mirjana Rajer

Published by InTech
Janeza Trdine 9, 51000 Rijeka, Croatia

Publishing Process Manager Dajana Pemac
Technical Editor SPi Global
Cover InTech Design team

First published February, 2017
Printed in Croatia
Legal deposit, Croatia: National and University Library in Zagreb

Additional hard copies can be obtained from orders@intechopen.com

A Global Scientific Vision - Prevention, Diagnosis, and Treatment of Lung Cancer, Edited by Marta Adonis
p. cm.
Print ISBN 978-953-51-2965-3
Online ISBN 978-953-51-2966-0

For EU product safety concerns:
IN TECH d.o.o., Prolaz Marije Krucifikse Kozulić 3, 51000 Rijeka, Croatia,
info@intechopen.com or visit our website at intechopen.com.

Meet the editor

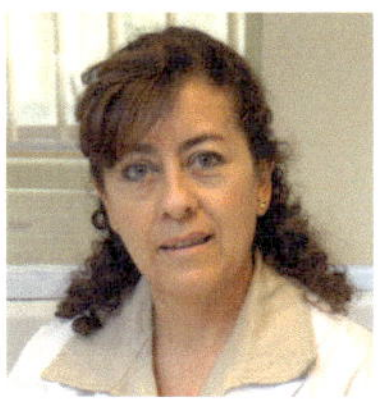

Dr. Marta Adonis has a wide experience as a director, leading and managing national and international research projects, as well as in human capacity building. At the research level, she has participated in different national and international projects, not only relevant at the scientific level but also with important public impact. Her role in each grant has been related with the formulation, development, human capacity building, and national and international diffusion through different media (scientific journals, newspapers, TV and radio interview, congress, workshops, etc.) Dr. Adonis has several publications not only in journals but also books, related mainly to science, technology, and medicine.

Contents

Preface

Probably, if our ancestors could come back to this life, they would be very surprised and amazed with each thing that invades all of our space and life: huge buildings, technology that includes cars, airplanes, cell phones, and many other things that we do not have a real awareness of. Within all the advances that are part of our daily life, it is important to mention the huge effort, without limit, that we make to prolong life. My parents who are 86 years old are part, as many people, of the advances and at this age when people and family dream "to be together for many years and that the grandparents get to know their grandchildren and the children get to know their grandparents." Thanks to the technology, people are more informed not only in relation to what to eat, but also in relation to what to do and how to prevent any risk factor. Many scientists work endlessly in order to have a safer car or airplane and others work to get to the technology to cure diseases so that people can lead a more healthy life. And I am one of those scientists working for many years to identify people with high lung cancer risk and trying to find signals that can show if something is wrong and if it is related with abnormalities that can put at risk a life. Possibly, for cancer, including lung cancer, the final aim is to find ways to make this devastating disease a chronic disease and that people could not only prevent the pathology but also live with the disease without any major problems.

My research is dedicated to lung cancer, not only for being the number one cause of cancer deaths around the world, but also because lung cancer occurs not only in people who smoke but also in people who are poor, who use polluted cooking and heating sources, and in people who are exposed naturally to toxic compounds present in indoor and outdoor environments such as arsenic (As) and radon (Rn). Additionally, it is important to point out that close to 14% of all new cancers in the world are lung cancer, and when detected at an earlier stage, the survival rate is up to 5 years. Although smoking is the first risk factor for lung cancer, 20% of people who die of lung cancer in the United States every year are nonsmokers. As per the information released for lung cancer, it can be inferred that lung cancer is not only a very complex disease, but it also does not depend on race, gender, country, or life style. The pathology can find a new victim in any place and in any moment of life.

Coming back to the main objective of life, leaving behind all the personal ambitions and only trying to prolong our own life and the lives of our beloved as long as possible, the scientists have too much work to do. At the moment, research related with the prevention is to identify people with medium- or high-risk to lung cancer that will allow to diminish the risk factors and help to detect the pathology in early stages. This research is not only needed but also crucial if we want to increase the survival to 5 years for each patient diagnosed with lung cancer. Diagnosis and early detection obviously need advances in technologies and professionals working as multidisciplinary teams to offer better ways to patients.

Prevention and early detection shall go hand in hand in providing the best possible treatment or personalized treatment with less toxicity, better outcomes, and why not with high precision that allows to consider each tumor and each patient as a particular individual.

What should science offer to the lung cancer patients in a near future or for what should the lung cancer patients wait from the science? Personalized treatment? Most time to enjoy the life? To consider the lung cancer as a chronic disease? Probably, science is still far away to give the patients and their family these answers; however, if each lung cancer patient demands more time to love, to enjoy, or to live, the aim of each scientist working on lung cancer should give hope to the patients to fight against this disease. The world, mainly the family of lung cancer patients, needs to understand that the contribution of science to this pathology is the product of many scientists working together, who spend many hours each day to improve the prevention, diagnose mainly in early stages, treat, and mainly survive this disease.

This book is a demonstration of the scientists who are working for a better life, trying to improve the quality of life of humans. The work and chapter of each author shows the compromise with improvement not only the diagnosis, treatment of lung cancer and also the quality of life of each patients and the pain produced to their families and friends. This book will provide interesting information and reference sources to professionals from different areas and specializations. This book will contribute positively to the knowledge and advances in the prevention, diagnosis, and treatment of lung cancer.

I appreciate the invitation of InTech to work with them as editor of this book. For me, being a scientist has been a great experience. I have learned each author's thoughts from their chapter, and I have felt their love for their work. I appreciate the contribution of each author, and I really enjoyed reading their chapters. They have done a great work and I value their help and diligence. I think that people will find each lecture of this book as an interesting and useful material.

Marta Adonis
CeTeCancer
Faculty of Medicine, University of Chile
Independencia 1027, Santiago, Chile

Section 1

Lung Cancer and Smoking Habit

Chapter 1

The Epidemiology of Tobacco and Lung Cancer: Some Conclusions from a Lifetime of Research

Peter N. Lee

Additional information is available at the end of the chapter

http://dx.doi.org/10.5772/67167

Abstract

This review summarizes evidence on the smoking/lung cancer relationship, based on the author's 50 years' experience. It starts by illustrating variations in national rates by time and sex. It then demonstrates that the relationship of smoking to overall lung cancer risk is strong, consistently seen and dose-related with amount smoked, duration, age of start and time of quitting. Relative risks vary markedly by country, but little by sex, age, race, occupation, genetics and other factors. Though precisely estimating the smoking risk is difficult, the relationship is clearly causal, not explained by bias or confounding. The risk from smoking is reduced in lower tar filter cigarettes, and essentially independent of mentholation and type of curing. Lung cancer risk is not increased by smokeless tobacco use. The relative risk is much greater for squamous/small-cell carcinoma than for adeno/large-cell carcinoma. The argument that the increasing ratio of squamous to adenocarcinoma results from changes in cigarettes is shown to be weak, the increase also being seen in never smokers, starting before filters were introduced, and associated with diagnostic changes. Most of the weak association of lung cancer with passive smoking is explicable by confounding and by misclassification of some ever smokers as never smokers.

Keywords: smoking, lung cancer, trends, dose response, quitting smoking, confounding, bias, cigarettes, tar reduction, compensation, mentholation, flue-cured, blended, histological type, passive smoking

1. Introduction

While, at the beginning of the twentieth century, lung cancer was a rare disease, it was diagnosed progressively more often over the next 50 years, and various suggestions were made during this period that cigarette smoking might be the cause, deriving mainly from the simple fact that the incidence and cigarette consumption were increasing concomitantly [1]. Although earlier case-control studies had been conducted in Germany [2, 3], it was not until studies in the UK [4] and in the USA [5] published in the 1950s that serious attention was given to the possibility that smoking might cause lung cancer. Following additional evidence from a number of large prospective studies, the US Surgeon General concluded [6] that 'cigarette smoking is a cause of lung cancer in men, and a suspected cause of lung cancer in women', and later reports [7–9] have confirmed and extended the conclusions.

Following a section which concerns trends in lung cancer rates, this review summarizes the evidence on a number of aspects of the relationship of smoking with lung cancer, and also considers the evidence on environmental tobacco smoke (ETS) or 'passive smoking'. In general, less attention is given to those aspects that are well-known and non-contentious, while dealing more fully with areas where the evidence is more open to interpretation. Concentration also tends to be in areas where the author and his colleagues have been involved in detailed reviews of the evidence. As the author has some 50 years of experience, this covers quite a wide range of topics, though not all.

2. Trends in lung cancer rates

Figure 1 shows trends in lung cancer rates in eight countries over the period 1946–2010. They are presented separately for males and females and for age 15+, weighted according to the age distribution of the European standard population. As can be seen, rates in males always substantially exceed rates in females. While in each country rates in males have risen to a peak and then declined, rates of females have tended to rise over the whole period, though there is evidence of flattening out in some countries. The differing trends in the two sexes are consistent with differing trends in the take up of smoking, which can be clearly seen in the detailed data presented in International Smoking Statistics [10].

For both sexes, there is striking variation by country in the trends seen. Points to note are the relatively low rates in Sweden and in Japan, and the rapidly accelerating rates in Hungary, so that in males, rates are now almost double those elsewhere. It is interesting that the lung cancer rates in Canada and the USA are so similar, given the type of tobacco predominantly used in Canada is made only from flue-cured tobacco, while American cigarettes are blended, a topic discussed further in Section 3.5.

Trends in the UK are markedly different from those in other countries, particularly in males. In the 1950s, rates in males were much higher than in other countries, but following a much earlier and steeper decline than elsewhere, are now below those in all countries except Japan and Sweden. In 1998, Lee and Forey [11] attempted to determine whether the trends could be fully explained by trends in cigarette consumption, concluding that they could not, with factors other than cigarette smoking contributing importantly to risk. A contributor to the declining trend may have been the introduction of the Clean Air Act in the UK in 1956.

The trends in the UK are very different from those in the USA. Thus, UK rates, once much higher than in the USA, are now lower in both sexes. To some extent, this may have coloured differing national opinions on the benefits (or otherwise) of changes from high tar plain

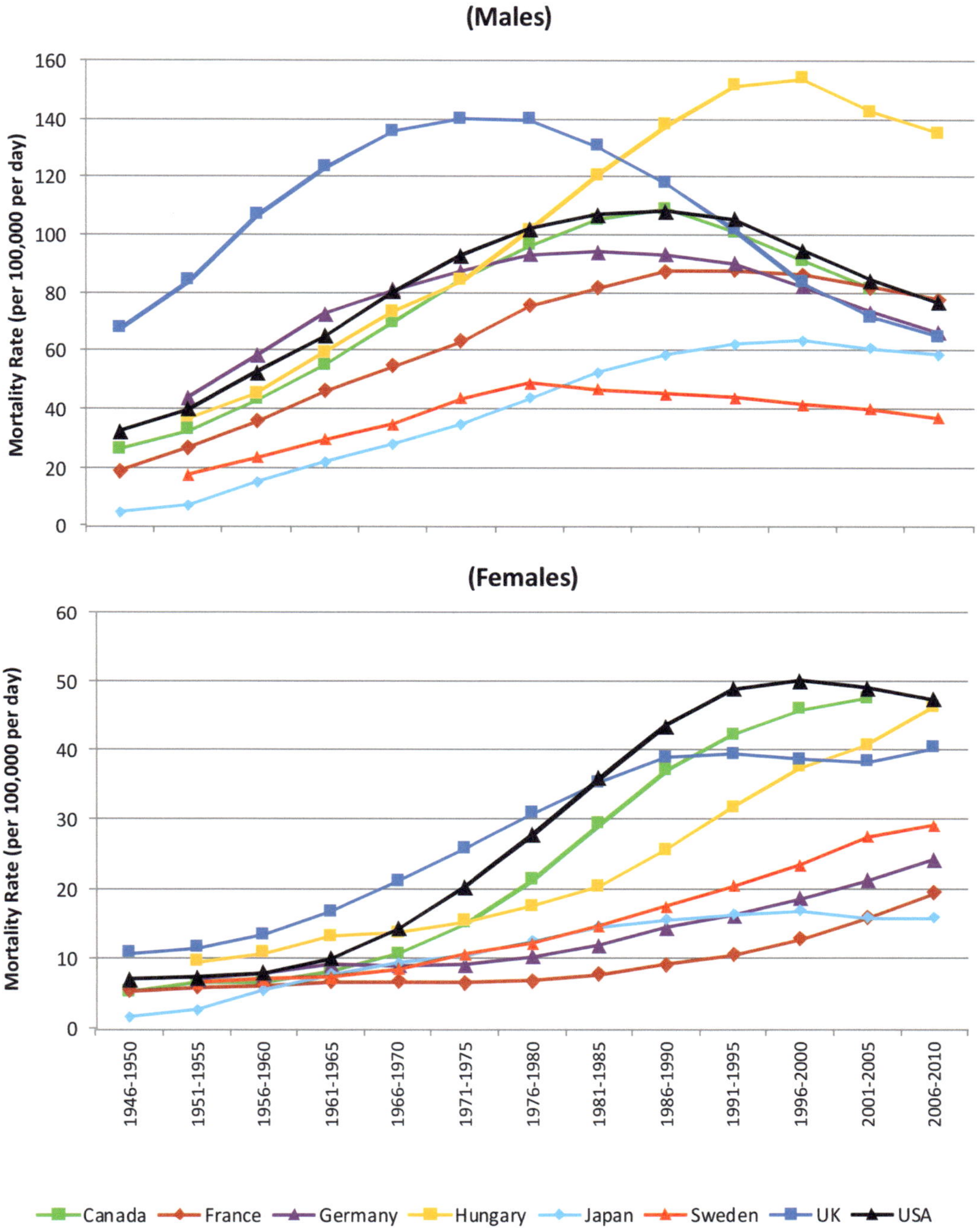

Figure 1. Lung cancer mortality rates by country and period.

cigarettes to low-tar filtered cigarettes. In 2003, Lee and Forey [12] looked in detail at the question as to why the trends in the US and UK are so different. Their analyses took into account detailed data on trends in the age of starting and stopping smoking, amount smoked per smoker and tar levels, and demonstrated clearly that the differing trends in lung cancer rates could not be explained by these factors. They concluded that the explanation must lie in changes over time in aspects of smoking not considered in the analyses and/or exposure to risk factors other than smoking. Evidence relating to a number of possible such smoking variables or other risk factors was considered, but no clear explanation of the differing trends could be found. Lee and Forey [12] also criticised views expressed in NCI Monograph 13 [13], in particular that tar reduction has been ineffective in lowering lung cancer risk, and that trends in US lung cancer rates fit in well with trends in smoking habits.

3. Relationship of smoking to overall lung cancer risk

In order to describe the main characteristics of the relationship, this section leans heavily on a recently published systematic review with meta-analysis by Lee et al. [14]. This involved all epidemiological studies published before 2000 which included at least 100 lung cancer cases, and which provided relevant information on risks associated with smoking. The meta-analyses involved almost 300 studies, far more than in any other published meta-analysis.

3.1. Dose-related increase in risk in current and former smokers

Although the relative risk (RR) estimates vary considerably between studies, the evidence of an association is extremely clear from the meta-analyses [14], with overall random-effects relative risk estimates of 5.50 (95% confidence interval [CI] 5.07–5.96) for ever smokers, 8.43 (7.63–9.31) for current smokers and 4.30 (3.93–4.71) for ex-smokers, these *RRs* all being expressed relative to those who have never smoked. Although the individual RR estimates are variable in magnitude, they are highly consistent in direction. Thus, of 195 sex-specific RR estimates for current smoking, every single one is greater than 1.0, and all but seven are individually statistically significant at $p < 0.05$, with as many as 27 of the *RRs* exceeding 20. These estimates are for smoking of any product or for cigarettes if results for any product were not available. Estimates for cigarette only smokers were less commonly available but were somewhat higher, with a combined estimate of 8.95 (7.76–10.33) for current smokers.

That there is a tendency for the RR to increase with number of cigarettes smoked per day is abundantly clear. Because studies vary in the groupings used to categorize amount smoked, analyses were included in the systematic review [14] comparing ever smoking *RRs* for three groups: 'about 5 cigs/day' (the category for which results provided includes 5 but not 20 cigs/day), 'about 20 cigs/day' (includes 20 but not 5 or 45 cigs/day), and 'about 45 cigs/day' (includes 45 but not 20 cigs/day). The *RRs* increased steadily with increasing amount smoked, being 3.49 (95% CI 3.13–3.89), 7.33 (6.29–8.54) and 13.69 (11.80–15.89) for the three groups.

Later Fry et al. [15], based on model-fitting techniques, successfully fitted the linear with baseline model $\log_e RR = 0.833 \log_e (1 + 0.81c)$ to 97 independent data blocks, where c is cigarettes smoked per day. This model predicted quite a linear relationship between c and *RR*, with the *RR* estimated as 3.86, 6.30, 10.71, 14.77, 18.62 and 22.31 for, respectively, 5, 10, 20, 30, 40 and 50 cigs/day (see **Figure 2**).

http://dx.doi.org/10.5772/67167

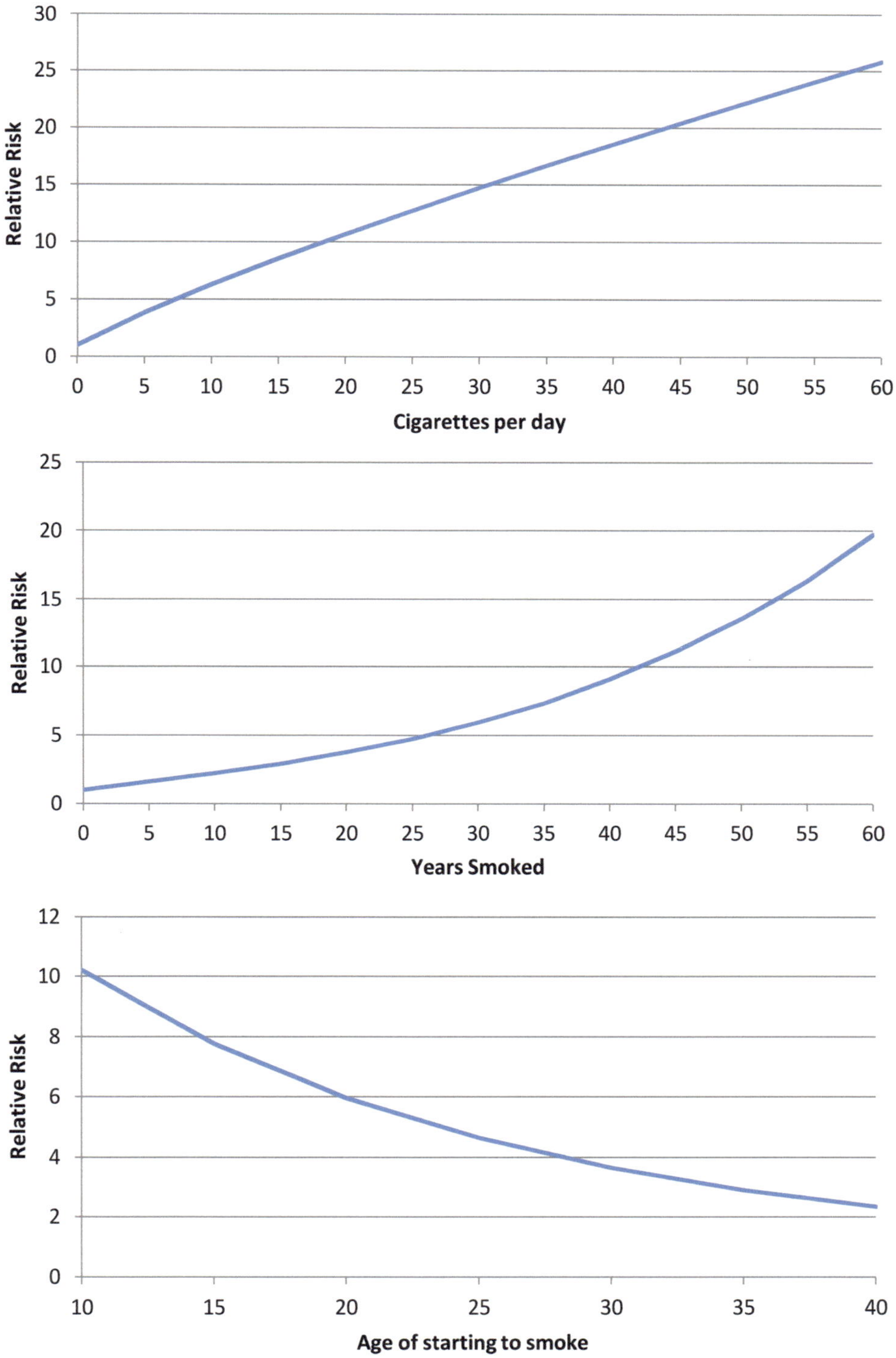

Figure 2. Dose-response relationships for current smoking fitted to 97, 35 and 27 independent data blocks for amount smoked, duration of smoking and age of starting to smoke.

For years smoked, the shape of the dose response was best fitted by a power model $\log_e RR = 0.792\ (y/10)^{0.74}$, where *y* is years smoked. When applied to 35 data sets, this predicted *RRs* of 2.21, 3.75, 5.96, 9.11 and 13.54 for, respectively, 10, 20, 30, 40 and 50 years smoked (**Figure 2**). Model-fitting techniques were also applied to data by age of starting to smoke, the best model being $\log_e RR = 0.176\ (7 - a/10)^{1.44}$, where *a* is age of start. Here, based on 27 data sets, the *RRs* declined sharply with increasing age of start, being 8.94, 7.80, 6.83, 5.99, 4.66 and 3.66 for, respectively, 12.5, 15, 17.5, 20, 25 and 30 years (**Figure 2**).

Although there is uncertainty as to the actual shape of the true dose-relationship, and misclassification of smoking status and dose may bias the fitted relationships to some extent, it is abundantly clear that risk of lung cancer increases markedly with increasing dose, whether quantified by increased daily amount smoked, increased duration of smoking, or earlier age of starting to smoke.

It is also clear that risk declines, relative to continuing smokers, in those who quit smoking. This is evident, not only from the lower *RRs* in ex-smokers than in current smokers noted above, but also from those studies that report results by time quit. In a review of studies published in the 1900s [14] it was estimated that, compared to current smokers, those who had quit for 'about 12 years' (the category for which results are provided includes 12 but not 7 years), 'about 7 years' (includes 7 but not 3 or 12 years), and 'about 3 years' (includes 3 but not 7 years) had, respectively, *RRs* of 0.28 (0.24–0.32), 0.57 (0.50–0.64) and 0.95 (0.84–1.08). The lack of any clear reduction in the short-term quitters is considered to be due to 'reverse causation' with some smokers quitting due to incipient disease.

A later paper [16], investigated whether the decline in RR of lung cancer following quitting (expressed relative to never smokers) could be adequately fitted by a simple, negative exponential, model. In this model, the excess relative risk ER (= *RR* – 1) following *t* years of quitting was estimated by multiplying the ER for a continuing smoker by the factor $\exp(-\frac{t \log_e 2}{H})$, where *H* is the estimated half-life. Thus, for example, if *H* is 10 years, and the *RR* for a continuing smoker is 11 (*ER* = 10), the *RR* for a quitter will be 6 after 10 years of quitting (the *ER* of 10 being halved to 5), 3.5 after 20 years, and 2.25 after 30 years, and will still be doubled after 35 years. Based on 106 independent data sets from 85 studies, published up to 2011, it was found that if reverse causation was ignored, the model fit was poor, but the fit was much improved if reverse causation was allowed for, either by ignoring short-term quitters, or by considering them to be smokers. For the best-fitting analysis (ignoring short-term quitters), *H* was estimated as 9.93 (95% 9.31–10.60), but varied by sex (females 7.92, males 10.71) and age (increasing from 6.98 for age <50 years to 12.99 for age 70+ years). It was concluded that the model adequately described the decline in ER, although precise estimates of *H* may be biased by misclassification of smoking status and failure to update smoking habits during follow-up in long-term prospective studies. The large value of *H* illustrates clearly the persistent effects of smoking.

As shown subsequently [17], the negative exponential model can quite simply be adapted to predict risk following changes in exposure more generally. The adaptation was shown to satisfactorily predict results from those (relatively few) studies that have investigated the effect of reducing cigarette consumption, and suggests it may be useful for predicting changes in risk following switching to a reduced exposure product.

3.2. Factors affecting risk

The age-specific absolute risk of lung cancer is known to be related to many factors other than smoking. These include alcohol, occupation, air pollution, diet, viruses and genetic factors [18].

However, the evidence considered in this section relates not to which factors modify the risk of lung cancer, but to which affect the RR associated with smoking.

3.2.1. Sex

There has been considerable discussion about whether smoking increases the risk of lung cancer more in women than in men, e.g. [19]. Based on the systematic review of Lee et al. [14], there was little evidence of any difference, though RR estimates generally tended to be higher for men than for women. This conclusion was supported by additional analyses comparing *RRs* within individual studies using the same definition of exposure and similar levels of amount smoked. The slightly higher *RRs* in men do not necessarily indicate any greater susceptibility, as they may reflect increased exposure to occupational carcinogens, differences in duration of smoking or increased use of higher tar and plain cigarettes. Note, however, that in prospective studies in which smoking habits are determined at baseline, the greater tendency of males to quit during follow-up may tend to understate the male/female ratio. Though it is difficult to get a precise answer on the male/female difference, these results appear to agree with the conclusion of Bain et al. [20] that 'women do not appear to have a greater susceptibility to lung cancer than men, given equal smoking exposure'.

3.2.2. Age

Though the absolute risk of lung cancer rises steeply with age, both in never and ever smokers, it is far less clear whether the RR also does, particularly when the great majority of published studies do not give results by age. However, a number of studies considered in the systematic review [14] did provide RR estimates for ever or current smoking separately by age, and it was possible to carry out meta-analyses based on the ratio within study of the estimate for the oldest age group for which data were available, compared to that for the youngest. While the meta-analysis did show a significantly higher risk in the oldest age group, the estimated average ratio (1.17, 95% CI 1.10–1.25) was quite modest. Clearly, any variation in RR by age is much smaller than the RR itself.

3.2.3. Location

There is a striking variation between study locations in the estimated RR associated with smoking. For current smoking, where the overall RR estimate for the sexes combined from meta-analyses [14], based on 195 estimates, was 8.43 (95% CI 7.63–9.31), the estimate was higher than this for studies based in North America (11.68, 10.61–12.85), and markedly lower than this for studies in China (2.94, 2.23–3.88), Japan (3.55, 3.05–4.14), and other parts of Asia (2.90, 2.04–4.13), with estimates intermediate in the United Kingdom (7.53, 5.40–10.50), Scandinavia (8.68, 7.14–10.54) and other parts of Europe (8.65, 5.98–12.51). The pattern of variation by location is similar if comparisons are based on ever rather than current smoking. The extent to which these quite clear differences are due to the product smoked, amount smoked, genetics or other factors, is a question which deserves further attention.

3.2.4. *Time*

The systematic review [14] generally showed a tendency for *RRs* to be lower in studies which started a long time ago. Thus, current smoker *RR* estimates rose continuously from 6.39 (95% CI 4.70–8.69) for studies starting before 1960 to 12.81 (8.70–18.85) for studies starting in the 1990s. Indeed, in the meta-regression analyses, start year of study and location were the most highly significant ($p < 0.001$) independent predictors of the current smoker RR. There are a number of possible reasons for the time trend, including changes in the use of cigarettes relative to pipes and cigars, and improvement in the quality of studies. However, the most plausible reason seems to be changes in patterns of uptake of smoking, with smokers in the earliest studies, born around the turn of the nineteenth century, being less likely to have had a lengthy smoking career than later-born smokers in more recent studies. Note that this increase occurs despite evidence, discussed in Section 3.4, that cigarettes have become somewhat less harmful due to reductions in tar and the switch to filters.

3.2.5. *Race*

Few studies considered in the systematic review [14] provided comparable *RRs* for ever or current smoking by race, and these results gave no indication that *RRs* for Whites differed systematically from those for Blacks (or non-Whites). Comparison of risks in Blacks and Whites is in any case made difficult by various differences in their smoking characteristics [21]. Thus, while in the USA. Blacks are more often current smokers, are less likely to quit smoking, smoke higher-tar cigarettes and have higher cotinine levels, all characteristics which would predict a higher risk of lung cancer, they are also less likely to have ever smoked, have lower daily cigarette consumption, and start smoking later, all characteristics predictive of a lower risk.

Other risk factors were not considered in detail in the systematic review [14]. However, reference is briefly made below to some of these.

3.2.6. *Asbestos and other occupational exposures*

It is well-known that asbestos exposure increases risk of lung cancer, though the increase depends materially on the type of asbestos. In an early large study of US insulation workers [22] *RRs*, compared to men who had never smoked cigarettes and who were unexposed to asbestos, were 5.17 for those exposed only to asbestos, 10.85 for those who had ever smoked only, and 53.24 for those exposed to both risk factors. These results, while suggesting a multiplicative relationship and an extremely high risk in those with both exposures, do not suggest that the smoking RR varies materially by asbestos exposure. A meta-analysis conducted in 2001 [23] involving 23 epidemiological studies confirmed that asbestos exposure and smoking have an approximate multiplicative relationship with lung cancer risk.

There are, of course, numerous occupational factors which affect risk of lung cancer. Nearly all, such as arsenic, chromium, nickel, chloromethyl ethers and polycyclic aromatic hydrocarbons increase risk, though a reduced risk has been reported for exposure to endotoxins [24]. The author is not aware of any occupation known to materially affect the RR associated with smoking. As smokers are more likely to work (or have worked) in 'dirty' occupations, there is a possible confounding effect of occupation. However, numerous epidemiological studies have adjusted for occupation (or indicators of it such as social grade) and the systematic review [14] found that the RR for smoking was hardly affected at all by the extent of adjustment for other risk factors.

3.2.7. Genetics and family history

A review by Lee in 1993 [25] considered the limited evidence then available on family history, concluding that risk was approximately doubled in those who have a relative with lung cancer. The association has been confirmed in a recent pooled analysis [26] of data from 24 studies, with the RR of lung cancer associated with having a first degree relative with lung cancer estimated as 1.51 (1.39–1.63). The *RR* was somewhat higher for ever smokers (1.55, 1.42–1.68) than for never smokers (1.25, 1.03–1.52). Similar results were reported in an earlier meta-analysis [27]. From the pooled meta-analysis results, one can estimate that the RR for ever versus never smoking is somewhat lower in those with a family history of lung cancer than in those without, by a factor which can be estimated as 1.25/1.55 = 0.81 (95% CI 0.65–1.00), a factor which is of considerably smaller magnitude than the *RR* for ever smoking of 5.50 (5.07–5.96), noted in Section 3.1.

The demonstration of an association of family history with lung cancer does not necessarily prove there is a genetic determinant of lung cancer, as family members may share aspects of smoking such as amount smoked, depth of inhalation and type of product smoked, or be exposed to common environmental factors other than smoking (e.g. heating and cooking practices). In recent years, there have been a very large number of studies aiming at looking more directly at how a whole range of genotypes are associated with lung cancer risk or with propensity to smoke. The author's impression of the literature is that associations reported are often non-significant and never strong. Even for well-studied relationships, such as chromosome 15q25, the evidence [28–31] only suggests that the variants are associated with an increased cigarette consumption of about one cigarette per day, and an increased lung cancer risk of about 30–50%. Furthermore, evidence obtained on whether the variants differentially affect lung cancer risk in never smokers is very limited. There seems to be no evidence that *RRs* associated with smoking are strongly affected by genetic factors.

3.3. Difficulties in the precise estimation of risk from smoking

3.3.1. Inaccuracy of diagnosis of lung cancer

A review in 1994 by Lee [32] demonstrated substantial evidence of disagreement between autopsy, clinical and death certificate diagnosis of lung cancer. Even though autopsy does not ensure 100% accuracy even if clinical history is taken into account, it offers the possibility of substantially improving the level of accuracy of death certificate data, which is affected by fashion and the particular interests and perceptions of certifying doctors. For example, knowledge that a person is a smoker affects diagnostic procedures so that lung cancer in a non-smoker is less likely to be detected clinically than in a non-smoker. The review also bemoaned the decline in autopsy rates, noting that advances in clinical diagnostic techniques seem not to be compensating for this in reducing inaccuracy.

While in many Western countries, autopsy rates are very low, this is not so in Hungary, or other countries in the old Austro-Hungarian empire. Autopsies were for many years routinely carried out there on all patients dying in hospital. A study there [33] showed a substantial discrepancy between pre- and post-autopsy diagnosis. In that study, 59% (36/61) of lung cancer seen at autopsy were not detected pre-autopsy, while 50% (25.50) of those diagnosed pre-autopsy were not confirmed at autopsy. Accuracy of diagnosis increased with the number of diagnostic techniques applied, but was still far from perfect in the absence of necropsy. Under-diagnosis was commoner in non-smokers and over-diagnosis commoner in smokers. Although improved diagnostic procedures could have increased accuracy of diagnosis, the results certainly imply the possibility of considerable bias to the estimated RR for lung cancer and smoking.

3.3.2. Inaccuracy in determining smoking habits

In comparing the risk of ever smokers and never smokers, random misclassification of smoking habits tends to dilute any true association with lung cancer risk. Thus, if the true *RR* is 10, and there are 50% ever and 50% never smokers random misclassification of 5% of the population into the wrong group would lead to the observed *RR* being $(47.5 \times 10 + 2.5 \times 1)/(47.5 \times 1 + 2.5 \times 10) = 6.59$. The major determinant of the bias is misclassification of ever as never smokers rather than the reverse. The association would also be diluted, if cases deny or understate their smoking, though this would not be relevant in prospective studies, where smoking habits are determined before onset of disease. Any tendency for current smokers to claim to be ex-smokers, as might happen in a situation where patients have been advised to stop smoking, would tend to increase the RR for ex-smokers and reduce the RR for current smokers. Generally, plausible levels of misclassification of smoking habits cannot explain the observed association of smoking with lung cancer.

3.3.3. Confounding factors

In the systematic review of Lee et al. [14] adjustment for age and other factors was found to have very little effect on the overall estimate of the RR associated with smoking. The conclusion of a minimal effect of confounding is consistent with that from an analysis of data from the very large US Cancer Prevention Study II [34]. It is in any case clear that the smoking RR is too large to be explained by confounding. For an RR which comfortably exceeds 10 for heavy smokers to be an artefact of confounding would require there to be another risk factor which is both extremely strongly related to lung cancer and to which smokers are very much more commonly exposed than non-smokers. While some rare risk factors (e.g. bis(chloromethyl) ethyl exposure) increase lung cancer risk very markedly, and smokers and non-smokers do differ in a range of characteristics, no factor (or group of factors) has emerged which can come close to explaining the observed RR for smoking in terms of confounding. Certainly there is no good evidence to support early theories by Fisher [35] and Burch [36] that the association of smoking with lung cancer might be totally explained by genetic factors. This theory seems, in any case, to be refuted by the observation that in smoking-discordant identical twins, risk of lung cancer was much higher in the twin who smoked [37–38].

Confounding is a more relevant issue when considering the dose-related aspects of smoking. As shown in the systematic review [14], adjustment for other aspects of smoking (typically including amount smoked) consistently reduces associations of lung cancer risk with age of starting to smoke, duration of smoking, years quit and tar level. This is because earlier starters and high tar smokers tend to smoke more heavily than do later starters and low-tar smokers, and lighter smokers tend to be more ready to quit smoking.

3.3.4. *Publication bias*

The tendency for researchers to be more likely to want to publish, and editors more likely to accept for publication, studies finding a statistically significant association may cause important bias for some relatively weak associations of exposure to disease [39, 40]. However, the association of smoking with lung cancer is too strong and consistently reported for publication bias to be a material explanation of the strong relationship.

3.3.5. *Recall bias*

In case-control studies, the smoking habits reported by a case may be affected by knowledge of the disease, particularly where the disease is widely reported to be caused by smoking. However, the fact that smoking *RRs* are quite similarly elevated in prospective studies (where such recall bias is not a possibility, smoking habits being reported before onset of the cancer) as in case-control studies (where it is a theoretical possibility) appears to rule out recall bias as an explanation for the observed association.

3.3.6. *Assessment of conclusions*

While there are a number of factors that affect precise estimation of the risk of lung cancer from smoking, it is very clear that smoking is an important determinant of risk. Looking back at the Bradford Hill criteria for determining whether an association is due to causation [41] the available evidence discussed above clearly demonstrates strength, consistency, temporality (with the exposure preceding the disease) and biological gradient (or dose response). The relationship also satisfies plausibility, given the numerous known carcinogens in tobacco smoke, and coherence, the evidence not conflicting with known facts concerning the natural history and biology of lung cancer. There is also experimental evidence, partly in humans in relation to the decline of risk following quitting, and partly in animals, with exposure to tobacco for having been shown to increase risk of skin cancer in mice and exposure to tobacco smoke having been shown to elicit lung tumours in rodents [9]. One could also argue analogy with regular inhalation of other pollutants increasing risk of lung cancer. Of the nine Bradford Hill criteria, the only one it fails is specificity. Smoking is clearly not a necessary condition for lung cancer to arise, inasmuch as there are other causes of lung cancer. Nor is it sufficient, as many smokers do not contract the disease. Though some old dictionary definitions appear to equate 'cause' to 'necessary and sufficient cause', this is not what is meant by saying that smoking causes lung cancer.

3.4. Types of product

While in most countries the majority of cigarette smokers smoke manufactured cigarettes, with relatively few smokers using hand-rolled cigarettes, in some countries, e.g. the Netherlands and Norway, hand-rolled smoking is relatively common [10]. The systematic review of studies in the 1900s [14] included 20 independent within-study estimates of the ratio of risk in hand-rolled versus manufactured cigarette smokers, which produced a combined *RR* estimate of 1.29 (95% CI 1.12–1.49), based mainly on lung cancers in men. The conclusion of a somewhat higher risk for hand-rolled cigarette smokers is consistent with that in an earlier review relating lung cancer to type of cigarette smoked [42].

That systematic review [14] also included results indicating that the RR of lung cancer was substantially lower for smokers of pipes and cigars than for cigarette smokers. Thus, for current smoking, while the *RRs* for cigarette only and for mixed cigarette and pipe/cigar smokers were, respectively, 9.57 (95% CI 7.90–11.59) and 9.60 (8.37–11.00), they were consistently lower for smokers of pipes only (5.20, 3.50–7.73), cigars only (4.67, 3.49–6.25) and smokers of pipes and/or cigars only (4.76, 3.44–6.59). Lower risks for smokers of pipes and cigars were also evident when results for ex-smokers or ever smokers were considered. Data on the types of cigars or pipes smoked were not considered, but the increased risk was evident in each continent. However, it is doubtless true that risk does vary to some extent by the type of pipe and cigar smoked.

There has been considerable research into the health risks of smokeless tobacco in Western populations, mainly based on data for Sweden, where a type of moist snuff known as snus is the dominant product, and for the USA, where chewing tobacco is common, and moist and dry snuff are also used [43–45]. The results provide no indication of any increased risk of lung cancer associated with smokeless tobacco use. They may help to explain the relatively low risk of lung cancer in Sweden (see **Figure 1**), where snus use is a common alternative to cigarette smoking.

3.5. Type of manufactured cigarette

Over the second half of the last century, the characteristics of manufactured cigarettes have changed substantially [10]. In the mid-1950s, cigarettes were typically of the non-filter plain variety with average tar levels exceeding 30 mg/cigarette. By now, nearly all cigarettes smoked have filters and average tar levels are around 10 mg/cigarette in many countries. Nicotine yields per cigarette have reduced by a similar factor.

An important question is whether these changes, introduced in order to reduce risk, have actually done so. Two points are worth making at the outset. The first is that, though the observed rise in RR for current smokers over the second half of the last century which was noted above would appear to suggest that the risk of cigarettes might have increased, this is not necessarily so, as changes in average duration of smoking by smokers have clearly had a major effect, and may mask any effects of the switch to lower tar filter cigarettes.

The second is that there is clear evidence of what is commonly termed 'compensation'. Thus, whereas one might expect smokers switching from cigarettes with a nicotine yield (machine-measured under standard smoking conditions) of, say, 2 mg/cigarette, to cigarettes with a nicotine yield of 1 mg/cigarette to halve their nicotine uptake, the reduction in measured dose is typically much less than this. This may, in theory, be because smokers increase their daily consumption or because they change how they smoke the cigarettes, the second possibility being more plausible given that consumption per smoker has changed little over the years in most countries [10].

Scherer and Lee [46] recently reviewed the available evidence on the extent of compensation, based partly on brand-switching and partly on cross-sectional studies. Using estimates based on nicotine biomarkers, commonly cotinine, they estimated a weighted mean compensation index of 0.781 (95% CI 0.720–0.842), where a value of 1 indicates complete and 0 no compensation. The index is estimated from a formula in which the biomarker, *B*, is related to the yield, *Y*, the formula $B = \mu Y^{1-C}$ where μ is a constant and *C* is the index. Thus, if *C* = 1, the biomarker is independent of the yield, while if *C* = 0, the biomarker is directly proportional to it. Using their estimated value of *C* of 0.781 would imply that a 50% reduction in yield would only produce a 14% reduction in dose, as assessed by the biomarker. This suggests that any effects of a reduction in nicotine yield on lung cancer risk are likely to be much less than would be suggested by the reduction in yield.

Various reviews have assessed the evidence on risk associated with the switch to lower tar filter cigarettes. In one of the earliest reviews [42], it was calculated, based on 43 sex-specific estimates, that the risk of lung cancer was 36% lower (95% CI 27–44%) in filter than in plain cigarettes, and 23% lower (95% CI 27–44%) for lower than higher tar cigarettes. The estimated reduction, seen in both sexes, equated to 2–3% risk reduction per mg tar per cigarette. Following publication of a report by the National Cancer Institute [13] claiming that the apparent benefits of lower delivery cigarettes may be illusory if *RRs* are adjusted for daily consumption, Lee and Sanders [47] investigated the claim by comparing *RRs* unadjusted and adjusted for consumption. They found clear reductions in risk associated with both filter and lower tar cigarette consumption, regardless of adjustment, reductions which were evident regardless of sex, study location, time period or study design. Their 2012 systematic review [14] also included a number of relevant results, among which were an estimated *RR* of 0.69 (95% CI 0.61–0.78) for only filter versus only plain smoking, and of 1.42 (1.18–1.71) for higher versus lower tar smoking.

It should be noted that the evidence considered is limited by the range of tar levels tested in any one study being often quite small (as all long-term smokers have experienced reducing tar levels), and also by there being essentially no evidence on risk of ultra-low (≤3 mg) tar cigarettes. Also, there are various other limitations, including difficulties in obtaining individual results in a comparable format, inadequate reporting of results, possible unreliability of the data recorded on cigarette type, and lack of adjustment in some studies for potential confounding variables. However, the results clearly suggest that the switch to lower tar filter cigarettes has been beneficial, though the benefit has been substantially reduced by compensation.

That cigarette mentholation might increase risk of lung cancer has some plausibility. First, the acute respiratory effects of menthol might affect inhalation of cigarette smoke, and secondly, in the USA, Black men (who have a very strong preference for mentholated cigarettes) have lung cancer rates that are substantially higher than those for White men. However, a systematic review by Lee [21] concluded that the epidemiological evidence is actually consistent with mentholation having no effect on the lung carcinogenicity of cigarettes. That review identified eight generally good quality studies, all but one conducted in the USA, which gave a combined RR estimate for ever versus never use of mentholated cigarettes of 0.93 (95% CI 0.84–1.02), with no significant evidence of any effect in males or females, or in Blacks or Whites. Noting also that, in the USA, Black women (who also have a very strong menthol preference) have lung cancer rates which are no higher than in Whites, the high rates in Black men cannot be explained by their greater preference for mentholated cigarettes.

Based on the tobacco they include, most cigarettes sold can be divided into two categories; flue-cured (or 100% Virginia) cigarettes, and blended (or American blended) cigarettes. The tobacco in flue-cured cigarettes is cured over a short period (about a week) at high temperatures, while blended cigarettes are based on three types of tobacco (flue-cured, Burley or Oriental) blended together [48]. Burley and Oriental tobaccos are air-cured over a period of about 6 weeks, the three tobacco types being genetically different. Different countries tend to predominantly use the different types of cigarettes. For example Austria, Denmark, Germany and the US use mainly blended cigarettes, while Australia, Canada and UK use mainly flue-cured cigarettes [10]. Comparing lung cancer risk for smokers of flue-cured and blended cigarettes is not straightforward since epidemiological studies are typically conducted in a single country where the smokers are likely to all (or virtually all) use one cigarette type or the other. An alternative approach tried by Lee et al. [49] was to compare lung cancer risk (for 1971–2000) by sex, age and period for those four countries listed above which traditionally use blended cigarettes, and those three listed countries which use flue-cured cigarettes. The comparisons were made both unadjusted and adjusted for prevalence of current and former smoking and for consumption per smoker. This approach was not particularly sensitive, due to the limited number of countries which (a) could both be clearly categorized by type, (b) had relevant data available and (c) did not have a large proportion of smokers of products other than cigarettes. However, it did not suggest any material effect of cigarette type on risk. Particularly noteworthy are the quite similar lung cancer rates and trends in the USA and in Canada shown in **Figure 1**, with one country using blended and the other flue-cured cigarettes.

4. Differential effect of smoking on histological type of lung cancer

4.1. Classification and diagnosis of histological type

The classification of lung cancer based on its microscopic characteristics, formulated nearly 100 years ago [50], has changed little in general structure, with the great majority of lung cancers classified into one of four basic types—squamous cell carcinoma, adenocarcinoma, small-cell carcinoma and large-cell carcinoma. However, successive WHO classifications [51–53] have differed in how tumours should be ascribed to these types, and there are considerable difficulties in ensuring an accurate and consistent diagnosis, with evidence of intra- and inter-observer variability of classification [54–56]. Part of the problem lies in the morphological heterogeneity of lung cancers with some tumours, and occasionally even in a single tissue block, presenting evidence of more than one type of lung cancer [57]. It is also clear that the morphological type of tumour is influenced by its site within the lung and by how the specimen was obtained.

4.2. Variation in relative risk of lung cancer by histological type

In their systematic review of studies published in the twentieth century [14], Lee et al. presented a range of RR estimates, not only for all lung cancer but also for squamous cell carcinoma. More limited results are also shown for small-cell and large-cell carcinoma. For current smoking overall *RRs* were strikingly higher for small-cell carcinoma (18.17, 95% CI 12.92–25.56) and squamous cell carcinoma (16.43, 12.66–21.32) than for adenocarcinoma (4.05, 3.15–5.22), with that for large-cell carcinoma (8.56, 5.29–13.86) being intermediate. The same pattern was seen for ever smoking.

For all lung cancer types *RRs* varied substantially by location, being much higher for North America than for China, with no clear pattern seen for other regions, some with sparse data. Evidence that risk increases with increasing amount smoked and duration of smoking and earlier age of starting to smoke was seen for both squamous cell carcinoma and for adenocarcinoma, though RR estimates were much higher for squamous cell carcinoma. Indeed, for squamous cell carcinoma, combined *RRs*, each based on a substantial number of estimates, were of order 30 for heavy smokers (about 45 cigs/day), long-term smokers (about 50 years) and early starting smokers (about age 14 years). *RRs* for ex-smokers were also substantially higher for squamous cell carcinoma (8.74, 95% CI 6.94–11.01) than for adenocarcinoma (2.85, 2.20–3.70). In a separate publication [58], based on data from 85 studies comparing cancer risks in current smokers, quitters (by time quit) and never smokers, it was found that the rate of decline in RR following quitting was somewhat less rapid for adenocarcinoma than for squamous cell carcinoma, where the half-lives were estimated, respectively, as 14.45 (11.92–17.45) and 11.68 (10.22–13.34). The slower decline in risk for adenocarcinoma was evident in subgroups by sex, age and other factors.

4.3. Possible explanations for the time shift in the relative frequency of adenocarcinoma and squamous cell carcinoma

A shift in the relative frequency of adenocarcinoma to squamous cell carcinoma over time has been clearly evident in many countries [59], and in 2014, the US Surgeon General [7] argued that the increasing incidence and relative frequency of adenocarcinoma has resulted 'from changes in the design and consumption of cigarettes since the 1950s'. The argument that the switch from higher tar, plain cigarettes to lower tar, filtered cigarettes is responsible for the rise in adenocarcinoma had been made previously [60–62] and supported by various researchers [63, 64]. However, there are a number of reasons which indicate that this conclusion is, to say the least, over-simplistic.

One reason for doubting the claim is that the observed shift in the relative frequency of adenocarcinoma to squamous cell carcinoma began well before the increase in consumption of low-tar filtered cigarettes started [65].

Had there been an adverse effect of low-tar filter cigarettes on risk of adenocarcinoma, one might have expected to see that for adenocarcinoma, the filter versus plain RR would be significantly increased. However, this is not the case [14, 42, 47], the systematic review [14] giving *RRs* close to 1, whether comparison was made between only filter and only plain smokers (0.84, 95% CI 0.66–1.08), ever filter and only plain smokers (0.99, 0.84–1.16) or only filter versus ever plain (0.98, 0.80–1.21). In contrast, significantly reduced risks were seen for the same three comparisons for squamous cell carcinoma 0.52 (0.40–0.68), 0.55 (0.41–0.74) and 0.69 (0.57–0.83), respectively. That the switch to lower tar filtered cigarettes has not resulted in an increase in risk for adenocarcinoma is also consistent with evidence from more recent studies [63, 66, 67]. Note that the reduced *RRs* for filtered cigarette smoking for squamous cell carcinoma suggests that the switch has been beneficial, not adverse, though the magnitude of effect is not enough to explain the observed large rise seen in the relative frequency of adenocarcinoma to squamous cell carcinoma.

Although the US Surgeon General [7] dismissed changes in diagnostic procedures as unimportant, there is quite clear evidence they are relevant, as indicated by three facts. First, schemes for classifying histological type of lung cancer have changed over time, notable being the reallocation of one of the four classes of large-cell carcinoma in the WHO classification [51] to adenocarcinoma in the 1981 classification [52]. Secondly, large studies where diagnoses of histological type made some years earlier were reviewed later by pathologists using later classification schemes generally report an increase in numbers of adenocarcinoma [68]. Finally, studies using standard criteria to review cases collected over a period of at least 10 years found no increase in the proportion of lung cancers classified as adenocarcinoma [68, 69]. Interestingly one of those studies [69] reported a substantial rise in the rate of bronchioloalveolar carcinoma, which affected smokers and non-smokers alike, and which the authors suggested may have a viral origin.

A huge weakness in the Surgeon General's argument [7] is that it would predict that the shift from squamous cell carcinoma to adenocarcinoma would be confined to smokers. Two pieces of work clearly indicate that there has been a clear change in never smokers. An analysis in 2013 [70] indirectly estimated absolute lung cancer mortality rates by smoking habit, time period- and histological-type-based studies published in the twentieth century, coupled with WHO mortality data for the same country and period. Thus, while in never smoker rates of squamous cell carcinoma per 100,000 per year were estimated to vary little by time period (7.6, 12.6, 12.7, 10.2 and 11.6 for, respectively, 1930–1960, 1961–1970, 1971–1980, 1981–1990 and 1991–1999) the corresponding rates for adenocarcinoma increased sharply for the same time period, (6.9, 17.0, 18.1, 29.0 and 33.9).

The change in never smokers is illustrated more clearly in a recent publication [68] which examined how the proportion of adenocarcinoma in never smokers varied by time, sex and region, based on 219 sex- and period-specific blocks of data drawn from 157 publications. Compared to the period 1950–1960, the ratio of adenocarcinoma to squamous cell carcinoma was higher by factors of 1.67, 1.97, 2.35 and 3.93 for, respectively, 1970–1979, 1980–1989, 1990–1999 and 2000 onwards. This publication presents arguments that the time trends could not be explained by changes in ETS exposure, or misclassification of ever smokers as never smokers.

While the switch to lower tar filtered cigarettes may have affected the relative frequency of adenocarcinoma to squamous cell carcinoma, the epidemiological evidence suggests that this is because changes in cigarettes have reduced risk of squamous cell carcinoma, not because they have increased risk of adenocarcinoma. The evidence also suggests that the differing trends by histological type are due partly to changes in diagnosis and classification and partly to other factors that have affected both non-smokers and smokers. What these factors are requires further research.

5. Relationship of ETS exposure to lung cancer risk

As active smoking causes lung cancer, and as ETS contains many of the carcinogens in tobacco smoke, one might expect there to be some increased risk from ETS exposure. However, exposure to smoke constituents from ETS is very much less than exposure from active smoking, with studies based on cotinine (the major metabolite of nicotine) suggesting relative exposure factors of order 0.06% [71]–0.4% [72]. For particulate matter, a series of studies conducted in different countries by Phillips et al., e.g. [73, 74], suggests a lower factor still, of about 0.005–0.02%. Given that the chemical compositions of ETS and of tobacco smoke are not identical, and given doubts about the shape of the dose response at low doses, it is not clear what increase in risk one might expect to be associated with ETS exposure. However, two things are evident. First, any increase in risk is likely to be quite low, if it exists at all, making it extremely difficult to detect reliably using epidemiological methods. Second, any increase in risk is only likely to be demonstrable in never smokers or in those with a smoking history that is very limited or ceased a long time ago [75].

Since the first publications in the early 1980s [76–79], reports of studies of ETS and lung cancer in never smokers have proliferated, and a recent meta-analysis [80] presented a systematic review of 102 studies. Except where noted, the conclusions reached are based on this review.

5.1. Relative risk by source of exposure

The early studies were mainly conducted in women, comparing risk in never smokers married to smokers and in never smokers married to non-smokers. There were good reasons for this: a much larger proportion of women than men had, at that time, never smoked; whether a spouse smoked or not could be determined quite reliably; and studies showed that cotinine levels in never smokers married to smokers were clearly (about three times) higher than in never smokers married to non-smokers [81]. However, over the years, evidence has been collected on a wide range of markers of ETS exposure, with some studies collecting extremely detailed histories of exposure.

Based on the meta-analyses [80] using random-effects estimates to account for the substantial between-study heterogeneity, significant ($p < 0.05$) positive associations were found with all the most commonly studied indices of exposure. The estimated *RRs* were 1.22 (95% CI 1.14–1.31) for smoking by the husband (or nearest equivalent exposure for which results were available), 1.14 (1.01–1.29) for smoking by the wife, 1.22 (1.15–1.30) for workplace exposure, 1.15 (1.02–1.29) for childhood exposure and 1.31 (1.10–1.45) for total exposure, each RR being based on a substantial number of studies. Based on very much less evidence no significant association was seen with ETS exposure in travel or in social situations, and interestingly a significant negative relationship was seen for ETS exposure in childhood specifically from the parents, with the relative risk of 0.78 (0.64–0.94). The *RR* for smoking by the husband could also be expressed as 1.10 (1.07–1.14) per 10 cigarettes smoked, using available dose-response data.

5.2. Factors affecting relative risk estimates

In order to study heterogeneity further the review [80] looked at the 119 relative risk estimates for smoking by the husband or wife (or nearest equivalent), where the overall estimate was 1.21 (95% CI 1.14–1.29), and found evidence that the largest relative risks were seen in small studies of fewer than 50 cases (1.47, 1.15–1.88), in the earliest studies, published before 1990 (1.38, 1.24–1.54), and in studies that did not adjust for age (1.42, 1.18–1.71). However, with one minor exception, some increase was seen in all the subgroups studied (which included location and study design).

There was also evidence of an increase, for spousal smoking, both for squamous cell carcinoma and adenocarcinoma.

5.3. Difficulties in interpreting the association

Whereas the RR for active smoking is large and cannot plausibly be attributed to bias or confounding, that for ETS exposure is substantially smaller, making a causal conclusion difficult to establish with any certainty. In the recent review [80], various potential sources of bias were discussed. Some sources were dismissed as being unlikely to be very relevant. These include publication bias, because large studies, which contribute most to the overall estimates, seem likely to publish their findings regardless of the results; recall bias, because the overall estimates varied little according to whether the study design was prospective (where recall bias is not an issue) or case-control (where it is), or according to diagnostic inaccuracy, because estimates were quite similar for studies that did or did not require full histological confirmation. Bias due to the reference group (never smokers married to never smokers) actually having some ETS exposure was considered, with comments made in the review [80] on the 'background correction' of Hackshaw et al. [81] aimed at converting an RR for marriage to a smoker to an RR expressed relative to never smokers with no ETS exposure at all. It was noted that this background correction only makes sense when the original association, with marriage to a smoker, derives from a causal relationship, and only applies to the *RRs* for marriage to a smoker, and does not affect the estimates of the increase in risk for amount smoked by the husband.

However, the review [80] did demonstrate clearly that confounding and misclassification of active smoking were extremely important issues which had a profound effect on the interpretation of the observed association of ETS exposure with lung cancer risk. The evidence that confounding may be a material issue derived from observations made some years ago [82, 83] strongly suggesting that, for a wide range of risk factors, exposure to the risk factor is higher in non-smokers exposed to ETS than in those not exposed to ETS. For some of these risk factors, available data are inadequate to provide any sort of reliable quantitative estimate of their relationship to lung cancer risk in non-smokers, but for four, increased dietary fat consumption, reduced fruit consumption, reduced vegetable consumption and fewer years of education, it was established that they were associated both with increased lung cancer risk and with increased ETS exposure in non-smokers. The review [80] found that adjustment for confounding reduced the *RR* for husband smoking from 1.219 (95% CI 1.138–1.305) to 1.139 (1.062–1.221), and for 10 cigs/day smoked by the husband from 1.102 (1.065–1.140) to 1.062 (1.027–1.099). Taking into account that adjustment is only for some risk factors, this illustrates the considerable potential for bias.

Bias from misclassification of active smoking arises partly because some current or former smokers are known to deny having smoked, so being wrongly described as never smokers [84, 85], and partly as smokers tend to marry smokers [75, 81]. Taken together, these two tendencies, if ignored, will bias the observed association of smoking by the husband to lung cancer risk in never smokers [81, 86, 87]. Based on what were regarded as reasonable estimates of the extent to which misclassification occurs and of the magnitude of the concordance between spouse's smoking habits it was found that correction for misclassification of smoking habits further reduced the confounder-adjusted estimates to 1.077 (0.999–1.162) for husband smoking and to 1.032 (0.994–1.071) for 10 cigs/day.

Given that adjustment for confounding and misclassification correction substantially weakens the association of lung cancer with the index of ETS exposure that is most usually considered (smoking by the husband) and renders it non-significant, and given that these adjustments and corrections may be incomplete, it seems that one cannot reliably conclude that any true causal effect of ETS exposure on lung cancer risk has been demonstrated. If there were any true relationship, it would certainly be much weaker than suggested by meta-analyses that do not adjust for confounding and misclassification.

6. Final comments

Some of the conclusions expressed here may disagree with those of other researchers. These include the risks of smoking being similar in men and women; the modest benefits of the switch to lower tar filter cigarettes; the inaccuracy of many diagnoses of lung cancer; the lack of evidence that cigarettes made from blended tobaccos (as used in the USA) are more harmful than cigarettes made from flue-cured tobacco (as used in the UK); the rise in the relative frequency of adenocarcinoma to squamous cell carcinoma (seen in never smokers, and affected by changes in diagnosis and classification) not being explained by changes in cigarettes; and the observed association of ETS exposure to lung cancer risk being to a large extent due to bias and confounding. However, it should be emphasised that all the conclusions arrived at from a detailed and careful study of the evidence, including as far as possible all relevant papers that have been published on these subjects, with in some cases reference back to the raw data.

Acknowledgements

I thank Japan Tobacco International who supported my time in preparing their paper. I also thank them and the numerous other tobacco companies and organizations who have supported my work over the last 50 years. The late Dr. Francis Roe provided inspiration for much of my work. Particular thanks are also due to the staff of my company P.N. Lee Statistics and Computing Ltd. who have, over many years, made an invaluable contribution to my research. These include Barbara Forey, John Fry, Jan Hamling, Alison Thornton and Katharine Coombs who have all featured as co-authors in many of my papers, and Diana Morris, Pauline Wassell and Yvonne Cooper who typed my manuscripts and obtained relevant references.

Author details

Peter N. Lee

Address all correspondence to: PeterLee@pnlee.co.uk

P.N. Lee Statistics and Computing Limited, Sutton, Surrey, England, UK

References

[1] Doll, R. Uncovering the effects of smoking: historical perspective. Statistical Methods in Medical Research. 1998;**7**:87–117.

[2] Müller, F.H. Tabakmißbrauch und Lungencarcinom (Tobacco abuse and lung carcinoma). Z. Krebsforsch. 1939;**49**:57–85.

[3] Schairer, E., Schöniger, E. Lung cancer and tobacco consumption. Zeitschrift für Krebsforschung. 1943;**54**:261–71.

[4] Doll, R., Hill, A.B. Smoking and carcinoma of the lung. Preliminary report. British Medical Journal. 1950;**2**:739–48.

[5] Wynder, E.L., Graham, E.A. Tobacco smoking as a possible etiologic factor in bronchiogenic carcinoma. A study of 684 proved cases. JAMA. 1950;**143**:329–36.

[6] Advisory Committee to the Surgeon General of the Public Health Service. Smoking and health. Report of the Advisory Committee to the Surgeon General of the Public Health Service. Washington DC: US Department of Health, Education, and Welfare; Public Health Service; 1964. 387 p.

[7] US Surgeon General. The health consequences of smoking—50 years of progress: a report of the Surgeon General. Atlanta, Georgia: US Department of Health and Human Services, Centers for Disease Control and Prevention, National Center for Chronic Disease Prevention and Health Promotion, Office on Smoking and Health; 2014. 944 p.

[8] US Surgeon General. Reducing the health consequences of smoking. 25 years of progress. A report of the Surgeon General. Rockville, Maryland: US Department of Health and Human Services; Public Health Services; 1989. 703 p.

[9] International Agency for Research on Cancer. Tobacco smoke and involuntary smoking—IARC Monographs on the evaluation of carcinogenic risks to humans. Lyon, France: IARC; 2004. 1452 p. IARC2004

[10] Forey, B., Hamling, J., Hamling, J., Thornton, A., Lee, P., editors. International Smoking Statistics. A collection of worldwide historical data. Web edition ed. Sutton, Surrey: P N Lee Statistics and Computing Ltd; 2006–2016.

[11] Lee, P.N., Forey, B.A. Trends in cigarette consumption cannot fully explain trends in British lung cancer rates. Journal of Epidemiology and Community Health. 1998;**52**(2):82–92.

[12] Lee, P.N., Forey, B.A. Why are lung cancer rate trends so different in the United States and United Kingdom? Inhalation Toxicology. 2003;**15**:909–49.

[13] National Cancer Institute. Risks associated with smoking cigarettes with low machine-measured yields of tar and nicotine. Smoking and Tobacco Control. Monograph No. 13 ed. Bethesda, MD: US Department of Health and Human Services, National Institutes of Health, National Cancer Institute; 2001. 235 p.

[14] Lee, P.N., Forey, B.A., Coombs, K.J. Systematic review with meta-analysis of the epidemiological evidence in the 1900s relating smoking to lung cancer. BMC Cancer. 2012;**12**:385. DOI: 10.1186/1471-2407-12-385

[15] Fry, J.S., Lee, P.N., Forey, B.A., Coombs, K.J. Dose–response relationship of lung cancer to amount smoked, duration and age starting. World Journal of Meta-Analysis. 2013;**1**(2):57–77.

[16] Fry, J.S., Lee, P.N., Forey, B.A., Coombs, K.J. How rapidly does the excess risk of lung cancer decline following quitting smoking? A quantitative review using the negative exponential model. Regulatory Toxicolology Pharmacology. 2013;**67**:13–26. DOI: 10.1016/j.yrtph.2013.06.001

[17] Lee, P.N., Hamling, J., Fry, J., Forey, B. Using the negative exponential model to describe changes in risk of smoking-related diseases following changes in exposure to tobacco. Advances in Epidemiology. 2015;Article ID 487876: 13 pages. DOI: 10.1155/2015/487876

[18] Schottenfeld, D., Fraumeni, J.F., Jr., editors. Cancer epidemiology and prevention. 3rd editionrd ed. New York: Oxford University Press; 2006. 1392 p.

[19] De Matteis, S., Consonni, D., Pesatori, A.C., Bergen, A.W., Bertazzi, P.A., Caporaso, N.E., Lubin, J.H., Wacholder, S., Landi, M.T. Are women who smoke at higher risk for lung cancer than men who smoke? American Journal of Epidemiology. 2013;**177**(7):601–12.

[20] Bain, C., Feskanich, D., Speizer, F.E., Thun, M., Hertzmark, E., Rosner, B.A., Colditz, G.A. Lung cancer rates in men and women with comparable histories of smoking. JNCI. 2004;**98**(11):826–34.

[21] Lee, P.N. Systematic review of the epidemiological evidence comparing lung cancer risk in smokers of mentholated and unmentholated cigarettes. BMC Pulmonary Medicine. 2011;**11**:18. DOI: 10.1186/1471-2466-11-18.

[22] Hammond, E.C., Selikoff, I.J., Seidman, H. Asbestos exposure, cigarette smoking and death rates. Annals of the New York Academy of Sciences. 1979;**330**:473–90.

[23] Lee, P.N. Relation between exposure to asbestos and smoking jointly and the risk of lung cancer. Occupational and Environmental Medicine. 2001;**58**(3):145–53.

[24] Enterline, P.E., Keleti, G., Sykora, J.L., Lange, J.H. Endotoxins, cotton dust, and cancer. Lancet. 1985;**2**(October 26):934–35.

[25] Lee, P.N. Epidemiological studies relating to family history of lung cancer to risk of the disease. Indoor Environment. 1993;**2**:129–42.

[26] Coté, M.L., Liu, M., Bonassi, S., Neri, M., Schwartz, A.G., Christiani, D.C., et. al. Increased risk of lung cancer in individuals with a family history of the disease: a pooled analysis from the International Lung Cancer Consortium. European Journal of Cancer. 2012;**48**(13):1957–68.

[27] Lissowska, J., Foretova, L., Dąbek, J., Zaridze, D., Szeszenia-Dabrowska, N., Rudnai, P. Family history and lung cancer risk: international multicentre case–control study in Eastern and Central Europe and meta-analyses. Cancer Causes Control. 2010;**21**(7):1091–104.

[28] Wang, Y., Broderick, P., Matakidou, A, Eisen, T., Houlston, R.S. Chromosome 15q25 (CHRNA3-CHRNA5) variation impacts indirectly on lung cancer risk. PLoS ONE. 2011;**6**(4):e19085.

[29] Timofeeva, M.N., McKay, J.D., Davey Smith, G., Johansson, M., Byrnes, G.B., Chabrier, A., et al. Genetic polymorphisms in 15q25 and 19q13 loci, cotinine levels, and risk of lung cancer in EPIC. Cancer Epidemiology Biomarkers & Prevention. 2011;**20**(10):2250–61.

[30] Munafò, M.R., Timofeeva, M.N., Morris, R.W., Prieto-Merino, D., Sattar, N., Brennan, P., et al. Association between genetic variants on chromosome 15q25 locus and objective measures of tobacco exposure. Journal of National Cancer Institute. 2012;**104**(10):740–8.

[31] Gabrielsen, M.E., Romundstad, P., Langhammer, A., Krokan, H.E., Skorpen, F. Association between a 15q25 gene variant, nicotine-related habits, lung cancer and COPD among 56307 individuals from the HUNT study in Norway. European Journal of Human Genetics. 2013;**21**(11):1293–99.

[32] Lee, P.N. Comparison of autopsy, clinical and death certificate diagnosis with particular reference to lung cancer. A review of the published data. APMIS. 1994;**102 (Suppl 45)**:42.

[33] Kendrey, G., Szende, B., Lapis, K., Marton, T., Hargitai, B., Roe, F.J.C., et al. Misdiagnosis of lung cancer in a 2000 consecutive autopsy study in Budapest. General and Diagnostic Pathology. 1995;**141**:169–78.

[34] Thun, M.J., Apicella, L.F., Henley, S.J. Smoking vs other risk factors as the cause of smoking-attributable deaths. Confounding in the courtroom. JAMA. 2000;**284**(6):706–12.

[35] Fisher, R.A. Dangers of cigarette-smoking. British Medical Journal. 1957;**2**:297–8.

[36] Burch, P.R.J. Does smoking cause lung cancer? New Scientist. 1974;**61**:458–67.

[37] Floderus, B., Cederlöf, R., Friberg, L. Smoking and mortality: a 21-year follow-up based on the Swedish Twin Registry. International Journal of Epidemiology. 1988;**17**(2):332–40.

[38] Kaprio, J., Koskenvuo, M.. Cigarette smoking as a cause of lung cancer and coronary heart disease. A study of smoking-discordant twin pairs. Acta Geneticae Medicae et Gemellologiae. 1990;**39**:25–34.

[39] Easterbrook, P.J., Berlin, J.A., Gopalan, R., Matthews, D.R. Publication bias in clinical research. Lancet. 1991;**337**(8746):867–72. DOI: 10.1016/0140-6736(91)90201-Y

[40] Thornton, A., Lee, P. Publication bias in meta-analysis: its causes and consequences. Journal of Clinical Epidemiology. 2000;**53**:207–16.

[41] Hill, A.B. The environment and disease: association or causation? Proceedings of the Royal Society of Medicine. 1965;**58**(5):295–300.

[42] Lee, P.N. Lung cancer and type of cigarette smoked. Inhalation Toxicology. 2001;**13**:951–76.

[43] Lee, P.N., Hamling, J.S. Systematic review of the relation between smokeless tobacco and cancer in Europe and North America. BMC Medicine. 2009;**7**:36. DOI: 10.1186/1741-7015-7-36

[44] Lee, P.N. Summary of the epidemiological evidence relating snus to health. Regulatory Toxicology and Pharmacology. 2011;**59**:197–214.

[45] Lee, P.N. Epidemiological evidence relating snus to health—an updated review based on recent publications. Harm Reduction Journal. 2013;**10**(1):36. DOI: 10.1186/1477-7517-10-36

[46] Scherer, G., Lee, P.N. Smoking behaviour and compensation: a review of the literature with meta-analysis. Regulatory Toxicology and Pharmacology. 2014;**70**(3):615–28. DOI: 10.1016/j.yrtph.2014.09.008

[47] Lee, P.N., Sanders, E. Does increased cigarette consumption nullify any reduction in lung cancer risk associated with low-tar filter cigarettes? Inhalation Toxicology. 2004;**16**:817–33.

[48] Tso, T.C. Maturity, harvesting, and curing. In: Production, physiology, and biochemistry of tobacco plant. Beltsville, Maryland: IDEALS, Inc; 1992. pp. 105–24.

[49] Lee, P.N., Forey, B.A., Fry, J.S., Hamling, J.S., Hamling, J.F., Sanders, E.B., Carchman, R.A. Does use of flue-cured rather than blended cigarettes affect international variation in mortality from lung cancer and COPD? Inhalation Toxicology. 2009;**21**(5):404–30.

[50] Marchesani, W. Über den primären bronchialkrebs. Frankfurt Z. Path. 1924;**30**:158–90.

[51] Kreyberg, L. Histological typing of lung tumors—International histological classification of tumours. Geneva: World Health Organization; 1967. 28 p.

[52] World Health Organization. The World Health Organization histological typing of lung tumours. Second edition. American Journal of Clinical & Patholology. 1982;**77**(2):123–36.

[53] Travis, W.D., Colby, T.V., Corrin, B., Shimosato, Y., Brambilla, E. Histological typing of lung and pleural tumours. Third Edition ed. Berlin Heidelberg: Springer; 1999. 156 p.

[54] Feinstein, A.R., Gelfman, N.A., Yesner, R., Auerbach, O., Hackel, D.B., Pratt, P.C. Observer variability in the histopathologic diagnosis of lung cancer. American Review of Respiratory Disease. 1970;**101**:671–84.

[55] Auerbach, O., Garfinkel, L., Parks, V.R. Histologic type of lung cancer in relation to smoking habits, year of diagnosis and sites of metastases. Chest. 1975;**67**:382–7.

[56] Cane, P., Linklater, K.M., Nicholson, A.G., Peake, M.D., Gosney, J. Morphological and genetic classification of lung cancer: variation in practice and implications for tailored treatment. Histopathology. 2015;**67**(2):216–24. DOI: 10.1111/his.12638

[57] Roggli, V.L., Vollmer, R.T., Greenberg, S.D., McGavran, M.H., Spjut, H.J., Yesner, R. Lung cancer heterogeneity: a blinded and randomized study of 100 consecutive cases. Human Patholology. 1985;**16**(6):569–79.

[58] Fry, J.S., Lee, P.N., Forey, B.A., Coombs, K.J. Is the shape of the decline in risk following quitting smoking similar for squamous cell carcinoma and adenocarcinoma of the lung? A quantitative review using the negative exponential model. Regulatory Toxicology and Pharmacology. 2015;**72**:49–57. DOI: 10.1016/j.yrtph.2015.02.010

[59] Devesa, S.S., Bray, F., Vizcaino, A.P., Parkin, D.M. International lung cancer trends by histologic type: male: female differences diminishing and adenocarcinoma rates rising. International Journal of Cancer. 2005;**117**(2):294–9.

[60] Burns, D.M., Anderson, C.M., Gray, N. Do changes in cigarette design influence the rise in adenocarcinoma of the lung?. Cancer Causes & Control. 2011;**22**:13–22.

[61] Thun, M.J., Burns, D.M. Health impact of "reduced yield" cigarettes: a critical assessment of the epidemiological evidence. Tobacco Control. 2001;**10(Suppl I)**:i4–i11.

[62] Thun, M.J., Lally, C.A., Flannery, J.T., Calle, E.E., Flanders, W.D., Heath, C.W., Jr. Cigarette smoking and changes in the histopathology of lung cancer. Journal of the National Cancer Institute. 1997;**89**(21):1580–6.

[63] Brooks, D.R., Austin, J.H.M., Heelan, R.T., Ginsberg, M.S., Shin, V., Olson, S.H., Muscat, J.E., Stellman, S.D. Influence of type of cigarette on peripheral versus central lung cancer. Cancer Epidemiology Biomarkers & Prevention. 2005;**14**:576–81.

[64] Ito, H., Matsuo, K., Tanaka, H., Koestler, D.C., Ombao, H., Fulton, J., et al. Nonfilter and filter cigarette consumption and the incidence of lung cancer by histological type in Japan and the United States: analysis of 30-year data from population-based cancer registries. International Journal of Cancer. 2011;**128**(8):1918–28.

[65] Chen, F., Bina, W.F., Cole, P. Declining incidence rate of lung adenocarcinoma in the United States. Chest. 2007;**131**:1000–5.

[66] Marugame, T., Sobue, T., Nakayama, T., Suzuki, T., Kuniyoshi, H., Sunagawa, K., et al. Filter cigarette smoking and lung cancer risk; a hospital-based case–control study in Japan. British Journal of Cancer. 2004;**90**:646–51.

[67] Papadopoulos, A., Guida, F., Cénée, S., Cyr, D., Schmaus, A., Radoï, L., et al. Cigarette smoking and lung cancer in women: results of the French ICARE case–control study. Lung Cancer. 2011;**74**(3):369–77.

[68] Lee, P.N., Forey, B.A., Coombs, K.J., Lipowicz, P.J., Appleton, S. Time trends in never smokers in the relative frequency of the different histological types of lung cancer, in particular adenocarcinoma. Regulatory Toxicology and Pharmacology. 2016;**74**:12–22. DOI: 10.1016/j.yrtph.2015.11.016

[69] Barsky, S.H., Cameron, R., Osann, K.E., Tomita, D., Holmes, E.C. Rising incidence of bronchioloalveolar lung carcinoma and its unique clinicopathologic features. Cancer. 1994;**73**(4):1163–70.

[70] Lee, P.N., Forey, B.A. Indirectly estimated absolute lung cancer mortality rates by smoking status and histological type based on a systematic review. BMC Cancer. 2013;**13**(1):189–224. DOI: 10.1186/1471-2407-13-189

[71] Pirkle, J.L., Flegal, K.M., Bernert, J.T., Brody, D.J., Etzel, R.A., Maurer, K.R. Exposure of the US population to environmental tobacco smoke. The Third National Health and Nutrition Examination Survey, 1988 to 1991. JAMA. 1996;**275**:1233–40. DOI: 10.1001/jama.275.16.1233

[72] Office of Population Censuses and Surveys. Health survey for England 1994. Volume I: Findings. Volume II: Survey methodology & documentation. Series HS no. 4 ed. London: HMSO; 1996. 607 p.

[73] Phillips, K., Bentley, M.C., Howard, D.A., Alván, G. Assessment of air quality in Stockholm by personal monitoring of nonsmokers for respirable suspended particles and environmental tobacco smoke. Scandinavian Journal of Work, Environment and Health. 1996;**22(Suppl 1)**:1–24.

[74] Phillips, K., Howard, D.A., Bentley, M.C., Alván, G. Assessment of air quality in Turin by personal monitoring of nonsmokers for respirable suspended particles and

environmental tobacco smoke. Environment International. 1997;**23**:851–71. DOI: 10.1016/S0160-4120(97)00097-4

[75] Lee, P.N. Environmental tobacco smoke and mortality. A detailed review of epidemiological evidence relating environmental tobacco smoke to the risk of cancer, heart disease and other causes of death in adults who have never smoked. Basel: Karger; 1992. 224 p.

[76] Hirayama, T. Non-smoking wives of heavy smokers have a higher risk of lung cancer: a study from Japan. British Medical Journal. 1981;**282**:183–5. DOI: 10.1136/bmj.282.6259.183

[77] Garfinkel, L. Time trends in lung cancer mortality among nonsmokers and a note on passive smoking. Journal of the National Cancer Institute. 1981;**66**(6):1061–6. DOI: 10.1093/jnci/66.6.1061

[78] Trichopoulos, D., Kalandidi, A., Tzonou, A. Incidence and distribution of lung cancer in Greece. Excerpta Medica International Congress Series. 1982;**558**:10–7.

[79] Chan, W.C., Fung, S.C. Lung cancer in non-smokers in Hong Kong. In: Grundmann, E., editors. Cancer Epidemiology. Stuttgart, New York: Gustav Fischer Verlag; 1982. pp. 199–202.

[80] Lee, P.N., Fry, J.S., Forey, B., Hamling, J.S., Thornton, A.J. Environmental tobacco smoke exposure and lung cancer: a systematic review. World Journal of Meta-Analysis. 2016;**4**(2):10–43. DOI: 10.13105/wjma.v4.i2.10

[81] Hackshaw, A.K., Law, M.R., Wald, N.J. The accumulated evidence on lung cancer and environmental tobacco smoke. BMJ. 1997;**315**:980–8. DOI: 10.1136/bmj.315.7114.980

[82] Thornton, A., Lee, P., Fry, J. Differences between smokers, ex-smokers, passive smokers and non-smokers. Journal of Clinical Epidemiology. 1994;**47**(10):1143–62. DOI: 10.1016/0895-4356(94)90101-5

[83] Matanoski, G., Kanchanaraksa, S., Lantry, D., Chang, Y. Characteristics of nonsmoking women in NHANES I and NHANES I epidemiologic follow-up study with exposure to spouses who smoke. American Journal of Epidemiology. 1995;**142**(2):149–57.

[84] Lee, P.N., Forey, B.A. Misclassification of smoking habits as determined by cotinine or by repeated self-report—a summary of evidence from 42 studies. Jouranal Smoking-Related Disease.. 1995;**6**:109–29.

[85] Connor-Gorber, S., Schofield-Hurwitz, S., Hardt, J., Levasseur, G., Tremblay, M. The accuracy of self-reported smoking: a systematic review of the relationship between self-reported and cotinine-assessed smoking status. Nicotine & Tobacco Research. 2009;**11**(1):12–24. DOI: 10.1093/ntr/ntn010

[86] Lee, P.N., Forey, B.A. Misclassification of smoking habits as a source of bias in the study of environmental tobacco smoke and lung cancer. Statistics in Medicine. 1996;**15**(6):581–605. DOI: 10.1002/(SICI)1097-0258(19960330)15

[87] Lehnert, G., Garfinkel, L., Hirayama, T., Schmähl, D., Uberla, K., Wynder, E.L., Lee, P. Roundtable discussion. Preventive Medicine. 1984;**13**(6):730–46.

Chapter 2

How Effective is Fear of Lung Cancer as a Smoking Cessation Motivator?

John A.A. Nichols

Additional information is available at the end of the chapter

http://dx.doi.org/10.5772/67235

Abstract

A risk score for lung cancer derived from genetic and clinical data has been shown to motivate smokers to quit. However, smokers with a relatively low (but not insignificant) risk score are more likely to carry on smoking. To understand this observation, the balance between smoking cessation motivators and de-motivators must be understood. A relatively low risk score can act as a de-motivator. Other de-motivators that have been recorded and were observed by researchers involved in this project were: nicotine addiction and fear of withdrawal symptoms, optimism bias, confirmation bias, attentional bias, post-traumatic stress disorder (PTSD), anxieties about smoking cessation and weight gain, side effects of smoking cessation therapy, fatalism, peer pressure and lack of family cohesion. This long list of de-motivators serves to emphasize the complexity of the psychological make-up of the individual smoker. This is illustrated by a set of case histories (anonymised for confidentiality). The future use of a risk score as a smoking cessation motivator is discussed and suggestions are made as to how a risk score could be made more effective including inclusion of scoring for cardiovascular risk.

Keywords: smoking cessation, genetic testing, lung neoplasms, primary health care

1. Introduction

The reasons why smokers either continue to smoke or stop smoking are diverse and every case is probably unique. However, there is a basic truth in that there is a constant seesaw between smoking cessation motivators and the rather less well understood de-motivators. The importance of de-motivators is illustrated by the simple fact that over 60% of smokers say they would like to quit but most seem somehow unable to do so [1, 2]. The obvious explanation is that this is due to nicotine addiction but this may be only one of many de-motivators.

In 2014, my colleagues and I at the University of Surrey, United Kingdom (UK), carried out research into smoking cessation. We recruited 67 smokers who wanted to quit from a primary care database of 32,000 (**Table 1**) and randomized them to either a control group or a test group. The test group had an additional motivator to quit. This was the Respiragene risk score for lung cancer derived from a genetic test (19 single-nucleotide polymorphisms (SNPs) and one deletion mutation) and clinical criteria including history of chronic obstructive pulmonary disease, family history of lung cancer, and age. Both groups attended 8 weekly smoking cessation clinics which took place at the same primary care venue but with test group and control group attended on different weekdays. We published our protocol and outcome measures a priori [3]. Primary outcome was smoking cessation after 6 months.

Demographic/smoking feature	Test group (n=36)	Control group (n=31)	p-Values (test)
Gender: female	55.6%	53.3%	0.747 (Chi-square)
Mean age (at start of study)	49.7	49.0	0.812 (Unpaired t)
Mean age at completion of education	18.4	18.5	0.971 (Unpaired t)
Years in education (excluding interruptions)	22.8	26.2	0.517 (Unpaired t)
Pack years	32.0	28.9	0.396 (Unpaired t)
Cigarettes/day at start	18.1	18.1	0.993 (Unpaired t)

Table 1. Demographic and baseline smoking data for Respiragene trial.

During our research, we found that 36% of smokers had stopped smoking and were still not smoking after 6 months. Of the 64% who were still smoking at 6 months, all but two participants planned to stop smoking at some time in the future and 30% had cut down substantially (by 10 or more cigarettes/day) [4].So why don't they just quit?

Our hypothesis was that when participants were told their lung cancer risk, this would tend to outbalance any de-motivators such as issues around nicotine addiction (**Figure 1**) and give a high 6-month quit rate. However, we were probably underestimating the potency of known and unknown de-motivators. It certainly cannot be entirely due to nicotine addiction because varenicline blocks the physical addiction and prevents most withdrawal symptoms and yet 50–75% of subjects taking varenicline will still be smoking 6 months later [5, 6]. There must, therefore, be more to it than nicotine addiction.

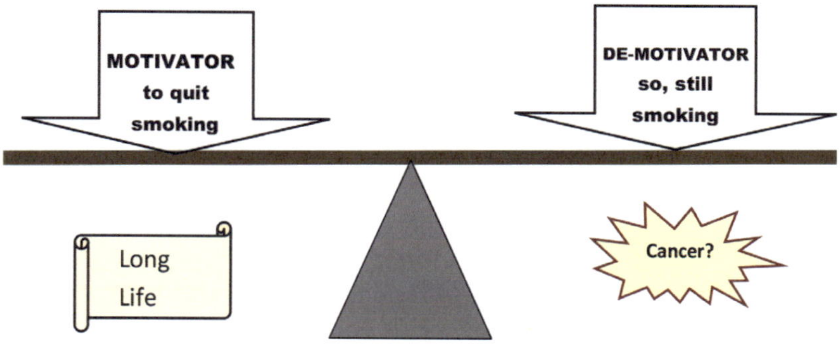

Figure 1. For smokers: the seesaw of destiny. The balance between motivators and de-motivators determines success or failure for smokers trying to quit.

2. The Respiragene project

As already reported [4], the 6-month quit rate in our Respiragene trial was more dependent on the risk score than we had expected. The laboratory reported the Respiragene risk score as three categories: average risk of lung cancer, high risk of lung cancer, and very high risk of lung cancer. Only non-smokers and ex-smokers can achieve the category "low risk". We were also able to estimate lifetime risk as a percentage (i.e., a 50% lifetime risk meant that the risk of lung cancer was like tossing a life/death coin). The 6-month quit rate results are summarized in **Figure 2**. However, assessing the balance of motivators and de-motivators was included in secondary outcomes. The relative importance of ten smoking cessation motivators was estimated using a feedback questionnaire at 8 weeks and again at 6 months. The results show the perceived importance of these motivators (**Figure 3**).

From taking notes on comments from patients during counselling and from responses to open-ended questions in feedback questionnaires that participants completed, we were able to clarify the roles of some of these de-motivating factors. Most smokers have two main de-motivators:

1. **Nicotine addiction and fear of withdrawal symptoms** [7–9]. Nicotine has been shown to be as addictive as illegal drugs such as morphine and cocaine.
2. **Optimism bias** [10–13].Tendency to underestimate the health risks of smoking and the feeling "It'll never happen to me".

We expected that our study would confirm the hypothesis that being told a risk score for lung cancer would cancel out both nicotine addiction and optimism bias in at least 50% of participants. An earlier study (n = 99) using the Respiragene risk score had shown that smokers were more likely to quit compared with a control group whatever risk score they were given [14]. However, these participants were recruited from a hospital in New Zealand. We carried out a similar trial in a UK primary care setting. A surprise finding from our trial was that although all but one of the participants with a very high risk score had stopped smoking at 6 months, participants with an average risk score were more likely to be smoking than controls (**Figure 2**).

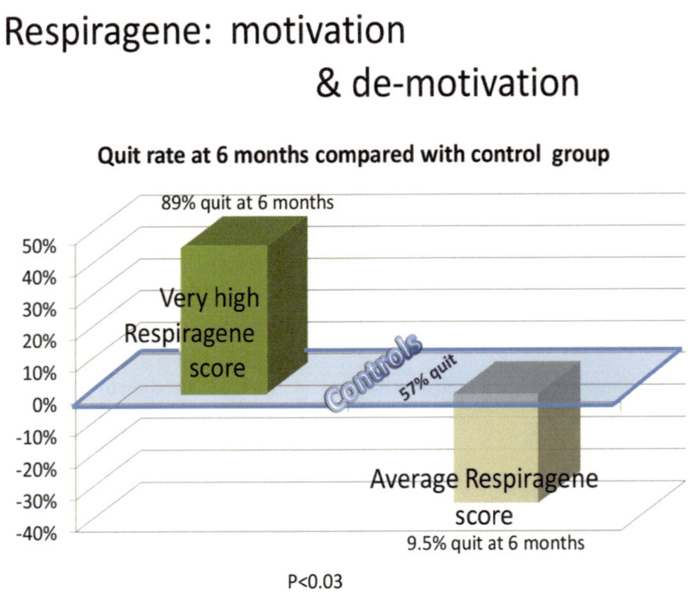

Figure 2. The blue "glass ceiling" represents the quit rate for the control group. Quit rate at 6 months for controls was 57%. Subjects with an average risk score for lung cancer (only non-smokers and ex-smokers are assessed as "low risk score") had a lower quit rate than controls, and a "moderately high" quit rate was no better but difficult to judge due to small numbers (only 4). However, all but one of the nine subjects with a "very high" risk score (equivalent to 50% lifetime risk of lung cancer) had quit at 6 months giving an 89% quit rate.

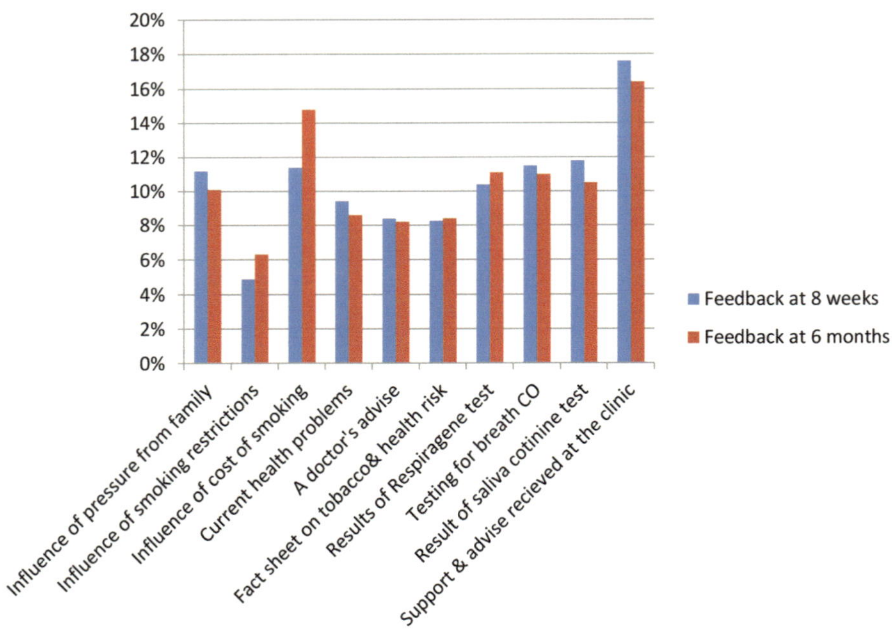

Figure 3. Mean values for motivators and influences that have helped to reduce or stop smoking: "Please score each of the items below according to how strong an influence they have been in helping you to quit smoking". Scores for motivators for individual participants were calculated as percentages of the sum of total scores of the individual and mean values calculated from these percentage scores.

The test subjects with an average risk score demonstrated a quit rate that was significantly lower than the quit rate in the control group ($p = 0.03$) which suggests that they had been de-motivated and encouraged to think that it was safe to carry on smoking because their lifetime risk was perceived as "not so bad". Or to put it another way, their optimism bias has been reinforced by their average risk score! Psychologists refer to this phenomenon as **(No. (iii)) confirmation bias** [15] and explain that when a subject has two conflicting ideas in their head (i.e., smoking is too risky versus the risk of smoking is exaggerated), this is intolerable—a phenomenon known as cognitive dissonance [16]. This mental discomfort can only be solved by ditching one idea and giving undue prominence to the other. A classic example is the smoker who responds to a challenge about the risks of his habit by saying: "Uncle Charlie smoked like a trouper and lived to be 90". Any evidence to the contrary, such as other smokers in the family who died young, is conveniently ignored.

Other possible factors that make it difficult to quit that we noted in our participants and which have been previously recognized by other researchers in this field were as follows:

1. **Attentional bias** [17, 18]. The smoker is plagued by recurrent thoughts about the pleasures of smoking that serve to increase craving for the next cigarette.

2. **Post-traumatic stress disorder (PTSD)** [19–21]. This is a mental health condition caused by a traumatic event such as rape, warfare experiences, and other near death experiences such as road traffic accidents and industrial accidents. The subjects experience distressing dreams and flashbacks, and they are more likely to become heavily addicted smokers.

3. **Anxieties about smoking cessation and weight gain** [22, 23]. This is an issue for many female smokers who start smoking when they are relatively young to control their weight. Later in life, they may try to quit but revert to smoking when they put on weight.

4. **Side effects of smoking cessation therapy** [24–26]. Patients using pharmaceuticals such as nicotine replacement therapy (NRT) patches or nicotine blocking drugs frequently report side effects. Once they have experienced a side effect, they usually revert to smoking.

5. **Fatalism** [27, 28]. This is the attitude that "What will be will be". These smokers either feel they have little or no control over outcomes such as lung cancer or they simply do not care if they are destined to develop a smoking-related disease.

6. **Peer pressure** [29, 30]. The influence of fellow workers on smoking can be a decisive factor. All the emphasis has been on peer pressure in adolescence and initiation of smoking, but peer pressure can be equally important in the adult work force.

7. **Lack of family cohesion** [31, 32]. Research has shown that family cohesion is associated with concerns about passive smoking and smoking cessation. Conversely, lack of family cohesion is associated with a significantly higher incidence of persistent smoking.

8. **Inadequacy of the risk score as a motivator**. Our own research, as described above, suggests that a risk score for a single disease (lung cancer in this case) is not a powerful enough motivator to cancel out de-motivators in 64% of smokers, especially if the risk score is "low average" when they may be falsely reassured and continue smoking.

2.1. Case histories

To preserve confidentiality, the case histories I present here have been altered (age, gender, and circumstantial details) so that the participants in our research project are unrecognizable. However, basic clinical details have been preserved as far as possible. These cases help to demonstrate why some smokers cannot quit, despite stating that they would like to.

2.1.1. Case no. 1.: lifetime risk of lung cancer = 35%

This participant was a young housewife who was stressed by having to care for two mildly hyperactive small boys aged 3 and 5 and was still smoking 15 cigarettes/day at 6 months. She seemed falsely reassured by the 35% lifetime risk commenting: "only 35% that's not so bad". When I gave her an analogy: "What if I told you that if you carried on living in your present house, you stood a 35% chance of being murdered in your bed, but if you moved to a house in the next road the risk would drop to 1%". She hesitated a moment then said: "But doctor, that's completely different".

2.1.1.1. Commentary

A 35% lifetime risk is less than the risk of tossing a life/death coin but close enough to be worrying. So why wasn't this patient worried? Her hesitation suggests cognitive dissonance [16]. That is two competing ideas buzzing around in your head. For stability and well-being, one of the competing ideas must give way. Her most comforting solution was to accept that the 35% risk of lung cancer was nothing like the risk of being murdered in your bed. Well, of course, it is a different scenario but the risk of death is identical. This is also a good example of confirmation bias [15]. She managed to confirm her feeling that a 35% risk was "not so bad" by rejecting my analogy.

2.1.2. Case no. 2.: lifetime risk of lung cancer = 10%

This participant had been a mature medical student who qualified in his mid 30s. Soon after qualifying, he was at BMA House, Tavistock Square, in 2007, when the suicide bomber detonated on the top deck of a bus in Tavistock Square, and he was the first doctor on the scene. Although he was a non-smoker at the time, he found the only way to cope with flash backs and other PTSD symptoms related to this horrific incident was to become a habitual smoker. He is now a part-time psychiatrist near retirement and was still smoking 10 cigarettes/day at the 6- month follow-up.

2.1.2.1. Commentary

This participant started smoking for the first time aged 40 years, which is unusual. However, the circumstances were also unusual. Although this is obviously linked to post-traumatic stress disorder (PTSD), there may be less dramatic and less obvious versions of PTSD that fuel the smoking habit such as unreported domestic abuse.

2.1.3. Case no. 3.: lifetime risk of lung cancer = 19%

This participant was a 23-year-old woman who worked as a stable maid. She had quit at 8 weeks and she had always seemed highly motivated. However, she sustained a compound fracture to her right tibia when she was kicked by a horse. As a result, she was stuck at home, off sick, with the injury for some time. All the pain and worry and the boredom of being at home all the time is what started her back on the cigarettes (10/day)—they made it all a bit more bearable.

2.1.3.1. Commentary

Although this participant cites pain and boredom as the reasons for relapsing to smoking, there were also features of PTSD. Her failure to quit was surprising as she was the "leading light" of the test group. She was the first in her group to quit and gently encouraged other participants. Perhaps this case illustrates how PTSD acts as a very powerful de-motivator.

2.1.4. Case no. 4.: control (no risk score)

This 58–year-old woman in the control group did not seem to have much of a problem quitting after a lifetime as a smoker (started aged 14 year) but she told me, at the 6-month follow-up that it was far from easy and described it as being like bereavement. It is, quite literally, as difficult to deal with as the death of someone very close to you. On the other hand, her lead motivator was concern about the affects of side-stream smoke on someone very dear to her—her new baby grandson.

2.1.4.1. Commentary

This participant was remarkably open and honest about her feelings, and it is certainly sobering to think that smoking cessation is as difficult to cope with as suffering a bereavement. However, the fact that her main motivator was concern for her grandchild is very significant. Researchers have shown that family cohesion is associated with a lower incidence of smoking and lack of family cohesion with a very high incidence (70%) of smoking [32]. Family cohesion and awareness and acceptance of the health hazards of side-stream smoke correlated ($p < 0.01$) in a paper from Texas in 2010 [31]. Two other participants mentioned the influence of grandchildren in relation to passive smoking and their decision to quit. Altogether, 8/67 (12%) of our participants mentioned passive smoking and family as a key motivator without prompting (in response to an open-ended question asking for "further comments").

2.1.5. Case no. 5.: lifetime risk of lung cancer >50%

This 48-year-old woman, who had recently been through a stressful divorce, was unable to work due to the debilitating effects of Crohn's disease. She was well aware that smoking cessation would probably improve her Crohn's symptoms. She started on varenicline but had to stop taking it after 3 days due to an acute exacerbation of Crohn's symptoms. She never returned to the clinic and was still smoking 12/day at the 6-month follow-up saying: "This is my only way of coping with boredom".

2.1.5.1. *Commentary*

The impression from this patient was that she had simply "given up". There are varying degrees of fatalism like this exhibited by smokers [27]. She might have been able to fight back with the help of varenicline, unfortunately she had gastrointestinal side effects that she interpreted as an exacerbation of her Crohn's disease so stopped taking varenicline after 3 days. In her case, the varenicline side effects seemed to a significant de-motivator.

2.1.6. *Case no. 6.: lifetime risk of lung cancer 58%*

This 35-year-old single man in a high-powered office job had managed to stop smoking for 5 years when his younger brother died of lung cancer. This was the third 1st degree relative to die from lung cancer. However, his current work ethos was one in which "everyone smoked" and now he was back on 15 cigarettes/day. Despite the family history and a high risk score he was still smoking 15 cigarettes/day at the 6-month follow-up. He blamed "work stress and peer pressure" for his inability to quit.

2.1.6.1. *Commentary*

This subject's inability to quit was really puzzling, and he himself was puzzled by it. There may have been several de-motivating issues but peer pressure at work was certainly very significant in his case.

3. Genetics and smoking behaviour

Nicotine, cannabinoids, and cocaine act as insecticides to protect plants from insect attack. Mammals that eat plants have evolved to tolerate these chemicals but only humans have developed the habit of burning and inhaling plants containing these toxic chemicals. Archaeologists have found evidence for this habit going back into prehistory [33]. There is even evidence of genetic adaptions to nicotine specific to humans [34]. Edward Hagan, professor of Anthropology at Washington State University, argues that there is a balance of benefits and costs to smoking tobacco. Nicotine must have some advantages that outweigh the health costs in some circumstances. Our ancestors may have found the effects of nicotine on the brain beneficial in times of stress and hunger but Hagan argues that nicotine's greatest evolutionary advantage may have been efficacy as an anti-helminth drug, especially in controlling those helminth parasites that migrate through the lungs [35].

It is no surprise, therefore, that there are human genes that relate to smoking behaviour. A recent review estimated that, according to twin studies, 75% of behavioural variation (variation in smoking initiation, persistence, and cessation rates) is genetically determined [36]. However, only about 5% of this variation can currently be explained by known gene variants, mainly single-nucleotide polymorphisms (SNPs) but 19% of the variation in smoking initiation can be explained by known SNPs. Research is ongoing in this area with the hope that identification of further SNPs and other gene variants will improve our understanding of smoking behaviour and smoking cessation demotivators leading to new effective treatments to aid smoking cessation [8, 36]. This research includes increasing our understanding of epigenetic off/on gene switching in determining various aspects of smoking behaviour and pathologies associated with smoking [8, 37].

An understanding of the genetics and epigenetics of PTSD is very relevant to helping smokers to quit, especially those who seem to be hardened nicotine addicts. Twin studies have shown that only 20–30% of subjects exposed to severe trauma develop PTSD [38]. Less than 50% of women who experience violent rape develop overt PTSD. Genetic studies have shown that a combination of four or more high-risk alleles (single gene variants) confer a sevenfold increase in the risk of PTSD following trauma [38]. However, lesser degrees of PTSD associated with cigarette smoking [19] may also have a genetic component. Further research in this area seems likely to overlap with research focused on the genetics of smoking behaviour and is likely to lead to new strategies in treatment of both PTSD and in helping to achieve smoking cessation.

4. Discussion

I had been unaware of the possibility that PTSD could be a common barrier to smoking cessation. Beckham et al. [20] showed that there is a significant difference between PTSD and non-PTSD smokers during attempts to quit with the PTSD subjects being more likely to lapse after 1 week (**Figure 4**). There is also a growing body of research that shows that we may only recognize the more obvious instances such as PTSD in war veterans and rape victims. The literature is unclear on the incidence of PTSD in the general population with reports ranging from 1 to 5%. If we take 3% as a median value, it is likely that a sample of lifelong non-smokers would exhibit a lower incidence (approx. 2%) so that the incidence of overt PTSD is 3 times higher in smokers. A paper by Matthews et al. [19] showed that 6.7% of smokers are suffering from overt PTSD but also showed that another 73% of their study group of current smokers (n = 342) had symptom scores suggestive of some degree of stress or as they termed it: "sub-threshold PTSD". There was no correlation between smoking and anhedonia. Only 20% of their sample was completely negative for their PTSD score. Perhaps sub-threshold PTSD includes unreported domestic abuse and bullying at work. Domestic violence has been recorded as a cause of PTSD-related smoking [39]. There is evidence from research by neuropsychiatry that nicotine inhibits negative symptoms experienced in PTSD and that the positive "feel good" effects of nicotine is relatively insignificant [19, 21]. Further research is needed to clarify the differences in PTSD scoring between smokers and non-smokers and to determine what can be done to help this category of refractory smokers.

Smokers who are concerned about weight gain will need special help but sometimes counselling and dietary advice are ineffective. Hurt et al. at The Mayo Clinic, USA, are currently researching the combined pharmacological approach of varenicline and lorcaserin (a new anti-obesity drug) for overweight smokers who want to quit. Early results are encouraging (personal communication from Hurt).

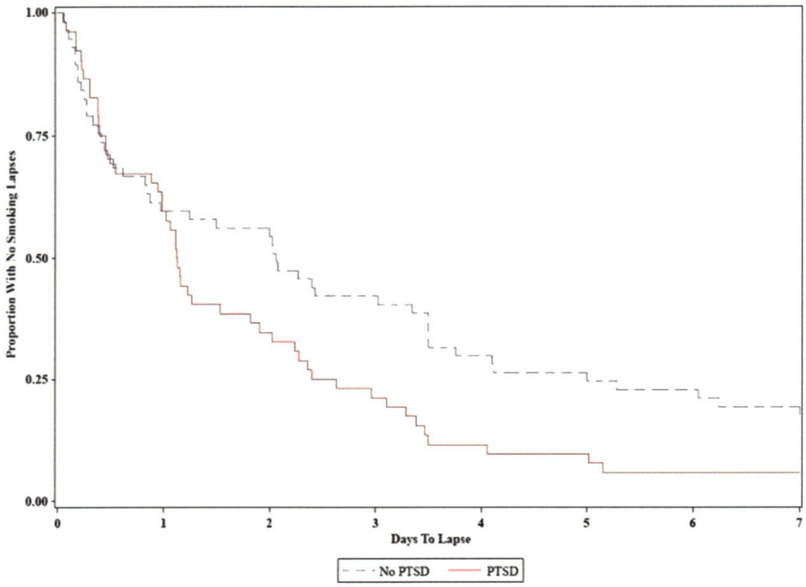

Figure 4. Survival curves for smoking lapse in PTSD (n = 55) versus non-PTSD (n = 52) in first week of a quit attempt showing that PTSD is associated with a higher smoking relapse rate (from Beckham et al. [16]).

Do smokers who experience side effects from smoking cessation drugs tend to give up trying to quit as seemed to be the case with case 5? The literature is unclear on this issue. However, the Respiragene project certainly showed a significant difference between those that had been able to persist with their original smoking cessation prescription (varenicline or nicotine replacement therapy) and those who had stopped due to side effects (**Table 2**) with quit rates at 6 months of 42.6 and 15.3%, respectively (p = 0.01).

	Stopped smoking at 6-month follow-up			Total
	Lost to follow-up	Yes	No	
Prescription history unknown	2	0	5	7
Persisted with first prescription	3	20	24	47
Stopped first prescription	0	2	11	13
Total	5	22	40	67

χ^2 = 6.6, p = 0.01.

Table 2. Smoking cessation outcome for subjects who stopped smoking cessation therapy due to side effects compared with subjects who had persisted with smoking cessation therapy.

Studies linking work stress to smoking are equally balanced between those that do and do not show a link. One of the best studies, however, from Finland shows an odds ratio of 1.28 (p < 0.01) for smoking where there is a high imbalance between effort and reward consistent with work stress [40]. Concerns about passive smoking in the family home have received a

http://dx.doi.org/10.5772/67235

good deal of publicity recently despite attempts by the tobacco industry to play down the risks [41]. Finding that 12% of our participants mentioned this as a key smoking cessation motivator was not, therefore, unexpected. Just as family cohesion is a factor here, conversely lack of family cohesion is emerging as a significant de-motivator [31, 32].

Fatalism and peer pressure are well known as factors that encourage smoking but the precise role of adult peer pressure in the workplace needs further research. A review of smoking cessation in the workplace has outlined strategies for influencing the workplace ethos to improve attitudes and introducing workplace smoking cessation programmes and smoking cessation inducements [42].

The efficacy of a risk score such as the Respiragene risk score as a smoking cessation motivator could, perhaps, be improved if it included cardiovascular risk as well as lung cancer risk. A recent paper estimated that smokers double the risk of an early death from cardiovascular events but that risk reverts to normal after 2 years of smoking cessation [43]. Personalized data on cardiovascular risk could be included in the risk score in future. This might include genetic risk factors such as the apolipoprotein E4 gene but clinical factors such as family history, blood pressure, body mass index, lipid profile, and HbA1C would be equally important.

5. Conclusions

Fear of lung cancer can certainly act as a powerful motivator as demonstrated by the high quit rate for subjects with a very high Respiragene risk score. However, the problem with a personalized risk score is that if the risk is relatively low, it may act as a de-motivator. Including a personalized risk score for life-threatening cardiovascular events (stroke and myocardial infarction) might help to counter this problem, especially as most smokers will be given a risk score round about the mean of 100% increase in risk of a fatal event. However, even the most persuasive smoking cessation motivator is unlikely to overcome powerful de-motivators such as PTSD or weight control issues in about 20% of smokers. If a smoker in this category who may have attempted to quit 2 or 3 times already is still determined to quit, the de-motivator that is standing in the way of success must be addressed and this may need intense one to one counselling and/or a pharmacological intervention. New and better pharmacological approaches are likely to result from genetic studies on smoking behaviour.

Acknowledgements

I am indebted to my colleagues Paul Grob, Wendy Kite, Peter Williams, and Simon de Lusignan at the University of Surrey who helped me in the planning and implementation of the Respiragene project and were my co-authors for the main paper reporting the results of this research [4]. I could not have completed this research without the help of: A Telaranta-Keerie and the staff of Lab 21, Cambridge, who processed and analyzed the buccal swabs for genetic testing; A Roscoe and the staff of the Integrated Care Partnership, Epsom, for help with recruitment and premises;

and Surrey Smoking Cessation Practitioners J Golding and H Phillips for their expertise. We are grateful for grants from Lab 21 and Synergenz Bioscience Ltd without which this research could not have been completed.

Author details

John A.A. Nichols

Address all correspondence to: drjaan@ntlworld.com

Department of Clinical and Experimental Medicine, University of Surrey, Guilford, UK

References

[1] Quitting Smoking Among Adults—United States, 2001–2010. CDC Morbitity and Mortality Weekly. 2011;60(44):1513–1519.

[2] Manning DM. Why won't our patients stop smoking? Diabetes Care. 2009;32(S2):S426–S428.

[3] Nichols JA, Grob P, Kite W, de Lusignan S, Williams P. Genetic test to stop smoking (GeTSS) trial protocol: randomised controlled trial of a genetic test (Respiragene) and Auckland formula to assess lung cancer risk. BMC Pulmonary Medicine. 2014;14:77.

[4] Nichols JAA, Grob PR, Kite W, Williams P, de Lusignan S. Using a genetic/clinical risk score to stop smoking (GeTSS): randomised controlled trial. (submitted for publication 2016).

[5] Swan GE, McClure JB, Jack LM. Behavioral counseling and vareniclinetreatment for smoking cessation. The American Journal of Preventive Medicine. 2010;38(5):482–490.

[6] Lee JH, Philip Jones G, Bybee K, O'Keefe JH. A longer course of varenicline therapy improves smoking cessation rates. Preventive Cardiology. 2008;11:210–214.

[7] Benowitz NL. Neurobiology of nicotine addiction: implications for smoking cessation treatment. The American Journal of Medicine. 2008;121(4A): S3–S10.

[8] Gardner PD, Tapper AR, King JA, DiFranza JR, Ziedonis DM. The neurobiology of nicotine addiction: clinical and public policy implications. Journal of Drug Issues. 2009;39(2):417–441.

[9] Sharma A, Brody AL. In vivo brain imaging of human exposure to nicotine and tobacco. Handbook of Experimental Pharmacology. 2009;192:145–171.

[10] Masiero M, Lucchiari C, Pravettoni G. Personal fable: optimistic bias in cigarette smokers. International Journal of High Risk Behaviors and Addiction. 2015;4(1):e20939.

[11] Weinstein ND, Marcus SE, Moser RP. Smokers' unrealistic optimism about their risk. Tobacco Control. 2005;**14**:55e9.

[12] Young RP, Hopkins RJ, Smith M, Hogarth DK. Smoking cessation: the potential role of risk assessment tools as motivational triggers [Review]. Postgraduate Medical Journal. 2010;**86**(1011):26–33.

[13] Smith SM, Campbell MC, Macleod U. Factors contributing to the time taken to consult with symptoms of lung cancer: a cross sectional study. Thorax. 2009;**64**:523–531.

[14] Hopkins RJ, Young RP, Hay B, et al. Gene-based lung cancer risk score triggers smoking cessation in randomly recruited smokers. American Journal of Respiratory and Critical Medicine. 2011;**183**:A5441.

[15] Jones M, Sugden R. Positive confirmation bias in the acquisition of information. Theory and Decision. 2001;**50**:59–99.

[16] Fotuhi O, Fong GT, Zanna MP, Borland R, Yong HH, Cummings KM. Patterns of cognitive dissonance-reducing beliefs among smokers: a longitudinal analysis from the International Tobacco Control (ITC) Four Country Survey. Journal of Tobacco Control. 2013;**22**(1): 52–58.

[17] Waters AJ, Shiffman S, Bradley BP, Mogg K. Attentional shifts to smoking cues in smokers. Addiction. 2003;**98**(10):1409–1417.

[18] McClernon FJ, Addicott MA, Sweitzer MM. Smoking abstinence and neurocognition: implications for cessation and relapse. Current Topics in Behavioral Neurosciences. 2015;**23**:193–227.

[19] Mathew AR, Cook JW, Japuntich SJ, Leventhal AM. Post-traumatic stress disorder symptoms, underlying affective vulnerabilities, and smoking for affect regulation. The American Journal on Addictions. 2015;**24**:39–46.

[20] Beckham JC, Calhoun PS, Dennis MF, Wilson SM, Dedert EA. Predictors of lapse in first week of smoking abstinence in PTSD and Non-PTSD Smokers. Nicotine and Tobacco Research. 2012;**15**:1122–1129.

[21] Froeliger B, Beckham JC, Dennis MF, Kozink RV, McClernon FJ. Effects of nicotine on emotional reactivity in PTSD and non-PTSD smokers: results of a pilot fMRI Study. Advances in Pharmacological Sciences. 2012:6 (Article ID 265724).

[22] Weekley CK, Klesges RC, Reylea G. Smoking as a weight-control strategy and its relationship to smoking status. Addictive Behaviors. 1992;**17**(3):259–271.

[23] Seeley RJ, Sandoval DA. Neuroscience: weight loss through smoking. Nature. 2011;**475**(7355):176–177.

[24] Morphett K, Partridge B, Gartner C, Carter A, Hall W. Why don't smokers want help to quit? A qualitative study of smokers' attitudes towards assisted vs. unassisted quitting. International Journal of Environmental Research and Public Health. 2015;**12**:6591–6607.

[25] Leung LK, Patafio FM, Rosser WW. Gastrointestinal adverse effects of varenicline at maintenance dose: a meta-analysis [Review]. BMC Clinical Pharmacology. 2011;**11**:15.

[26] Anthenelli RM, Benowitz NL, West R, St Aubin L, McRae T, Lawrence D, Ascher J, Russ C, Krishen A, Evins AE. Neuropsychiatric safety and efficacy of varenicline, bupropion, and nicotine patch in smokers with and without psychiatric disorders (EAGLES): a double-blind, randomised, placebo-controlled clinical trial. Lancet. 2016;**387**(10037):2507–2520.

[27] Lewis PA, Charny M, Lambert D, Coombes J. A fatalistic attitude to health amongst smokers in Cardiff. Health Education Research. 1989:**4**(3):361–365.

[28] Chatwin J, Povey A, Kennedy A, Frank T, Firth A, Booton R, Barber P, Sanders C. The mediation of social influences on smoking cessation and awareness of the early signs of lung cancer. BMC Public Health. 2014;**14**:1043.

[29] Kim YJ. Impact of work environments and occupational hazards on smoking intensity in korean workers. Journal of Workplace Health and Safety. 2015;**64**(3):103–113.

[30] Rowe K, Macleod Clark J. Why nurses smoke: a review of the literature [Review]. International Journal of Nursing Studies. 2000;**37**(2):173–181.

[31] Law J, Kelly M, Garcia P, Taylor T. An evaluation of Mi Familia No Fuma: family cohesion and impact on second hand smoking. American Journal of Health Education. 2010;**41**(5):265–273.

[32] Coonrod DV, Balcazar H, Brady J, Garcia S, Van Tine M. Smoking, acculturation and family cohesion in Mexican-American women. Ethnicity and Disease. 1999;**9**(3):434–440.

[33] Merlin MD. Archaeological evidence for the tradition of psychoactive plant use in the old world. Economic Botany. 2003;**57**(3):295–323.

[34] Xiu X, Puskar NL, Shanata JAP, Lester HA, Dougherty DA. Nicotine binding to brain receptors requires a strong cation-π interaction. Nature. 2009;**458**:534–537.

[35] Hagen EH, Roulette CJ, Sullivan RJ. Explaining human recreational use of 'pesticides': the neurotoxin regulation model of substance use vs. the hijack model and implications for age and sex differences in drug consumption. Frontiers in Psychiatry. 2013;**4**(142):1–21.

[36] Ware JJ, Munafò MR. Genetics of Smoking Behaviour. In: Balfour DJK, Munafò MR, editors. The Neurobiology and Genetics of Nicotine and Tobacco. Springer International Publishing, Switzerland; 2015. p. 19–36. doi:10.1007/978-3-319-13665-3_2

[37] Kabesch M, Adcock IM. Epigenetics in asthma and COPD. Biochimie. 2012;**94**:2231–2241.

[38] Almli LM, Fani N, Smith AK, Ressler KJ. Genetic approaches to understanding post-traumatic stress disorder. The International Journal of Neuropsychopharmacology. 2014;**17**(2):355–370.

[39] Crane CA, Hawes SW, Weinberger AH. Intimate partner violence victimization and cigarette smoking: a meta-analytic review. Trauma Violence and Abuse. 2013;**14**(4):305–315.

[40] Kouvonen A, Kivimaki M, Virtanen M, Pentti J, Vahtera J. Work stress, smoking status, and smoking intensity: an observational study of 46,190 employees. Journal of Epidemiology and Community Health. 2005;**9**(1):63–69.

[41] Kennedy GE, Bero LA. Print media coverage of research on passive smoking. Tobacco Control. 1999;**8**:254–260.

[42] Fishwick D, Carroll C, McGregor M, Drury M, Webster J, Bradshaw L, Rick J, Leaviss J. Smoking cessation in the workplace. Occupational Medicine. 2013;**63**:526–536.

[43] Mallaina P, Lionis C, Rol H, Imperiali R, Burgess A, Nixon M, Malvestiti FM. Smoking cessation and the risk of cardiovascular disease outcomes predicted from established risk scores: results of the Cardiovascular Risk Assessment among Smokers in Primary Care in Europe (CV-ASPIRE) study. BMC Public Health. 2013;**13**:362.

Section 2

The Role of the Imaging Methods in Diagnosis of Lung Cancer: A Global Vision

Chapter 3

Low-Dose Computed Tomography Screening for Lung Cancer

Trevor Keith Rogers

Additional information is available at the end of the chapter

http://dx.doi.org/10.5772/66358

Abstract

In the landmark American National Lung Cancer Screening Trial (NLST), low-dose CT (LDCT) screening produced a relative mortality reduction of 20%. These results have not been replicated in any of the European studies, although these are of limited statistical power. Besides doubt about the general applicability of the NLST findings, if LDCT screening is to be successfully implemented, a number of developments are still required, including better characterisation of entry criteria and refinement of screening and nodule management protocols. The high incidence of false-positive findings increases costs and morbidity. Even when histologically malignant tumours are identified, frequently these would not have manifested as disease, i.e. they are "overdiagnosed". These patients are liable to receive unnecessary treatment. LDCT screening is relatively expensive in comparison with other cancer screening modalities. Whilst cost-effectiveness can be improved by integration with smoking cessation programmes, how this would be done in practice remains unclear. Furthermore, individuals at high-risk of lung cancer are virtually by definition risk prone, raising concerns about how attractive participation in a screening programme would be, especially given the very small reported absolute risk reduction in the NLST.

Keywords: lung cancer, screening, low-dose computed tomography, early diagnosis, cost-effectiveness, overdiagnosis

1. Introduction

Lung cancer is the commonest cause of cancer death in both men and women across the developed world, due to a combination of its high incidence and relatively short average survival after diagnosis. Most lung cancer patients present symptomatically and most already have incurable disease at presentation. These considerations have resulted in attempts to improve outcomes through screening.

Screening, though, is a challenging strategy for harm reduction. Screening programmes have been introduced for many cancers, often as a result of political pressures rather than on sound evidence. Indeed, the harms of many screening programmes have only become evident well after widespread implementation, and their utility has often become more rather than less controversial with time. Self-evidently, for screening to be effective, earlier disease identification needs to lead to improved treatment outcomes. This calls into question what we know about the natural history of early stage, asymptomatic tumours, which turns out to be surprisingly little. It is now becoming increasingly certain though that, whilst some tumours will progress and ultimately cause premature death, others may never cause harm. This leads to a bias known as overdiagnosis [1]. The other way in which overdiagnosis can occur is when a competing cause of death prevents clinical manifestations of a tumour that would otherwise have proved lethal [2]. Screening is particularly liable to overdiagnosis, because more aggressive tumours have short volume-doubling times and progress rapidly. Thus, the interval between the onset of a radiological abnormality and the emergence of symptoms is relatively short, and the opportunity for presymptomatic detection in a screening programme is small. Conversely, tumours that grow slowly will have a long phase when they exist without symptoms and are particularly liable to be identified through screening.

There is now convincing evidence that overdiagnosis does occur as an inherent harm in most, and probably all, cancer screening programmes, including mammography [3]. It is always harmful because it is unknown which of the tumours identified are the ones overdiagnosed, meaning that some patients will have treatment for a disease that would never have materialised. The resulting costs include financial (unnecessary investigations/treatments), physical (side effects and complications of treatments) and psychological and are all serious, irrespective of any benefits derived by those with "real" disease.

The other important bias of screening programmes is lead-time bias, which occurs when a disease is diagnosed earlier than it would have been without screening. Even if the natural history of the case is not improved, the patient appears to survive longer than otherwise they would have but dies at the same date. Because of this it is vital that for proper evaluation of a screening programme the endpoint taken should be mortality difference in comparison with a control group.

2. Lung cancer screening trials

Several large studies were conducted in the 1960s and 1970s using plain chest radiography, with or without sputum cytology [4–10]. These studies all had methodological weaknesses [11], including possessing limited power and, rather remarkably, even the control group in several having three-year radiographs. No study provided evidence that mortality was reduced. Recently, the PLCO study has reported [12] and has finally and convincingly shown an absence of any mortality benefit of plain chest radiography screening, compared to no screening.

The advent of low-dose CT (LDCT) scanning provided a new modality applicable to lung cancer screening. Initial studies indicated that LDCT was able to identify early lung cancers with a high rate of resectability [13]. The landmark National Lung Screening Trial (NLST) was a large and adequately powered, randomised, controlled trial of screening with LDCT against plain chest radiography, undertaken in the USA. The headline result was a reduction in lung cancer mortality, by the apparently impressive figure of 20% [14]. Does this mean that CT screening immediately to be implemented for lung cancer or that lung cancer mortality could be reduced by anything like this amount? I believe that the answer is no to both.

2.1. The National Lung Screening Trial (NLST)

Eligible participants were identified as current or former smokers between the ages of 55 and 75 years with no personal history of malignancy and at least a 30-pack-year smoking history [14]. Former smokers had to have quit less than 15 years prior to participating in the study. Volunteers who had previously received a diagnosis of lung cancer or who had undergone a chest CT scan within 18 months before enrolment, and those who had haemoptysis or unexplained weight loss of more than 6.8 kg in the preceding year were excluded. An impressive total of 53,454 volunteers were enrolled; 26,722 were randomly assigned to receive three annual screening examinations by either LDCT or chest radiography. They were then followed for an additional 5 years after the screening examinations were completed. No further screening was undertaken in subjects diagnosed with lung cancer. In both groups, the screening test was deemed positive if it showed a non-calcified pulmonary nodule 4 mm or larger in diameter or if there were other findings suspicious for cancer. When comparing the two groups after the completion of the three annual screenings, 24% of participants screened with LDCT had positive screening results compared with 6.9% of individuals who received chest radiography, confirming the superiority of LDCT in identifying nodules over plain chest radiography [14]. More than 75% of the participants with a positive screening result underwent further diagnostic evaluation, either with additional imaging or with invasive/surgical procedures. In this report, a "false positive" was defined as any case requiring further evaluation, including just repeat CT imaging. Using this definition, more than 90% of the positive findings were false positives, both in the controls and in the LDCT group.

Of the 26,722 volunteers screened with LDCT, 1060 participants were found to have lung cancer in comparison to 941 of the group screened with chest radiography. Overall, when comparing the two groups, the detection rate of lung cancer was 13% greater in the group screened with LDCT than with chest radiography. More early stage (IA and IB) cancers were diagnosed with CT. Most importantly in the evaluation of a screening study, there was evidence of reduced mortality: a total of 356 lung cancer deaths occurred in the LDCT vs. 443 deaths in the plain radiography group, over a median of 6.5 years of follow-up ($P = 0.004$). Whilst the *relative reduction* in mortality rate from lung cancer was 20% in individuals screened using LDCT, the *absolute risk reduction* in mortality was only 0.33% less over the study period in the LDCT group (87 avoided deaths over 26,722 screened participants), meaning 310 individuals needed to participate in screening for typically three rounds to prevent one lung cancer death. Given the conclusion of the PLCO trial that plain radiography screening is ineffective, it can be assumed that this represents a similar benefit to eligible participants in comparison with no screening. However this is evaluated in terms of cost-effectiveness, this study does indicate that there exists a subgroup of patients with lung cancer that can be cured if it is identified earlier and, conversely, who will die from their disease if it is not. Despite the large number of participants who underwent further diagnostic testing, the authors noted that the testing resulted in only a small number of adverse events.

2.2. European studies

An important issue is to what extent the findings of the NSLT might hold for a non-US population. There are important differences in epidemiology in Europe, including a difference in distribution of histological subtypes and a much lower frequency of non-calcified pulmonary nodules arising from fungal pathogens. In the UK, squamous cancers represent about 40% of cancers and adenocarcinomas 18%, whilst in the USA, squamous cancers only represent 27% with adenocarcinoma being the most prevalent type at 31% [15]. As squamous cancers tend to arise in proximal airways, they are less amenable to identification as a lung nodule on CT, unlike adenocarcinomas, which more often present as intrapulmonary nodules.

The DANTE and DLCST studies each compared five annual rounds of LDCT screening to usual care and were both considerably smaller than the NLST. The DANTE study randomised 2811 and the DLCST randomised 4104 men and women who were healthy, heavy and current or former smokers to LDCT screening or no screening. After medians of 34 and 58 months of follow-up, respectively, not even a trend towards reduced mortality was found: (DANTE, relative risk [RR], 0.97; 95% CI, 0.71–1.32; $P = 0.84$) (DLCST, RR, 1.15; 95% CI, 0.83–1.61; $P = 0.430$) [16, 17]. The NELSON study is the largest European study so far performed, with 15,822 participants, and has employed a volumetry-based LDCT screening protocol with longer intervals between screening rounds [18, 19]. These investigators greatly reduced their reported false-positive rate when compared with the figure reported in NLST (23.3% in NLST vs. 3.6% in NELSON) by changing the definition of "false positive" to include only those nodules that had a baseline appearance or interval growth that supported malignancy. This is probably justified, given that whilst being recalled for a repeat CT may generate some anxiety and distress, this would be anticipated to be much less than the need for urgent evaluation and is likely to be short-lived.

A comparison of the larger European and LDCT screening trails with the NLST with the trials of the plain chest X-ray in screening [4, 12] is shown in **Table 1**, particularly in respect of their effects on mortality. It should be emphasised that the only trial producing a statistically significant result was the NLST.

2.3. Downsides of LDCT screening

Any benefits of CT screening need to be weighed against the harms. Besides the relatively small direct risk of cancers that are caused directly by the radiation exposure from the

Trial	Modality	Recruits	No. of lung cancers detected (%)	No. at stage 1 (%)	No. of deaths from lung cancer (%)	Relative mortality reduction from screening	Absolute mortality reduction from screening
						Negative figures denote mortality increase	
NLST (14)	Chest X-ray	26,035	941 (3.61)	131 (0.5)	443 (1.70)	+20%	+0.33%
	LDCT	26,309	1060 (4.03)	400 (0.52)	356 (1.35)		
DANTE (17)	Clinical	1186	73 (6.07)	16 (1.35)	55 (4.64)	−0.65%	−0.03%
	LDCT	1264	104 (8.23)	47 (3.72)	59 (4.67)		
DLCST (16)	Usual	2052	24 (1.17)	5 (0.24)	11 (0.54)	−35%	−0.19%
	LDCT	2052	70 (3.41)	47 (2.29)	15 (0.73)		
PLCO (12)	Usual	77,456	1620 (2.09)	462 (0.6)	1230 (1.59)	+1.26%	−0.02%
	Chest X-ray	77,445	1696 (2.19)	374 (0.48)	1213 (1.57)		
MLP (4)	Usual	4593	160 (3.48)	31 (0.67)	115 (2.50)	−6%	−0.14%
	Chest X-ray	4618	206 (4.46)	68 (1.47)	122 (2.64)		

Table 1. Comparison of lung cancer screening trials, showing rates of identification of early stage disease and effects on mortality.

CT scans, CT screening suffers from all of the general limitations of screening in general. These include:

- Overdiagnosis—see above
- The costs—both psychological and financial arising particularly through the high rate of false-positive diagnoses or indeterminate findings
- Uncertainty regarding how such a programme would work in practice including its potential to reach/capture a reasonable proportion of incident cases

In the NLST, the substantial excess of cancers diagnosed in the CT group (1060 vs. 941) implies that overdiagnosis did occur. Patz and colleagues' [20] analysis of the NLST study suggested that up to 18% of the cancers identified in the NLST may have been indolent and likely to have been overdiagnosed and indicated that for each cancer death avoided, 1.38 cases may have been overdiagnosed. Moreover, the figures for overdiagnosis may have been even worse if the control arm had received no chest radiographs, which can also be assumed to have resulted in some overdiagnosis. The risk of overdiagnosis, as might be expected, depends on histological subtype and is most striking in patients with a diagnosis of bronchoalveolar cell carcinoma (now called minimally invasive adenocarcinoma), in whom the risk of overdiagnosis was estimated to be 85% after 7 years of follow-up or 49% with lifetime follow-up [20]. These data also raise the question as to the necessity and type of therapy required if a diagnosis of minimally invasive adenocarcinoma is established.

Because the major risk factor for lung cancer is the smoking of tobacco, in order to qualify for entrance into a screening programme, individuals need to have smoked significantly, and many will be current cigarette smokers. Consequently, the target population of a lung cancer screening programme may be expected to have a relative disregard for its own health and a tendency to accept of risk, potentially predisposing to poor acceptability of, and adherence to, screening. This is likely to be much more evident in real life in comparison to a highly motivated volunteer population. It has been shown that smokers in the USA are significantly more likely than never smokers to be male, non-white and less educated; to report poor health status; and to be less likely to be able to identify a usual source of healthcare [21]. This study also indicated that current smokers were less likely than never smokers to believe that early detection would result in a good chance of survival and expressed relative reluctance to consider computed tomography screening for lung cancer. Interestingly, only half of these smokers stated that they would opt for surgery for a cancer diagnosed as a result of screening, further calling into question the value of early diagnosis in this group.

Importantly, even if all subjects meeting the NLST criteria were to accept and adhere to screening, it has been estimated that only 27% of incident lung cancer patients would be included [22]. This implies that the potential to limit lung cancer mortality could only at the very best be 20 of 27% of cases, i.e. a 5.4% mortality reduction overall.

It can also be argued that a screening programme represents a collusion with self-harming behaviour, particularly in relation to current smokers, and throws into focus the interrelationship between smoking cessation and lung cancer screening, particularly as CT screening is only designed to mitigate one of the many potential harms of smoking. This is all the more relevant because recruitment into a lung cancer screening programme does not appear to increase the likelihood of smoking cessation [23–25] and reduce it [19]. Offering smoking cessation, which is one of the most cost-effective of all heath interventions, within a screening programme has been shown to improve the cost-effectiveness of the screening—by 20–45% [26, 27]. Is this "cheating"? It is only when expensive LDCT screening is combined with highly cost-effective smoking cessation that cost-utility ratios become comparable with those of other accepted cancer screening programmes!

No long-term psychological harm was found in the NELSON trial. In those with negative results, anxiety and distress fell from baseline; following an abnormal result, anxiety and distress were transient and tended to have returned to baseline by the next screening round [28]. However, the harms—psychological, physical and financial—suffered by those with overdiagnosed tumours have not been quantified and are likely to be substantial.

In the NLST, a major complication occurred in almost five of every 10,000 persons screened due to investigation of a benign lung nodule [14]. Whilst this is a low proportion, these were "normal" subjects in whom any harm is seriously to be regretted.

Based on the NSLT's own size cut-offs, the average nodule detection rate per round of screening was very high at 20%. In most LDCT screening studies, more than 90% of nodules prove to be benign. Whilst there is a tendency towards lower nodule detection rates in repeat screening rounds, this appears only to be due to the discounting of nodules that had been present in the prior round, so screening, if embarked upon, should probably continue. Furthermore, from the evidence of the fourth round of screening in the NELSON study, lengthening the duration of intervals between rounds beyond 2 years does not appear to be an effective strategy.

In most screening study protocols, a detected nodule triggers further imaging, but the approaches have been inconsistent between studies, and it has been suggested that follow-up imaging rates may have been underestimated [29]. The frequency of further CT imaging among screened individuals has ranged from 1% in the study by Veronesi et al. [30] to 44.6% in the study by Sobue et al. [31]. The frequency of further positron emission tomography (PET) imaging among screened individuals has exhibited less variation, ranging from 2.5% in the study by Bastarrika et al. [32] to 5.5% in the NLST.

The frequency of invasive evaluation of detected nodules, although generally low, has shown marked variation in reported studies. In the NLST, in the patients not found to have lung cancer, 1.2% underwent an invasive procedure such as needle biopsy or bronchoscopy, and 0.7% had a thoracoscopy, mediastinoscopy or thoracotomy. In the NELSON study, these numbers were very similar at 1.2% and 0.6%, respectively [18].

A workshop undertaken by the International Association for the Study of Lung Cancer (IASLC) [33] identified a number of areas where improvements are needed to be made in relation to future implementation of LDCT screening, indicating that, whilst LDCT screening may have potential value, the science around the process remains preliminary. The specific areas requiring clarification were identified as optimization of the identification of high-risk individuals, development of radiological guidelines, development of guidelines for the clinical workup of indeterminate nodules, development of guidelines for pathology reporting, definition of criteria for surgical and therapeutic interventions of suspicious nodules identified through lung cancer CT screening programmes and development of recommendations for the integration of smoking cessation practices into future national lung cancer CT screening programmes.

2.4. Cost-effectiveness

Incremental cost-effectiveness ratio (ICER) is defined as = $(C1 - C2)/(E1 - E2)$, where C1 and E1 are the cost and effect in the intervention and where C2 and E2 are the cost and effect in the control group. Costs are usually described in monetary units, whilst benefits/effect in health status is measured in terms of quality-adjusted life years (QALYs).

Using such methodology, lung cancer LDCT screening was found to be considerably more expensive than other US screening programmes with an ICER of between $126,000 and $169,000/LY [34]. In comparison, colorectal cancer screening has an ICER of $13,000 to $32,000/LY. When a basic smoking cessation intervention is included, which, as outlined above, subsidises an expensive intervention with a cheap one, but which also adds to the total costs, an ICER of $23,185 per QALY is gained, falling further to $16,198 to per QALY gained with a more intensive regimen [26]. Given the huge benefits of smoking cessation for a wide range of diseases, the case for offering smoking cessation to all anyway is strong. Setting up an LDCT screening programme first and adding on smoking cessation to that seems to be putting the cart before the horse: if employed at all for smokers, it should be an add-on to a smoking cessation intervention.

In the UKLST, the cost-effectiveness analyses used data from life tables and modelled data on quality-adjusted life year (QALY) from the NLST, the validity of which is unclear. Given that no effect on mortality could be shown, the reliability of cost-utility analysis is highly questionable, although was estimated at only £8466 (approximately $11,000 at today's exchange rate) per QALY gained. This figure is substantially less than that quoted in the NLST and is well within the threshold deemed acceptable by the National Institute for Health and Care Excellence.

2.5. Applicability of trial findings to routine clinical practice

Most of the NLST sites were designated National Cancer Institute centres, and more than 80% were large, multidisciplinary academic centres with more than 400 beds [29]. It seems unlikely that the results obtained by less specialised centres will be directly comparable. Furthermore, screening trials are likely to attract, if not healthy volunteers, at least a group who may be more likely than the average to adhere to the screening protocol. Indeed, adherence to the three screening rounds in the NLST was 90%, which is highly unlikely to be achievable in routine practice.

Great difficulty was experienced in recruiting participants to UKLS, given that a system comparable to that that may be used in a real-life screening programme was employed: of the 247,354 questionnaires sent out, response rates to the initial questionnaire were low, with an initial positive response rate of only 15% in current smokers and about 40% in never or former smokers. Even then, a high attrition rate occurred with potential participants being lost at every stage of the recruitment process. Finally, only 4061 subjects (46.5% of all high-risk positive responders) consented and were recruited into the trial.

Another positive from the CT screening studies is that they have provided evidence underpinning the rational approach to the investigation of solitary pulmonary nodules, including the very helpful algorithm developed by the BTS [35]. This includes appreciation that minimally invasive adenocarcinomas may be benign in behaviour and may allow a less aggressive approach to management in comorbid or frail patients.

3. Conclusions

The American NLST, in finding a 20% relative reduction in mortality from screening with LDCT, in comparison to plain chest radiography, which itself is ineffective, suggests that screening may be one strategy for improving lung cancer outcomes in a well-motivated American population. This benefit was achieved at a cost comparable to those of other established screening programmes but only when smoking cessation was included. However, the absolute reduction in mortality achieved is small: 87 avoided deaths in 26,722 screened participants, representing a 0.33% lower risk of dying from lung cancer for each individual participant. Besides the harms resulting from the unnecessary treatment of overdiagnosed

http://dx.doi.org/10.5772/66358

cases, 24% of participants were found to have a nodule over three rounds, leading to further diagnostic workup. Even in these large academic institutions, a major complication occurred in five of every 10,000 cases with a benign nodule. Many of the cancers diagnosed are small, minimally invasive adenocarcinomas, and these contribute significantly to overdiagnosed cases. Overall, for every cancer death avoided, 1.38 cases may have been overdiagnosed.

Disappointingly, none of the European studies (DANTE and DLCST and NELSON) have found evidence of any significant, or indeed even a trend towards, reduction in mortality, possibly reflecting different epidemiology of cancer subtypes. The use of volumetric techniques employed in the NELSON study seems attractive, but the efficacy of this approach remains completely unproven.

Concentration on harm reduction through screening potentially deflects attention from the need to improve diagnosis and treatment for the majority of cases falling outwith current screening eligibility criteria for smoking history and age. It is known that patients often tolerate lung cancer symptoms for long periods before presenting with them [36]. General practitioners also find identifying lung cancer cases challenging, and patients will often attend several times before the diagnosis is considered and a chest radiograph performed [37]. An early study revealed that educating the public and primary healthcare teams on the importance of cough as a lung cancer symptom resulted in a large increase in chest radiographs being performed and suggested earlier diagnosis [38]. This led on to the national "Be Clear on Cancer" campaign in the UK, the results of which were positive, leading to state funding of repeat programmes. Further work is taking place to look at the effects of lowering thresholds for the obtaining of chest radiographs for chest symptoms in primary care [39]. Facilitating earlier diagnosis of symptomatic disease should also minimise overdiagnosis.

I believe that screening in lung cancer is potentially able to improve lung cancer mortality, but our understanding of how to apply this in real populations, including those outside the USA, is in its infancy. Cost-effectiveness is much improved when screening is combined with smoking cessation, but this is in effect subsidising an otherwise unaffordable screening programme by combining it with another highly cost-effective intervention that could be provided anyway.

Besides the expense of screening, small but definite harms resulting from radiation exposure, investigations of benign lesions and the more significant difficulty of finding of inconsequential disease (overdiagnosis) also reduce its attractiveness. Until we have better understanding of these issues, I believe we should be concentrating more effort on the earlier diagnosis of symptomatic disease, at least in Europe.

Whatever we think of the weaknesses of the current attempts to reduce mortality though screening, the NLST does point to the potential for improving lung cancer outcomes through expeditious diagnosis. For now, at least in Europe, this must be based on improved identification of symptomatic disease. Initiatives to improve detection of early stage disease will rely on improving public and primary care awareness of lung cancer symptoms and reducing the impediments to diagnosis following recognition that lung cancer is a possible diagnosis.

Author details

Trevor Keith Rogers

Address all correspondence to: Trevor.Rogers@dbh.nhs.uk

Doncaster Royal Infirmary, Doncaster, UK

References

[1] Welch HG, Black WC. Overdiagnosis in cancer. Journal of the National Cancer Institute. 2010;102(9):605–13.

[2] Reich JM. A critical appraisal of overdiagnosis: estimates of its magnitude and implications for lung cancer screening. Thorax. 2008;63(4):377–83.

[3] Miller AB, Wall C, Baines CJ, Sun P, To T, Narod SA. Twenty five year follow-up for breast cancer incidence and mortality of the Canadian national breast screening study: randomised screening trial. BMJ. 2014 23:31:29;348.

[4] Fontana RS, Sanderson DR, Taylor WF, Woolner LB, Miller WE, Muhm JR, et al. Early lung cancer detection: results of the initial (prevalence) radiologic and cytologic screening in the Mayo clinic study. American Review of Respiratory Disease. 1984;130(4):561–5.

[5] Frost JK, Ball WC, Jr., Levin ML, Tockman MS, Baker RR, Carter D, et al. Early lung cancer detection: results of the initial (prevalence) radiologic and cytologic screening in the Johns Hopkins study. American Review of Respiratory Disease. 1984;130(4):549–54.

[6] Kubik A, Polak J. Lung cancer detection. Results of a randomized prospective study in Czechoslovakia. Cancer. 1986;57(12):2427–37.

[7] Melamed MR, Flehinger BJ. Detection of lung cancer: highlights of the memorial Sloan-Kettering Study in New York city. Schweizerische Medizinische Wochenschrift. 1987;117(39):1457–63.

[8] Kubik A, Parkin DM, Khlat M, Erban J, Polak J, Adamec M. Lack of benefit from semi-annual screening for cancer of the lung: follow-up report of a randomized controlled trial on a population of high-risk males in Czechoslovakia. International Journal of Cancer. 1990;45(1):26–33.

[9] Kubik AK, Parkin DM, Zatloukal P. Czech study on lung cancer screening: post-trial follow-up of lung cancer deaths up to year 15 since enrollment. Cancer. 2000;89(11:Suppl):2363–8.

[10] Melamed MR. Lung cancer screening results in the National Cancer Institute New York study. Cancer. 2000;89(11:Suppl);2356–62.

[11] Fontana RS, Sanderson DR, Woolner LB, Taylor WF, Miller WE, Muhm JR, et al. Screening for lung cancer. A critique of the Mayo Lung Project. Cancer. 1991;67(4 Suppl):1154–64.

[12] Oken MM, Hocking WG, Kvale PA, Andriole GL, Buys SS, Church TR, et al. Screening by chest radiograph and lung cancer mortality: the prostate, lung, colorectal, and ovarian (PLCO) randomized trial. JAMA. 2011;306(17):1865–73. PMID: 22031728.

[13] Survival of patients with stage I lung cancer detected on CT screening. New England Journal of Medicine. 2006;355(17):1763–71. PMID: 17065637.

[14] Aberle DR, Adams AM, Berg CD, Black WC, Clapp JD, Fagerstrom RM, et al. Reduced lung-cancer mortality with low-dose computed tomographic screening. The New England Journal of Medicine. 2011;365(5):395–409. PMID: 21714641. Epub 2011/07/01.

[15] Youlden DR, Cramb SM, Baade PD. The international epidemiology of lung cancer: geographical distribution and secular trends. Journal of Thoracic Oncology. 2008;3(8):819–31 10.1097/JTO.0b013e31818020eb.

[16] Saghir Z, Dirksen A, Ashraf H, Bach KS, Brodersen J, Clementsen PF, et al. CT screening for lung cancer brings forward early disease. The randomised Danish Lung Cancer Screening Trial: status after five annual screening rounds with low-dose CT. Thorax. 2012;67(4):296–301. PubMed PMID: 22286927.

[17] Infante M, Cavuto S, Lutman FR, Brambilla G, Chiesa G, Ceresoli G, et al. A randomized study of lung cancer screening with spiral computed tomography. American Journal of Respiratory and Critical Care Medicine. 2009;180(5):445–53.

[18] Horeweg N, van der Aalst CM, Thunnissen E, Nackaerts K, Weenink C, Groen HJ, et al. Characteristics of lung cancers detected by computer tomography screening in the randomized NELSON trial. American Journal of Respiratory & Critical Care Medicine. 2013;187(8):848–54. PMID: 23348977.

[19] Yousaf-Khan U, van der Aalst C, de Jong PA, Heuvelmans M, Scholten E, Lammers JW, et al. Final screening round of the NELSON lung cancer screening trial: the effect of a 2.5-year screening interval. Thorax. 2016.

[20] Patz EF, Pinsky P, Gatsonis C, Sicks JD, Kramer BS, Tammemägi MC, et al. Overdiagnosis in low-dose computed tomography screening for lung cancer. JAMA Internal Medicine. 2014;174(2):269–74. Epub 09/12/2013.

[21] Silvestri GA, Nietert PJ, Zoller J, Carter C, Bradford D. Attitudes towards screening for lung cancer among smokers and their non-smoking counterparts. Thorax. 2007;62(2):126–30.

[22] Pinsky PF, Berg CD. Applying the National Lung Screening Trial eligibility criteria to the US population: what percent of the population and of incident lung cancers would be covered? Journal of Medical Screening. 2012;19(3):154–6. PMID: 23060474.

[23] Park ER, Streck JM, Gareen IF, Ostroff JS, Hyland KA, Rigotti NA, et al. A qualitative study of lung cancer risk perceptions and smoking beliefs among national lung screening trial

participants. Nicotine & Tobacco Research: Official Journal of the Society for Research on Nicotine and Tobacco. 2014;16(2):166–73. PMID: 23999653. Epub 2013/09/04.

[24] Ashraf H, Tønnesen P, Holst Pedersen J, Dirksen A, Thorsen H, Døssing M. Effect of CT screening on smoking habits at 1-year follow-up in the Danish Lung Cancer Screening Trial (DLCST). Thorax. 2009;64(5):388–92.

[25] van der Aalst CM, van den Bergh KA, Willemsen MC, de Koning HJ, van Klaveren RJ. Lung cancer screening and smoking abstinence: 2 year follow-up data from the Dutch-Belgian randomised controlled lung cancer screening trial. Thorax. 2010;65(7):600–5. PMID: 20627916.

[26] Villanti AC, Jiang Y, Abrams DB, Pyenson BS. A cost-utility analysis of lung cancer screening and the additional benefits of incorporating smoking cessation interventions. PloS One. 2013;8(8):e71379. PMID: 23940744. Pubmed Central PMCID: PMC3737088. Epub 2013/08/14.

[27] Tota JE, Ramanakumar AV, Franco EL. Lung cancer screening: review and performance comparison under different risk scenarios. Lung. 2013. PMID: 24153450. Epub 2013/10/25.

[28] van den Bergh KA, Essink-Bot ML, Borsboom GJ, Scholten ET, van Klaveren RJ, de Koning HJ. Long-term effects of lung cancer computed tomography screening on health-related quality of life: the NELSON trial. European Respiratory Journal. 2011;38(1):154–61. PMID: 21148229.

[29] Bach PB, Mirkin JN, Oliver TK, Azzoli CG, Berry DA, Brawley OW, et al. Benefits and harms of CT screening for lung cancer: a systematic review. JAMA. 2012;307(22):2418–29. PMID: 22610500. Pubmed Central PMCID: PMC3709596. Epub 2012/05/23. eng.

[30] Veronesi G, Maisonneuve P, Rampinelli C, Bertolotti R, Petrella F, Spaggiari L, et al. Computed tomography screening for lung cancer: results of 10 years of annual screening and validation of cosmos prediction model. Lung Cancer. 2013;82(3):426–30. PMID: 24099665. Epub 2013/10/09.

[31] Sobue T, Moriyama N, Kaneko M, Kusumoto M, Kobayashi T, Tsuchiya R, et al. Screening for lung cancer with low-dose helical computed tomography: anti-lung cancer association project. Journal of Clinical Oncology. 2002;20(4):911–20.

[32] Bastarrika G, Garcia-Velloso MJ, Lozano MD, Montes U, Torre W, Spiteri N, et al. Early lung cancer detection using spiral computed tomography and positron emission tomography. American Journal of Respiratory and Critical Care Medicine. 2005;171(12):1378–83. PMID: 15790860.

[33] Field JK, Smith RA, Aberle DR, et al. International Association for the Study of Lung Cancer computed tomography screening workshop 2011 report. Journal of Thoracic Oncology: Official Publication of the International Association for the Study of Lung Cancer. 2012;7:10–9.

[34] McMahon PM, Kong CY, Bouzan C, Weinstein MC, Cipriano LE, Tramontano AC, et al. Cost-effectiveness of CT screening for lung cancer in the U.S. Journal of Thoracic Oncology: Official Publication of the International Association for the Study of Lung Cancer. 2011;6(11):1841–8. PMID: PMC3202298.

[35] Baldwin DR, Callister ME. The British Thoracic Society guidelines on the investigation and management of pulmonary nodules. Thorax 2015.

[36] Corner J, Hopkinson J, Fitzsimmons D, Barclay S, Muers M. Is late diagnosis of lung cancer inevitable? Interview study of patients' recollections of symptoms before diagnosis. Thorax. 2005;60(4):314–9.

[37] Bowen EF, Rayner CF. Patient and GP led delays in the recognition of symptoms suggestive of lung cancer. Lung Cancer. 2002;37(2):227–8.

[38] Athey VL, Suckling RJ, Tod AM, Walters SJ, Rogers TK. Early diagnosis of lung cancer: evaluation of a community-based social marketing intervention. Thorax. 2012 May;67(5):412–7. PMID: 22052579. Epub 2011/11/05.

[39] Hurt CN, Roberts K, Rogers TK, Griffiths GO, Hood K, Prout H, et al. A feasibility study examining the effect on lung cancer diagnosis of offering a chest X-ray to higher-risk patients with chest symptoms: protocol for a randomized controlled trial. Trials 2013;14:405. PMID: 24279296.

Chapter 4

Transthoracic Ultrasonography: Advantages and Limitations in the Assessment of Lung Cancer

Romeo Ioan Chira, Alexandra Chira and
Petru Adrian Mircea

Additional information is available at the end of the chapter

http://dx.doi.org/10.5772/67169

Abstract

Lung cancer (LC) represents the leading cause of cancer-related mortality worldwide, with most of the cases being still diagnosed in advanced stages. Recently published data estimates an increase of LC deaths worldwide from 1.6 million in 2012 to 3 million in 2035. In this context, ultrasonography (US) aspires to become the method of choice that can offer essential information concerning subpleural LC. Therefore, it is an urgent need for an objective evaluation of the role of US and US-guided biopsies as an accurate diagnosis method, as until now large studies to assess this have been seldom performed. Our main aim was to perform a review over the use of US and US-guided biopsy in the assessment of LC, and our second aim was to illustrate how US is a valuable tool in the approach of patients with LC. We also compared the advantages and disadvantages of different types of biopsy needles. Other non-invasive applications of US (contrast-enhanced US and elastography) and their usefulness for LC were also evaluated. Though transthoracic US is today underused for lung cancer diagnosis, it offers multiple advantages that seem extremely useful for the efficient management of such tumours.

Keywords: biopsy, lung cancer, transthoracic, ultrasonography

1. Introduction

Lung cancer (LC) represents the leading cause of cancer-related mortality worldwide [1–3], with most of the cases being still diagnosed in advanced stages. Recently published data estimates an increase of LC deaths worldwide from 1.6 million in 2012 to 3 million in 2035 [3]. The 5-year survival of LC patients is still very low—15% even in the wealthiest countries—so urgent strategies are needed in order to facilitate early diagnosis or to improve current diagnosis techniques. Ultrasonography (US), with its multiple advantages, has an already well-established role in the management of tumoral and non-tumoral abdominal pathology. Though a common technique, US was less used for some organs such as the lung. Ultrasonography can assess peripheral lung tumours, offering valuable information related to the tumour structure, vascularization, the stage of parietal invasion and sometimes lymph node invasion. Moreover, US can guide the biopsy of the peripheral tumours with very good sensibility/specificity and less complications and smaller costs than computed tomography (CT). More recently, transthoracic US (TUS), US-guided biopsy and other applications (contrast-enhanced US and elastography) have gained a larger field in the management of patients with peripheral pulmonary nodules or masses. In this context, US aspires to become the method of choice that can offer essential information concerning subpleural LC [4, 5]. Therefore, an objective evaluation of the role of US and US-guided biopsies as accurate diagnosis method is necessary because until now large studies to assess this have been seldom performed.

2. Transthoracic ultrasonography for the lung cancer

2.1. Standard ultrasonography and its applications for lung cancer

Ventilated lung reflects up to 99% of the sound waves, and, consequently, the peripheral lung tumours abutting the visceral pleura can be visualized. When pleural effusions or condensate lung are present, facilitation of the ultrasound beam can also allow examination of deeper lesions.

US examination of the lung is performed with convex transducers with frequencies of 3–6 MHz. For chest wall and lung surface assessment, a higher frequencies—10–13 MHz—and linear transducers are needed. When TUS is recommended for evaluation of a lung tumour, it follows usually a radiological examination of the chest—X-ray (Rx) or computed tomography (CT)—which have detected a lesion. Otherwise, it is indicated for a localized pain or other clinical signs, so it is a guided examination of an area of the chest. Sometimes, this 'focused' US can be followed by a global US chest examination, as we must search peripheral lung, pleura or chest wall for metastasis. It is also important to scan cervical lymph nodes and at least upper abdominal organs - adrenal glands [6] and the liver for metastasis.

Normal pleuropulmonary interface is visualized as a hyperechoic line situated beneath the chest wall structure, followed by reverberation artefacts (A-lines), being mobile with respiration in real-time examination which represent the 'gliding sign'. The presence of a subpleural pulmonary lesion interrupts this hyperechoic line, appearing as a hypoechoic image with different shapes, structures and contours according somehow to the type of the disease.

When a lung tumour is identified, TUS should try to solve several issues. One of the most important problems is represented by differential diagnosis between benign and malignant lesions [7]. TUS can describe certain characteristics of a peripheral lung lesion in order to suggest benign or malignant characteristic:

—Contour of the lung surface may be irregular in LC and regular in benign lesions.

—The margins of the tumours are sharp, delineated from the ventilated lung (**Figure 1**). They can be irregular or with finger-shaped ramification into the normal lung. Benign lesions are usually less sharp delimited from normal ventilated lung.

—Destruction of the adjacent lung. LC invades the adjacent parenchyma and either destroys or displaces the bronchi and normal vessels which normally present a radial, centrifugal distribution identifiable with colour Doppler US examination (**Figure 2**). Tumour neovascularization can be seen as tortuous vessels usually situated in the periphery and calibre variations [8, 9].

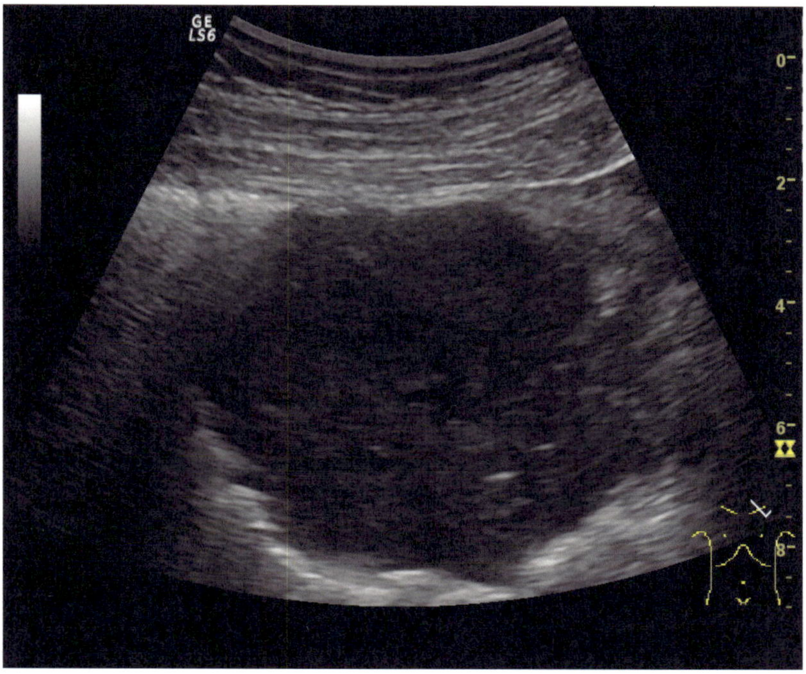

Figure 1. Ultrasonography aspect of a lung cancer abutting the pleura—hypoechoic mass, slight inhomogeneous, with irregular surface but sharp delimited from ventilated lung.

The most difficult situations are represented by chronic pneumonia and cicatricial peripheral lesion [10] which cannot be differentiated only by imagistic methods. In these cases, the histopathological exam is decisive.

If the diagnosis of malignancy is obvious, TUS can offer elements for staging of the lung cancer too. This information (assessment of resectability) can be critical for the decision of surgical treatment or other types of therapies. Contribution of TUS for staging LC should comprise the evaluation for the invasion of the adjacent structures (T3/T4), the extension to the lymph nodes which can be examined by US—supraclavicular, axillar, and sometimes intrathoracic—and the metastases in the liver, adrenal glands (mostly left side) or other sites.

Concerning chest wall invasion US has been proven to be at least as accurate as magnetic resonance imaging (MRI) and superior to CT by many studies (**Table 1**).

There are four criteria to be checked for the diagnosis of chest wall invasion: (a) absence of the gliding sign of the tumour over the chest wall, (b) interruption of the pleuropulmonary line, (c) direct invasion of the soft structures of the wall (**Figure 3**), and (d) direct invasion of the bony parts—mostly ribs by the tumour [14] (**Figure 4**). One of the last two criteria is diagnostic; the first two (respectively, a and b) are only suggesting invasion. A recent study also proposed a cut-off value of 4.5 cm for diameters of the LC predicting invasion of the chest wall [16]. Unfortunately, TUS is not used widely enough for these purposes, even though it has the well-known advantages over CT—availability, cost, time of examination and lack of irradiation. Invasion of the diaphragm and pericardium can be also assessed by TUS, considering the possibility of real-time evaluation to prove direct extension of the tumour and not only the contact between this and the structure of interest.

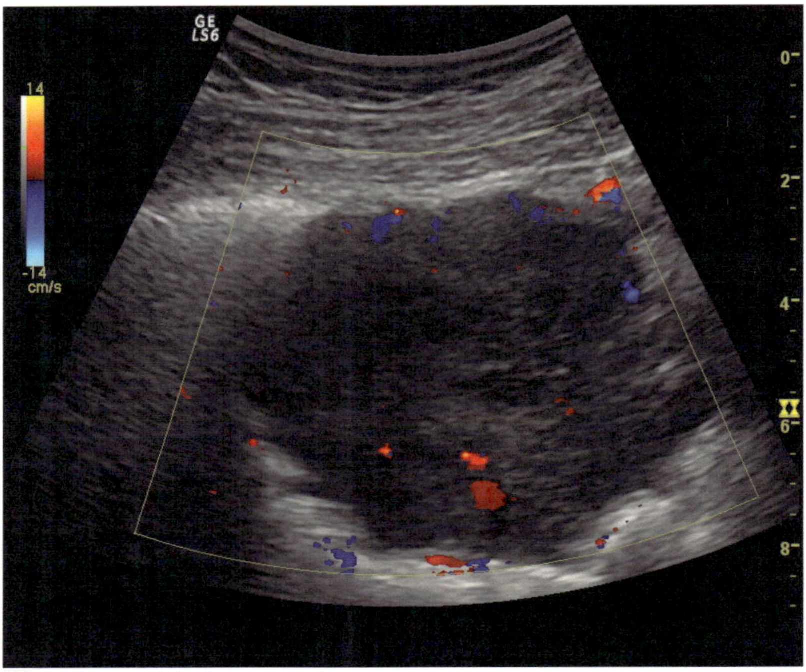

Figure 2. Colour Doppler US of a lung cancer showing hypovascularity without normal, radial distribution of vessels and bronchi (destruction of normal structure of the lung).

Author	Number of patients	TUS	CT
Sugama et al. [11]	65	Acc = 77%	Acc = 39%
Suzuki et al. [12]	120	Se = 100%	Se = 68%
Nakano et al. [13]	23	Se = 76.9%, Sp = 68.8%, Acc = 72.4%	Se = 69.2%, Sp = 75.0%, Acc = 72.4%
Bandi et al. [14]	90	Se = 89%, Sp = 95%	Se = 42%, Sp = 100%
Tahiri et al. [15]	28	Se = 90.9%, Sp = 85.7%	
Caroli et al. [16]	14	Se = 88.89%, Sp = 100%	

Acc - accuracy; Se - sensibility; Sp - specificity.

Table 1. Studies comparing diagnostic performances for chest wall invasion of LC for TUS and CT.

http://dx.doi.org/10.5772/67169

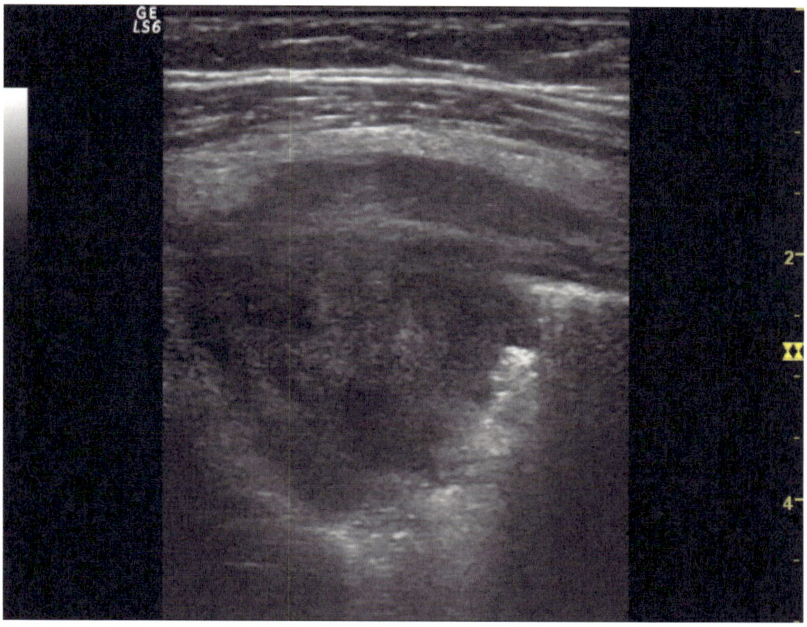

Figure 3. Peripheral hypoechoic and inhomogeneous LC with irregular contour, invading soft structures of the chest wall (extension of the tumour in the neighbouring layers of the wall).

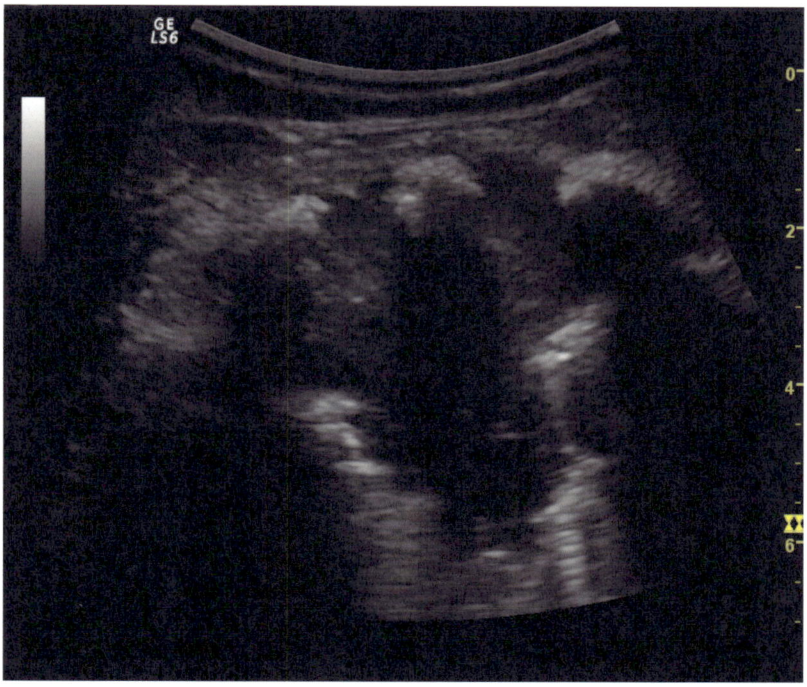

Figure 4. Peripheral hypoechoic LC invading the chest wall including ribs (three ovoid hyperechoic images with acoustic shadows partially included in the superficial tumoral area).

The presence of a pleural effusion signifies a T4 stage of the disease in an LC patient [17] or M1a (according to the 7th American Joint Committee on Cancer LC classification) although in rare cases it can have other causes (lymphatic drainage dysfunction, hypoproteinemia, atelectasis) [18]. In such situation, aspiration of fluid guided by TUS followed by cytological and biochemical analysis could solve the differential diagnosis of the effusions.

In the presence of atelectasis, TUS can delineate tumoral area from atelectatic lung even better than CT scans [19] based on structure, contour and vessel disposition in targeted areas (**Figure 5**). Also large LCs, usually more than 5 cm in diameter, demonstrate central necrosis. Those structural changes can be visualized as hypoechoic or transonic areas (**Figure 6**), and when communication with the bronchial tree or infection occurs, they appear as aerated hyperechoic irregular images surrounded by a thick wall hypoechoic masses (**Figure 7**). Those necrotic changes should always be precisely identified if a transthoracic-guided biopsy is taken into account. Thus, it is surprisingly how extended can be the necrosis inside larger tumours. In these cases, the best delimitation is realized by contrast-enhanced US (CEUS) where they appear as non-enhancing areas inside a late-enhancing tumoral tissue (see also the section dedicated to CEUS).

When a central tumour becomes obstructive, it will be associated with atelectasis or recurrent pneumonitis in the same region. Consolidation of the lung tissue allows better transmission of the ultrasound beam and visualization of the tumour through the non-ventilated lung. Other signs—as vascular distribution and fluid bronchogram—can be also seen inside the consolidated non-tumoral areas.

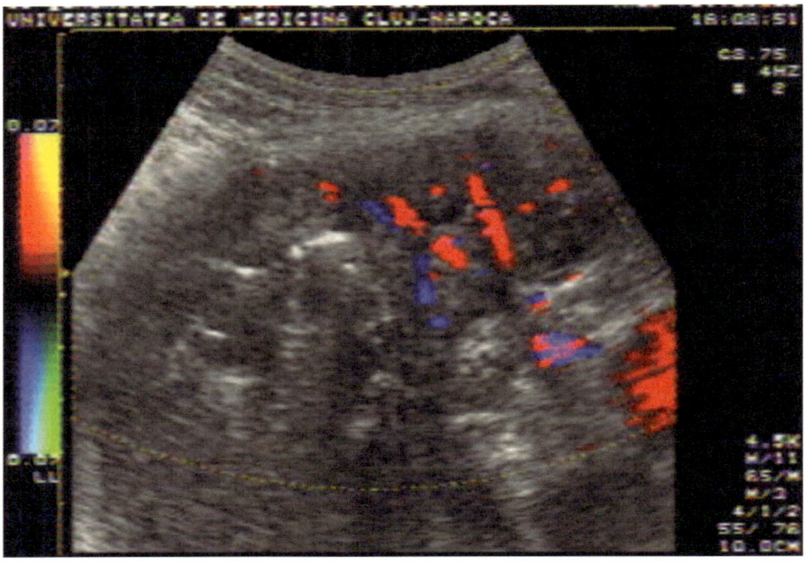

Figure 5. Large hypovascular lung cancer with central excavation containing gas (hyperechoic intratumoral images) and peritumoral atelectasis showing normal distribution of vessels (colour Doppler US examination).

http://dx.doi.org/10.5772/67169

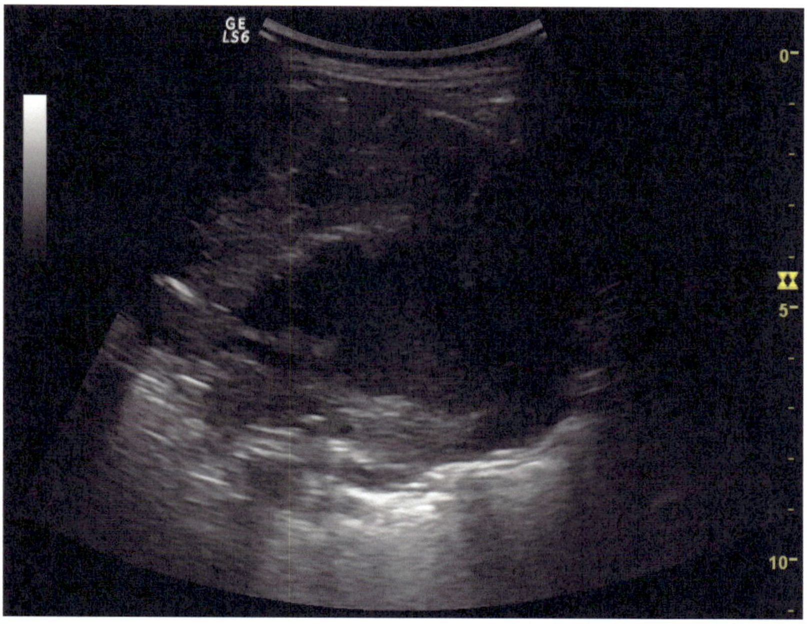

Figure 6. Large ovoid-shaped hypoechoic LC (squamous cell cancer) containing large central echo-free areas (necrosis).

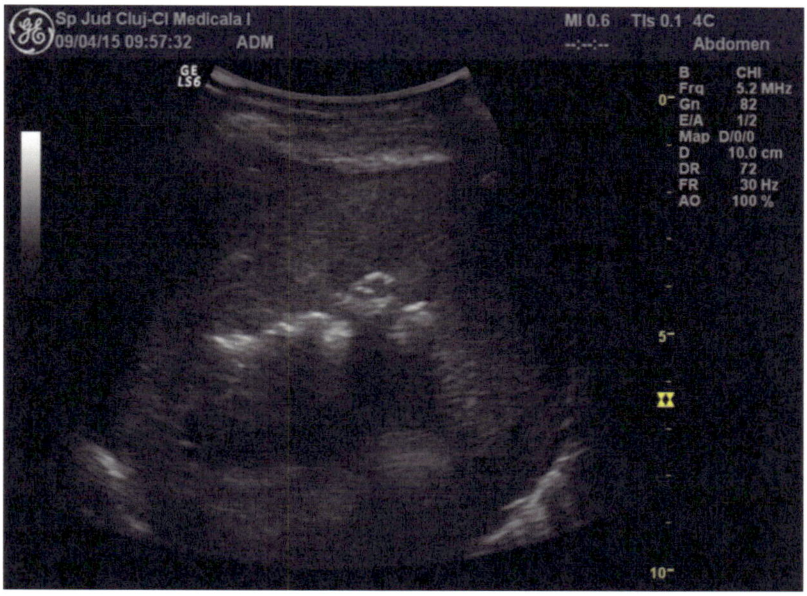

Figure 7. Large round-shaped hypoechoic LC (squamous cell cancer) containing hyperechoic central images corresponding to excavated necrotic core.

Colour Doppler examination of the neoplastic lung lesions reveals a reduced vascularization and disruption of normal vessel architecture [8, 9, 20]. In neoplastic lesions invasion of pulmonary arteries occurs in 56–87% of cases [21, 22], and vascularization is based mainly on neoangiogenesis originating in bronchial artery [23]. Moreover, central areas of the tumours are hypovascular due to stenosis/occlusions of pulmonary arteries. Duplex Doppler evaluation of impedance indices reveals monophasic low-resistance flow in the arterial vessels of the tumours [9] compared to high resistivity indices in pulmonary arteries present in benign lesions. Neoangiogenetic vessels can be suspected if they present a variable and convoluted/irregular position (**Figure 8**), variable flow direction and near-constant flow with reduced systolic-diastolic variations. It is important to know that almost 50% of the lung lesions present more than one type of vascularization [24] underlining the complexity of vascular distribution.

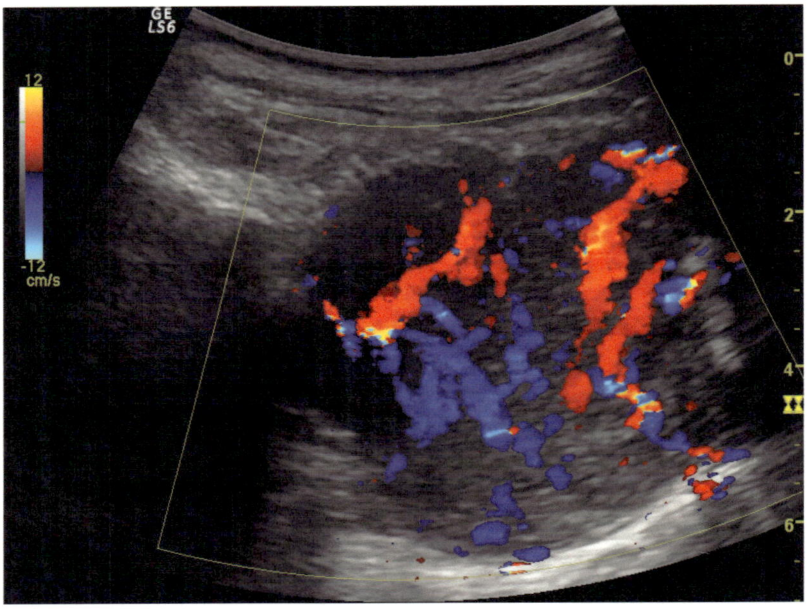

Figure 8. Hypervascular peripheral round-shaped hypoechoic LC with neovascularization—tortuous vessels with variable flow direction.

One of the most difficult diagnostic problems is represented by the peripheral adenocarcinoma with lepidic growth, which looks similar to a benign consolidation. The tumour can also preserve the normal bronchial tree and pseudo-normal distribution of vasculature (**Figure 9**) mimicking almost perfect pneumonic areas [25]. Minimal changes suggesting malignancy can be represented by irregular lung surface. In these cases, transthoracic US-guided biopsy refines the diagnosis.

In some cases, TUS can prove the extension of LC to hilar or mediastinal vessel. The invasion of pulmonary vessels can be visualized through the condensed or neoplastic lung in advanced cases. In these cases, TUS can also visualize metastatic hilar or mediastinal

http://dx.doi.org/10.5772/67169

lymph nodes, which are commonly impossible to assess by this method. The superior vena cava should be examined in order to diagnose compression or thrombosis of the locally advanced LC.

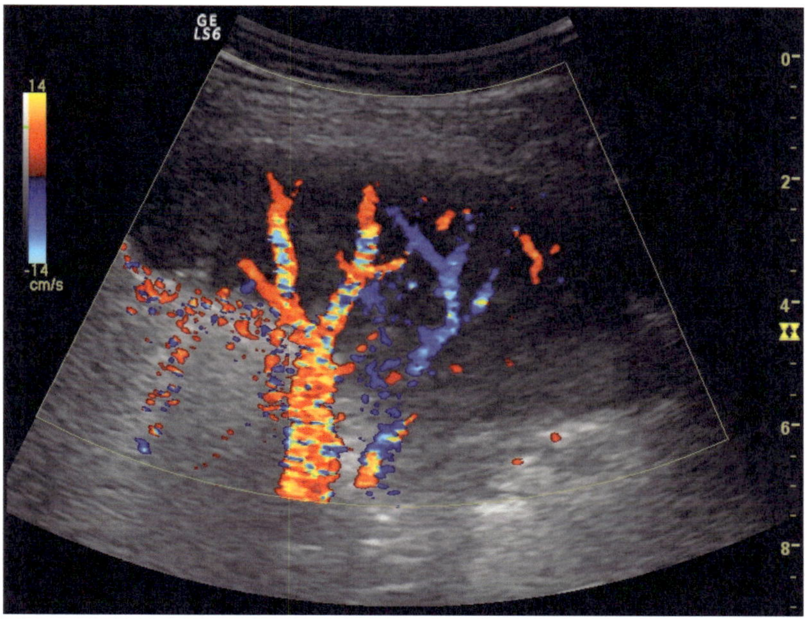

Figure 9. Adenocarcinoma with lepidic growth mimicking benign consolidation (pneumonia-like) with triangular-shaped and pseudonormal distribution of vascularization.

Another important component of US evaluation of an LC patient should include screening for the metastatic lymph nodes which cannot be clinically assessed with good accuracy—mainly supraclavicular stations. Metastases in cervical and supraclavicular nodes are present in 16–26% of cases, and US improves the identification of these affected stations with 31% [26, 27]. It surpasses three times the palpation performances and also CT scan with identification of 18–36% more cases of metastasis.

For the next step—histopathological diagnosis—TUS offers the possibility of guiding the percutaneous biopsy of the peripheral LC, with many advantages over radiological methods which were classically used. US guidance for transthoracic biopsies was done firstly more than four decades in the past, and since then, it has been successfully performed with various needle types [28, 29]. Indications and contraindications for percutaneous lung biopsy are according to the guidelines [30]. Most contraindications of transthoracic needle biopsy (TNB) are relative (platelet count < 100.000/ml, activated partial thromboplastin time (APTT) ratio or prothrombin time (PT) ratio > 1.4, contralateral pneumonectomy, Forced expiratory volume in the first second (FEV_1) < 35% or 1 l) and should be discussed in a multidisciplinary team [30]. Besides the contraindications, there are some limitations or particular situations such as the patients with pneumonectomy and nodule (either multiple or single) in the remaining lung [31]. Not seldom we encounter patients presenting multiple comorbidities that affect respiratory and/or circulatory systems such as chronic heart failure, chronic respiratory failure or association of the two. In patients with such severe disease, oxygen therapy during the procedure might be essential, since the approach of the lesions requires the patient to lay down either in dorsal or even in ventral decubitus in order to perform the biopsy.

Complications of TNB are theoretically numerous (chest wall haematoma, parietal pain, pneumothorax, haemoptysis, intrapulmonary haemorrhage, haemothorax, air embolism, empyema—mostly for infected lesions, tumour seeding along the needle tract, death (0.15%)) [30]. Among those two are more important: haemoptysis and pneumothorax. Haemoptysis is most of the time self-limited (in less than 1% significant) and not life-threatening. It appears seldom after US guidance—under 3% than under CT guidance, 5.3–15% [32]—also due to deeper lung tumour approach by CT. The risk of pneumothorax after US-guided TNB is significantly lower (1–3%) than after CT-guided biopsy (up to 20.5–25%), due to the real time visualization and direct approach of the tumors abutting the pleura during the US-guided biopsies. It is increased in the presence of emphysema and larger needle calibre [32]. The presence of pneumothorax must be routinely checked after TNB, and the presence of clinically significant pneumothorax must be followed by percutaneous drainage which can be done also under US guidance [30].

An original study that compared CT-guided biopsy versus US-guided biopsy concluded that US is a valuable option to CT for guidance of transthoracic biopsies [33]. Authors found that US guidance provided diagnosis in 91% cases, while CT in 71%. In the same study analyzing the average time for biopsy and the average time per passage, results indicated that they were both statistically significantly shorter for US guidance than for CT guidance of the biopsy ($P < 0.05$) [33]. Results obtained by Sconfienza et al. [34] also favour US for biopsy guidance, the authors reporting successful biopsies using US guidance in 97.1% versus the CT-guided biopsies in which technical success was obtained in 96.5%. Also, there was a statistically significant lower rate of pneumothoraxes ($P = 0.025$) and a shorter median time per intervention for US compared to the CT-guided biopsy [34]. A review published in 2015 [35] revealed important aspects summarizing data regarding US, CT and electromagnetic navigational-transthoracic needle aspiration. In this review data from 75 studies was analyzed with authors finding that the rate of post procedure pneumothorax was higher in CT (20.5%) than in US-guided biopsy (4.4%). The authors underline also the paucity of data regarding US-guided biopsy since they have found just ten studies that assessed it and forty-eight that have performed CT-guided biopsy. Authors have determined an overall pooled diagnostic accuracy for CT to be 92.1% and for US 88.7% with similar sensitivities for the detection of malignancies—92.1% for CT and, respectively, 91.5% for US [35].

Some authors did not found a statistically significant difference in the diagnostic yield of fine-needle aspiration (FNA) versus core biopsy or FNA + core biopsy ($P = 0.96$) [36]. Other authors found that cutting-needle biopsies are more sensitive than fine-needle aspiration for the diagnosis of malignancies including mesothelioma [37, 38]. It is considered now that there are some advantages for the cutting needles over fine needle consisting in a superior diagnostic

http://dx.doi.org/10.5772/67169

accuracy, a better differentiation of LC subtypes and a better sensibility for the diagnosis of lung benign lesion [39].

An older study compared a cutting needle (Trucut) versus an aspiration needle (Surecut—a modified Menghini) concluding that US-guided needle biopsy was accurate and safe while providing an adequate histological specimen with a diagnostic yield comparable for both of the needles [40]. An important study regarding the types of needle is the study performed by Tombesi et al. [41]. The authors compared Trucut-type and a Menghini-modified needles. They found that the Trucut needle was superior, as it achieved a correct diagnosis more than the Menghini modified results that reached statistical significance ($P = 0.0041$). The authors also compared the diagnostic yield and found that the Trucut improved the diagnostic yield significantly statistic for smaller lesions ≤2 cm ($P = 0.0139$). Also, the Trucut needle provided a lower number of inadequate specimens [41].

Comparison the data concerning biopsy needle diameter indicated that a larger diameter does not have a significantly higher benefit [38, 42, 43].

The size of the lesion is not a problem for US guidance, even small tumour (less than 2 cm) being amenable for this approach [36, 44].

For optimization of the biopsy accuracy, various strategies have been proposed regarding [45] the approach and incidence of the needle, the orientation of the probe or the use of probes which allow guidance by a central orifice [28, 46].

It is well known that US guidance of the transthoracic biopsy of neoplastic lesions improves the overall performance, even in the presence of the necrosis [47]. Necrotic areas in larger tumours can lower the accuracy of TNB with 9–26% [48, 49]. Contrast-enhanced US (CEUS) can solve this issue, by revealing the non-enhancing areas corresponding to necrosis [50].

Regarding the factors that affect diagnostic yield in US-guided transthoracic biopsy, Jeon et al. found that the only statistically significant factor was the lesion-pleura contact arc length [51]. Some authors have not found statistically significant correlations between the size of the pleural surface of the lesion and the outcome—an adequate biopsy specimen ($P = 0.106$) or the incidence of complications ($P = 0.23$) [52].

Fontalvo et al. [52] analyzed the US-guided biopsy performed in children and found that this technique is safe and adequate for sampling of lung tissue.

Though the rate of complications is low, constant efforts are made to optimize the US guidance of biopsies [45] as well as for training specialists [53, 54]. Still, there are discrepancies even when comparing data from studies; in some of the studies, biopsies were performed using the free-hand technique which is more operator dependent and other studies using automatized systems for guidance. Using a guidance system allows a more predictable path of the needle, as well as a shorten time for performing the biopsy [55]. The free-hand approach has also certain advantages, providing more freedom to the operator, and reduces the costs associated with the use of various systems for various transducers. Those advantages have led some authors and centres to prefer free-hand guidance [55]. Also, in our centre, we prefer and perform the free-hand approach.

After the complete diagnosis, the results of the chosen therapy (assessment of response and recurrence) can be followed up precisely by TUS and can save a lot of resources and irradiation for the patients with peripheral LC.

2.2. Newer ultrasonography techniques for lung diseases

2.2.1. Contrast-enhanced ultrasonography (CEUS)

The first results of the application of CEUS in lung tumours were represented by a better identification of necrotic areas in order to improve the performance of percutaneous US-guided biopsy [50]. The authors reported a successful percutaneous biopsy after using a contrast agent in a case with previous non-diagnostic US-guided biopsy. In recent studies, another authors showed much more frequent identification of necrosis in patients with tumours when they used CEUS (43.9%) compared with standard US (6.7%) and an improvement in diagnostic performance of biopsies after CEUS (93.6% compared to 80%) [56, 57].

Benign lung lesions have dual arterial supply (pulmonary and bronchial) compared to LC that usually has just a single arterial supply (bronchial). This peculiarity of LC perfusion can be demonstrated with the use of intravascular contrast agents. CEUS has added diagnostic value to standard US examination [58, 59] of the pleural-based lesions. The contrast substance commonly used is the second-generation agent hexafluoride sulphur (Sonovue®, Bracco Imaging srl, Milano, Italy). One of the preliminary studies using CEUS for the diagnosis of peripheral lung lesions (60 cases) has offered a sensitivity of for CEUS 95.0% compared with CT 96.66%, B-mode ultrasound 83.33% and conventional radiology 86.66% [60]. They found three signs suggesting neoplastic lesion (inhomogeneous enhancement, absence of pulmonary arteries and wash-out within the first 120 s) in 88.8% of cases [60]. Other studies (95 cases) proved that LC has a later enhancement—more than 2 s delay from normal lung or benign lung lesions [61]—or synchronous with the chest wall and a variable extent of enhancement (non-homogenous, with non-enhancing areas corresponding to necrosis). Also, these authors have proposed an arbitrary score of enhancement and wash-out parameters after contrast administration that has also offered significant sensibility (Se = 98.1%, Sp = 95.1%) [61].

2.2.2. Ultrasonographic elastography in lung cancer

There are few studies published assessing US elastography for lung tumours. One of them used colour-coded strain elastography on 95 patients, of which 61 have been diagnosed with lung cancer and the other 34 with pneumonic condensations [62]. The authors found that LC has a significantly statistic ($P < 0.001$) higher rigidity and high elastographic Itoh's score (of 4–5) [63] comparing it to pneumonia and lymphoma which demonstrated lower scores (≤3) [62]. Considering score 4 as a cut-off value for colour-coded elastography (in a scale of 0–5), this value has a sensibility of 87% and specificity of 99% for diagnosis of lung cancer. Also, squamous LC had the highest score, almost 5. These possibilities of differentiation malignant from benign lung lesions based on the elastography properties can be a useful adjunct for US method.

Another group tried to visualize through elastographic approach in pulmonary metastasis without pleural contact (invisible otherwise by US), and they succeed in a preliminary study to identify all lesions situated within 2.5 cm from the pleural space [64] in 18 patients. This new application tries to push further the borders of TUS application into a new area [65], and data presented by Adamietz et al. [64] proved its tremendous potential. The time will probably show if the peripheral tumours without pleural contact will be investigated by elastographic methods, but further rigorous studies to assess a greater number of patients to prove that the technique is reproducible are mandatory.

3. Advantages of transthoracic ultrasonography

Firstly, there are general advantages of US examination compared with other radiological examinations, considering availability, cost, time, lack of irradiation and bedside examination in critical patients. Careful and complete examination of a lung lesion by TUS can provide a lot of information for its benign or malignant character. For malignant lesions TUS provides very important details concerning size, local extension, association of atelectasis, necrosis, vascular invasion and sometimes intrathoracic lymph node metastasis. It can also diagnose pleural effusions with the highest sensitivity compared to other radiological methods. Also, for some information provided by TUS, accuracy is superior to that of CT scans and at least comparable to MRI. For example, diagnosis of chest wall invasion of LC by TUS has been already proven by many studies [14, 19, 66] to be more precise than those provided by CT. Being a dynamic exploration, TUS has advantages over CT scans, allowing a real-time examination of the pleuropulmonary interface during spontaneous respiration or cough.

Introduction of second-generation contrast agents for US added the possibility of perfusion analysis of lung lesion, with much less adverse reaction compared to other contrast agents used with CT (especially allergic, nephrotoxicity, etc.). CEUS improves the differential diagnostic between benign and malignant lesions, provides a better delineation of necrotic areas inside the tumours improving also the performance of US-guided lung biopsy. In the patients with allergic reaction or contraindications for administration of contrast agents, elastography can be used, and colour-coded information show a higher rigidity of the tumours compared to benign lesion (pneumonia being most studied). Also, we mentioned that, among cancers, squamous type showed the highest rigidity.

There are certain advantages for the US-guided biopsy over CT-guided biopsy:

—Comparable sensitivity and specificity with lower costs

—Less complications

—Less time

—No irradiation.

In patients with lung cancer US has to assess also extrathoracic lymph nodes, cervical, supraclavicular and eventually axillary, and at least the upper abdominal organ commonly affected by metastatic disease, the liver, adrenal glands (mainly left) and lymph nodes.

4. Limitations of transthoracic ultrasonography

TUS allows the assessment of pleural-based masses, providing information proportionally with the dimension of the contact of the tumour with the chest wall. When the pleural abutting is very small, only a part of the tumour can be seen even if it is large, but when the cancer invades the parietal pleura or the chest wall on large front, it can be characterized completely by TUS. Interposition of bony parts of the thorax and shoulder can also limit the visibility of some peripheral lesions (paravertebral, retroscapular, some apical tumours) by TUS and, consecutively, also the possibility of US-guided biopsy. Another limitation of TUS is the presence of chest wall pathology above the pulmonary region of interest—hematoma, fractures and parietal tumours—or pleural disease like calcifying pleuritis or fibrothorax which doesn't allow a proper examination of subsidiary lung areas. But fortunately, those situations are uncommon.

Contact of a tumour with the heart can be a limitation for TNB due to movement of the lesion. Limited pleural contact of an LC in patients with comorbidities and dyspnoea can increase the risk of post-TNB complications.

A problem for all imagistic methods is the differential diagnosis of primary LC from metastases. When metastases are abutting the visceral pleura, they can be visualized by TUS as rounded or ovoid hypoechoic lesions without aeric alveolograms. Their surfaces are sharp delineated from the surrounded lung with regular or irregular contours, and the vessels are usually displaced into the periphery. Single metastasis cannot be differentiated from primary LC, but when they are multiple or in a suggestive clinical context (other primary lesion diagnosed), they should be suspected.

5. Conclusions

Considering all advantages and limitations, TUS represents an essential investigation not only for the characterization of lung tumours, mainly subpleural, but also for guidance of various interventional procedures. It offers many advantages over CT including a better accuracy for identification of tumour necrosis, atelectasis, chest wall invasion and fewer complications after transthoracic US-guided biopsy with same accuracy as CT-guided biopsy.

Abbreviations

APTT	Activated partial thromboplastin time
CEUS	Contrast-enhanced ultrasonography
CT	Computed tomography
FEV_1	Forced expiratory volume in the first
FNA	Fine-needle aspiration
MRI	Magnetic resonance imaging

PT	Prothrombin time
SQC	Squamous cell lung carcinoma
TNB	Transthoracic needle biopsy
TUS	Transthoracic ultrasonography

Author details

Romeo Ioan Chira[1]*, Alexandra Chira[2] and Petru Adrian Mircea[1]

*Address all correspondence to: romeochira@yahoo.com

1 1st Medical Clinic, Department of Internal Medicine, "Iuliu Hatieganu" University of Medicine and Pharmacy, Cluj-Napoca, Romania

2 2nd Medical Clinic, Department of Internal Medicine, "Iuliu Hatieganu" University of Medicine and Pharmacy, Cluj-Napoca, Romania

References

[1] SEER Cancer Statistics Factsheets: Lung and Bronchus Cancer. Bethesda MNCI. [cited 2016 April 8]; Available from: http://seer.cancer.gov/statfacts/html/lungb.html.

[2] Dela Cruz CS, Tanoue LT, Matthay RA. Lung cancer: epidemiology, etiology, and prevention. Clin Chest Med. 2011;32(4):605–44. DOI: 10.1016/j.ccm.2011.09.001

[3] Didkowska J, Wojciechowska U, Manczuk M, Lobaszewski J. Lung cancer epidemiology: contemporary and future challenges worldwide. Ann Transl Med. 2016;4(8):150. DOI: 10.21037/atm.2016.03.11

[4] Wang S, Yang W, Zhang H, Xu Q, Yan K. The role of contrast-enhanced ultrasound in selection indication and improveing diagnosis for transthoracic biopsy in peripheral pulmonary and mediastinal lesions. Biomed Res Int. 2015;2015:231782. DOI: 10.1155/2015/231782

[5] Sartori S, Tombesi P. Emerging roles for transthoracic ultrasonography in pulmonary diseases. World J Radiol. 2010;2(6):203–14. DOI: 10.4329/wjr.v2.i6.203

[6] Allard P, Yankaskas BC, Fletcher RH, Parker LA, Halvorsen RA, Jr. Sensitivity and specificity of computed tomography for the detection of adrenal metastatic lesions among 91 autopsied lung cancer patients. Cancer. 1990;66(3):457–62.

[7] Beckh S. Neoplastic consolidations in the lung: primary lung tumors and metastases. In: Mathis G, editor. Chest Sonography. 3rd ed: Springer-Verlag Berlin Heidelberg 2011. pp. 69–77. DOI: 10.1007/978-3-642-21247-5

[8] Yuan A, Chang DB, Yu CJ, Kuo SH, Luh KT, Yang PC. Color Doppler sonography of benign and malignant pulmonary masses. AJR Am J Roentgenol. 1994;163(3):545–9. DOI: 10.2214/ajr.163.3.8079841

[9] Hsu WH, Ikezoe J, Chen CY, Kwan PC, Hsu CP, Hsu NY, et al. Color Doppler ultrasound signals of thoracic lesions. Correlation with resected histologic specimens. Am J Respir Crit Care Med. 1996;153(6 Pt 1):1938–51. DOI: 10.1164/ajrccm.153.6.8665059

[10] Mathis G. Thoraxsonography—part II: peripheral pulmonary consolidation. Ultrasound Med Biol. 1997;23(8):1141–53.

[11] Sugama Y, Tamaki S, Kitamura S, Kira S. Ultrasonographic evaluation of pleural and chest wall invasion of lung cancer. Chest. 1988;93(2):275–9.

[12] Suzuki N, Saitoh T, Kitamura S. Tumor invasion of the chest wall in lung cancer: diagnosis with US. Radiology. 1993;187(1):39–42. DOI: 10.1148/radiology.187.1.8451433

[13] Nakano N, Yasumitsu T, Kotake Y, Morino H, Ikezoe J. Preoperative histologic diagnosis of chest wall invasion by lung cancer using ultrasonically guided biopsy. J Thorac Cardiovasc Surg. 1994;107(3):891–5.

[14] Bandi V, Lunn W, Ernst A, Eberhardt R, Hoffmann H, Herth FJ. Ultrasound vs. CT in detecting chest wall invasion by tumor: a prospective study. Chest. 2008;133(4):881–6. DOI: 10.1378/chest.07-1656

[15] Tahiri M, Khereba M, Thiffault V, Ferraro P, Duranceau A, Martin J, et al. Preoperative assessment of chest wall invasion in non-small cell lung cancer using surgeon-performed ultrasound. Ann Thorac Surg. 2014;98(3):984–9. DOI: 10.1016/j.athoracsur.2014.04.111

[16] Caroli G, Dell'Amore A, Cassanelli N, Dolci G, Pipitone E, Asadi N, et al. Accuracy of transthoracic ultrasound for the prediction of chest wall infiltration by lung cancer and of lung infiltration by chest wall tumours. Heart Lung Circ. 2015;24(10):1020–6. DOI: 10.1016/j.hlc.2015.03.018

[17] Prosch H, Mathis G, Mostbeck GH. Percutaneous ultrasound in diagnosis and staging of lung cancer. Ultraschall Med. 2008;29(5):466–78; quiz 79–84. DOI: 10.1055/s-2008-1027672

[18] Rivera MP, Mehta AC. Initial diagnosis of lung cancer: ACCP evidence-based clinical practice guidelines (2nd edition). Chest. 2007;132(3 Suppl):131S–48S. DOI: 10.1378/chest.07-1357

[19] Chira R, Chira A, Mircea PA. Intrathoracic tumors in contact with the chest wall--ultrasonographic and computed tomography comparative evaluation. Med Ultrason. 2012;14(2):115–9.

[20] Civardi G, Fornari F, Cavanna L, Di Stasi M, Sbolli G, Rossi S, et al. Vascular signals from pleura-based lung lesions studied with pulsed Doppler ultrasonography. J Clin Ultrasound. 1993;21(9):617–22.

[21] Fisseler-Eckhoff A, Muller KM. The pathology of the pulmonary arteries in lung tumors. Dtsch Med Wochenschr. 1994;119(42):1415–20. DOI: 10.1055/s-2008-1058854

[22] Kolin A, Koutoulakis T. Role of arterial occlusion in pulmonary scar cancers. Hum Pathol. 1988;19(10):1161–7.

[23] Mitzner W, Lee W, Georgakopoulos D, Wagner E. Angiogenesis in the mouse lung. Am J Pathol. 2000;157(1):93–101. DOI: 10.1016/S0002-9440(10)64521-X

[24] Gorg C, Seifart U, Gorg K, Zugmaier G. Color Doppler sonographic mapping of pulmonary lesions: evidence of dual arterial supply by spectral analysis. J Ultrasound Med. 2003;22(10):1033–9.

[25] Gorg C, Seifart U, Holzinger I, Wolf M, Zugmaier G. Bronchioloalveolar carcinoma: sonographic pattern of 'pneumonia'. Eur J Ultrasound. 2002;15(3):109–17.

[26] Fultz PJ, Feins RH, Strang JG, Wandtke JC, Johnstone DW, Watson TJ, et al. Detection and diagnosis of nonpalpable supraclavicular lymph nodes in lung cancer at CT and US. Radiology. 2002;222(1):245–51. DOI: 10.1148/radiol.2221010431

[27] Prosch H, Strasser G, Sonka C, Oschatz E, Mashaal S, Mohn-Staudner A, et al. Cervical ultrasound (US) and US-guided lymph node biopsy as a routine procedure for staging of lung cancer. Ultraschall Med. 2007;28(6):598–603. DOI: 10.1055/s-2007-963215

[28] Goldberg BB, Pollack HM. Ultrasonic aspiration transducer. Radiology. 1972;102(1):187–9. DOI: 10.1148/102.1.187

[29] Chandrasekhar AJ, Reynes CJ, Churchill RJ. Ultrasonically guided percutaneous biopsy of peripheral pulmonary masses. Chest. 1976;70(5):627–30.

[30] Manhire A, Charig M, Clelland C, Gleeson F, Miller R, Moss H, et al. Guidelines for radiologically guided lung biopsy. Thorax. 2003;58(11):920–36.

[31] Klein JS, Zarka MA. Transthoracic needle biopsy. Radiol Clin North Am. 2000;38(2):235–66, vii.

[32] Ernst A, Silvestri GA, Johnstone D. Interventional pulmonary procedures: guidelines from the American College of Chest Physicians. Chest. 2003;123(5):1693–717.

[33] Sheth S, Hamper UM, Stanley DB, Wheeler JH, Smith PA. US guidance for thoracic biopsy: a valuable alternative to CT. Radiology. 1999;210(3):721–6. DOI: 10.1148/radiology.210.3.r99mr23721

[34] Sconfienza LM, Mauri G, Grossi F, Truini M, Serafini G, Sardanelli F, et al. Pleural and peripheral lung lesions: comparison of US- and CT-guided biopsy. Radiology. 2013;266(3):930–5. DOI: 10.1148/radiol.12112077

[35] DiBardino DM, Yarmus LB, Semaan RW. Transthoracic needle biopsy of the lung. J Thorac Dis. 2015;7(Suppl 4):S304–16. DOI: 10.3978/j.issn.2072-1439.2015.12.16

[36] Garcia-Ortega A, Briones-Gomez A, Fabregat S, Martinez-Tomas R, Martinez-Garcia MA, Cases E. Benefit of chest ultrasonography in the diagnosis of peripheral thoracic lesions in an interventional pulmonology unit. Arch Bronconeumol. 2016;52(5):244–9. DOI: 10.1016/j.arbres.2015.07.012

[37] Adams RF, Gleeson FV. Percutaneous image-guided cutting-needle biopsy of the pleura in the presence of a suspected malignant effusion. Radiology. 2001;219(2):510–4. DOI: 10.1148/radiology.219.2.r01ma07510

[38] Adams RF, Gray W, Davies RJ, Gleeson FV. Percutaneous image-guided cutting needle biopsy of the pleura in the diagnosis of malignant mesothelioma. Chest. 2001;120(6):1798–802.

[39] Diacon AH, Theron J, Schubert P, Brundyn K, Louw M, Wright CA, et al. Ultrasound-assisted transthoracic biopsy: fine-needle aspiration or cutting-needle biopsy?. Eur Respir J. 2007;29(2):357–62. DOI: 10.1183/09031936.00077706

[40] Pang JA, Tsang V, Hom BL, Metreweli C. Ultrasound-guided tissue-core biopsy of thoracic lesions with Trucut and Surecut needles. Chest. 1987;91(6):823–8.

[41] Tombesi P, Nielsen I, Tassinari D, Trevisani L, Abbasciano V, Sartori S. Transthoracic ultrasonography-guided core needle biopsy of pleural-based lung lesions: prospective randomized comparison between a Tru-cut-type needle and a modified Menghini-type needle. Ultraschall Med. 2009;30(4):390–5. DOI: 10.1055/s-0028-1109442

[42] Heilo A, Stenwig AE, Solheim OP. Malignant pleural mesothelioma: US-guided histologic core-needle biopsy. Radiology. 1999;211(3):657–9. DOI: 10.1148/radiology.211.3.r99jn03657

[43] Dixon G, de Fonseka D, Maskell N. Pleural controversies: image guided biopsy vs. thoracoscopy for undiagnosed pleural effusions?. J Thorac Dis. 2015;7(6):1041–51. DOI: 10.3978/j.issn.2072-1439.2015.01.36

[44] Liao WY, Chen MZ, Chang YL, Wu HD, Yu CJ, Kuo PH, et al. US-guided transthoracic cutting biopsy for peripheral thoracic lesions less than 3 cm in diameter. Radiology. 2000;217(3):685–91. DOI: 10.1148/radiology.217.3.r00dc21685

[45] Trovato GM, Sperandeo M, Catalano D. Optimization of thoracic US guidance for lung nodule biopsy. Radiology. 2014;270(1):308. DOI: 10.1148/radiol.13131527

[46] Joyner CR, Jr., Herman RJ, Reid JM. Reflected ultrasound in the detection and localization of pleural effusion. Jama. 1967;200(5):399–402.

[47] Pan JF, Yang PC, Chang DB, Lee YC, Kuo SH, Luh KT. Needle aspiration biopsy of malignant lung masses with necrotic centers. Improved sensitivity with ultrasonic guidance. Chest. 1993;103(5):1452–6.

[48] Trevisani L, Sartori S, Putinati S, Abbasciano V, Cervi PM. Needle aspiration biopsy and ultrasonic guidance. Chest. 1994;106(2):650.

[49] Sagar P, Gulati M, Gupta SK, Gupta S, Shankar S, Joshi K, et al. Ultrasound-guided transthoracic co-axial biopsy of thoracic mass lesions. Acta Radiol. 2000;41(6):529–32.

[50] Sartori S, Nielsen I, Trevisani L, Tombesi P, Ceccotti P, Abbasciano V. Contrast-enhanced sonography as guidance for transthoracic biopsy of a peripheral lung lesion with large necrotic areas. J Ultrasound Med. 2004;23(1):133–6.

[51] Jeon KN, Bae K, Park MJ, Choi HC, Shin HS, Shin S, et al. US-guided transthoracic biopsy of peripheral lung lesions: pleural contact length influences diagnostic yield. Acta Radiol. 2014;55(3):295–301. DOI: 10.1177/0284185113494984

[52] Fontalvo LF, Amaral JG, Temple M, Chait PG, John P, Krishnamuthy G, et al. Percutaneous US-guided biopsies of peripheral pulmonary lesions in children. Pediatr Radiol. 2006;36(6):491–7. DOI: 10.1007/s00247-005-0094-x

[53] Salamonsen M, McGrath D, Steiler G, Ware R, Colt H, Fielding D. A new instrument to assess physician skill at thoracic ultrasound, including pleural effusion markup. Chest. 2013;144(3):930–4. DOI: 10.1378/chest.12-2728

[54] Duncan DR, Morgenthaler TI, Ryu JH, Daniels CE. Reducing iatrogenic risk in thoracentesis: establishing best practice via experiential training in a zero-risk environment. Chest. 2009;135(5):1315–20. DOI: 10.1378/chest.08-1227

[55] Middleton WD, Teefey SA, Dahiya N. Ultrasound-guided chest biopsies. Ultrasound Q. 2006;22(4):241–52. DOI: 10.1097/01.ruq.0000237258.48756.94

[56] Wang J, Zhou D, Xie X, Shen P, Zeng Y. Utility of contrast-enhanced ultrasound with SonoVue in biopsy of small subpleural nodules. Int J Clin Exp Med. 2015;8(9):15991–8.

[57] Dong Y, Mao F, Wang WP, Ji ZB, Fan PL. Value of contrast-enhanced ultrasound in guidance of percutaneous biopsy in peripheral pulmonary lesions. Biomed Res Int. 2015;2015:531507. DOI: 10.1155/2015/531507

[58] Gorg C, Kring R, Bert T. Transcutaneous contrast-enhanced sonography of peripheral lung lesions. AJR Am J Roentgenol. 2006;187(4):W420–9. DOI: 10.2214/AJR.05.0890

[59] Sperandeo M, Sperandeo G, Varriale A, Filabozzi P, Decuzzi M, Dimitri L, et al. Contrast-enhanced ultrasound (CEUS) for the study of peripheral lung lesions: a preliminary study. Ultrasound Med Biol. 2006;32(10):1467–72. DOI: 10.1016/j.ultrasmedbio.2006.06.018

[60] Caremani M, Benci A, Lapini L, Tacconi D, Caremani A, Ciccotosto C, et al. Contrast enhanced ultrasonography (CEUS) in peripheral lung lesions: a study of 60 cases. J Ultrasound. 2008;11(3):89–96. DOI: 10.1016/j.jus.2008.05.008

[61] Sartori S, Postorivo S, Vece FD, Ermili F, Tassinari D, Tombesi P. Contrast-enhanced ultrasonography in peripheral lung consolidations: what's its actual role?. World J Radiol. 2013;5(10):372–80. DOI: 10.4329/wjr.v5.i10.372

[62] Sperandeo M, Rotondo A, Guglielmi G, Catalano D, Feragalli B, Trovato GM. Transthoracic ultrasound in the assessment of pleural and pulmonary diseases: use and limitations. Radiol Med. 2014;119(10):729–40. DOI: 10.1007/s11547-014-0385-0

[63] Itoh A, Ueno E, Tohno E, Kamma H, Takahashi H, Shiina T, et al. Breast disease: clinical application of US elastography for diagnosis. Radiology. 2006;239(2):341–50. DOI: 10.1148/radiol.2391041676

[64] Adamietz BR, Fasching PA, Jud S, Schulz-Wendtland R, Anders K, Uder M, et al. Ultrasound elastography of pulmonary lesions—a feasibility study. Ultraschall Med. 2014;35(1):33–7. DOI: 10.1055/s-0033-1355893

[65] Mostbeck G. Elastography everywhere—now even the lungs!. Ultraschall Med. 2014;35(1):5–8. DOI: 10.1055/s-0033-1356438

[66] Herth FJ, Becker HD, Ernst A. Ultrasound-guided transbronchial needle aspiration: an experience in 242 patients. Chest. 2003;123(2):604–7.

Section 3

A Molecular Vision of Lung Cancer: Prevention, Diagnosis and Treatment

Chapter 5

Clinical Lung Cancer Mutation Detection

Stephan C. Jahn and Petr Starostik

Additional information is available at the end of the chapter

http://dx.doi.org/10.5772/67168

Abstract

As the promise of personalized medicine in the treatment of cancer begins to be realized, the diagnostic techniques needed to drive that revolution have continued to evolve. What started as optical imaging of banded chromosomes for karyotyping has progressed to DNA sequencing and now next-generation sequencing capable of producing billions of reads. There are currently a large number of techniques that are used in the clinical laboratory for assessing the presence of mutations in lung tumors, all with their own strengths and weaknesses. Here, we survey the technology that is available and take a closer look at next-generation sequencing. We discuss the instruments that are currently on the market and demonstrate the common workflow from patient to data. Additionally, the outside factors that influence the use of these technologies, from government regulation to insurance reimbursement, are presented.

Keywords: detection, lung cancer, mutations, next-generation sequencing

1. Introduction

Ultimately, cancer is a genetic disease of the DNA. Changes in chromosomal sequences result in altered gene expression, protein structure, and enzyme activity, leading to increased cell growth, motility, and the associated clinical symptoms. Every cancer is different, and understanding the mutations present in each case is crucial in choosing the proper treatment.

The field of molecular diagnostics, the detection of DNA abnormalities, has come a long way since 1902 when Theodor Boveri first noted through microscopic observations that cancer likely came from abnormal chromosomes [1]. From the discovery that DNA consists of nucleotides, to the ability to sequence those nucleotides and the technology to do it more and more efficiently, our knowledge of cancerous mutations and their role in treating the disease has grown. We have progressed from manually generating one data point at a time to using automation to create billions of them in a matter of hours.

DNA abnormalities may be present in a number of forms. These range from the gain or loss of whole chromosomes to the substitution of one DNA nucleotide for another, leading to a change in the resulting protein. Between these extremes are chromosomal translocations, small or large deletions and insertions, amplifications, and inversions.

There are multiple generations of techniques currently being utilized in the clinical laboratory for the characterization of lung cancer. Each has its own inherent advantages and disadvantages that must be considered prior to ordering tests. The results of these diagnostics have profound impacts on the treatment of individual patients. They are also being used for research into better understanding the disease and have been responsible for the generation of the International Cancer Genome Consortium and The Cancer Genome Atlas [2]. Their impact on medicine will certainly only increase in the future.

2. Scope of mutation testing in lung cancer

The scope of mutation testing in lung cancer is determined by the mutation landscape described in these tumors. Considering which mutations need to be detected during diagnostic workup, two differentiations must be applied to mutations: driver mutations versus passenger mutations and therapeutically accessible *versus* inaccessible mutations. Driver mutations directly cause the development of cancer and allow it to grow and metastasize [3]. Other mutations that may either enhance the driver mutation or have no functional role in cancer progression are known as passenger mutations. As our knowledge of mutations is improving, the percentage of known driver mutations detected in lung cancer is increasing. The percentage of lung adenocarcinomas with no detected driver mutation dropped from 40% in 2013 to 24% in 2016 [4], increasing the number of known driver genes from 10 to 15 in the same time span. Some of the diver mutations are "actionable" in that they are therapeutically accessible and may be targeted in treatment. It is such mutations that are primary candidates for mutation screening assays. A nice summary of gene mutations, treatment options, and clinical trials in lung cancer is available from the mycancergenome.org website. Developing a lung cancer mutation assay with full coverage of the genes listed in the mycancergenome database would comprise a fairly comprehensive assay (**Table 1**). The absolute minimum of genes to be tested for mutations in lung cancer can be determined from the National Comprehensive Cancer Network (NCCN) Guidelines on Non-Small Cell Lung Cancer [5], which recommends at least EGFR mutation and ALK translocation testing.

The molecular characterization of lung cancer has focused primarily on those of the adenocarcinoma type for two main reasons. It is responsible for more deaths than any other form of cancer [6], and adenocarcinomas tend to be under the strong influence of identifiable driver mutations, making testing and treatment less nebulous than other cases. The three most common such mutations are of the epidermal growth factor receptor (EGFR), KRAS, and anaplastic lymphoma kinase (ALK), with ERBB2 mutations also being quite common [7]. Less common mutations in lung cancer are reviewed in Ref. [8].

Gene	Alteration	Frequency in NSCLC (%)	Available drugs
AKT1	Mutation	1	Drugs in clinical development
ALK	Rearrangement	3–7	Drugs approved in NSCLC
BRAF	Mutation	1–3	Drugs approved in other cancer
DDR2	Mutation	~4	Drugs approved in other cancer
EGFR	Mutation	10–35	Drugs approved in NSCLC
FGFR1	Amplification	20	Drugs in clinical development
ERBB2	Mutation	2–4	Drugs approved in other cancer
KRAS	Mutation	15–25	Drugs in clinical development
MEK1	Mutation	1	Drugs approved in other cancer
MET	Amplification	2–4	Drugs approved in NSCLC but for other molecular subtype
NRAS	Mutation	1	Drugs in clinical development
PIK3CA	Mutation	1–3	Drugs in clinical development
PTEN	Mutation	4–8	Drugs in clinical development
RET	Rearrangement	1	Drugs approved in other cancer
ROS1	Rearrangement	1	Drugs approved in NSCLC

Table 1. Frequency of mutations and availability of targeted therapies in NSCLC. Drug availability for the most frequent mutations detected in NSCLC is shown. Data are from mycancergenome.org.

EGFR-activating mutations represent a critical determinant for proper therapy selection in patients with lung cancer. There is a significant association between EGFR mutations, especially exon 19 deletions and exon 21 (L858R, L861), exon 18 (G719X, G719), and exon 20 (S768I) mutations, and sensitivity to EGFR inhibitors [9, 10]. A secondary mutation, T790M, is present in approximately 60% of tumors with acquired resistance to EGFR inhibitors [11] and confers resistance through steric interactions in the inhibitor binding site [12]. Primary resistance to EGFR-targeted therapy is associated with KRAS mutations. That is why some laboratories choose to add KRAS mutation testing to their assays, as concurrent EGFR and KRAS mutations occur in <1% of patients with lung cancer, and KRAS mutations are associated with intrinsic EGFR inhibitor resistance.

KRAS undergoes mutations resulting in single amino acid changes. In lung cancer, those mutations are most commonly present at the 12th amino acid position [13]. While KRAS mutations are the second most common mutation in lung cancer [7] and are especially prevalent in adenocarcinoma of the lung [13], their use as a prognostic marker or therapeutic guide in lung cancer has been limited. Studies have shown both a correlation between a KRAS mutation and a worse prognosis [14], but also no association with outcome [15]. ALK rearrangements represent the fusion between ALK and various partner genes, including echinoderm microtubule-associated protein-like 4 (EML4) [16]. ALK fusions have been identified in a subset of patients with NSCLC and represent a unique subset of NSCLC patients for whom ALK inhibitors may represent a very effective therapeutic strategy. That is the reason why ALK translocation testing should be included in any basic lung cancer mutation panel. For the most part, ALK translocations and EGFR mutations are mutually exclusive.

The parameters of tests employed in mutation analysis should fulfill the criteria suggested by professional organizations like the College of American Pathologists, International Association for the Study of Lung Cancer, and the Association for Molecular Pathology that have recently offered guidance on the use of molecular pathology in the screening of lung cancer patients. Their recommendations focus largely on the importance of EGFR mutations and ALK rearrangements. While they encourage testing for these abnormalities in patients with early stage lung adenocarcinoma, leaving the decision to the physician and laboratory, they require testing in advanced lung adenocarcinoma. Additionally, these tests may be performed on lung tumors other than adenocarcinoma if there is reason to believe an oncogenic driver is likely to be found.

3. Current technologies to detect mutations

There are multiple techniques that are currently used to detect mutations in clinical tumor samples. The specific technique used for each case is dependent on a number of factors including fundamental requirements such as the type of analysis to be performed (structural/copy number changes *vs* sequence mutations), the length of sequence required, and the type of nucleic acid being sequenced (DNA or RNA), as well as practical considerations including amount and quality of the sample, turnaround time (TAT), and cost to carry out the analysis. While the ability exists to sequence a patient's entire genome, most clinical assays are more targeted, focusing on one specific nucleotide, a chosen gene, or a number of genes due to the cost and labor involved.

3.1. Analysis of gross chromosomal changes

3.1.1. Cytogenetics

Still widely used today, karyotyping was the first clinical mutation assay and was responsible for the identification of the Philadelphia chromosome in 1960, which is the result of a translocation and is the defining aberration in chronic myeloid leukemia. When stained, generally with Giemsa stain, chromosomes develop a characteristic appearance of alternating light and dark "bands." This allows for the documentation of gross changes in chromosome number or structure. Structural changes able to be identified include large insertions or deletions, sequence inversions, and translocations. The technique has been considerably improved over the years, including the ability to digitally photograph the chromosomes; however, the preparatory work-up is still very labor intensive, and the analysis requires highly trained individuals. This limits the number of cells that can be analyzed for each sample, increasing the risk of false-negative results in samples that are highly heterogeneous. Additionally, as cells must be cultured to generate the necessary metaphase spreads, genotyping is mostly limited to rapidly dividing hematological malignancies and is only used sparingly in solid tumors such as lung cancer.

3.1.2. Fluorescence in situ hybridization

Rather than using a generic dye, fluorescence *in situ* hybridization (FISH) uses single-stranded, fluorophore-labeled DNA probes that hybridize to complementary regions in the genome and can be visualized as fluorescent spots on a metaphase spread or in an interphase nucleus. Due to the paired nature of human chromosomes, a FISH probe would be expected to identify two instances of the target sequence in each cell. Any numeric deviance from that indicates a loss or amplification of that locus (**Figure 1A**). Abnormal distances between probes targeting neighboring regions on the same chromosome can also indicate a translocation or an inversion has occurred.

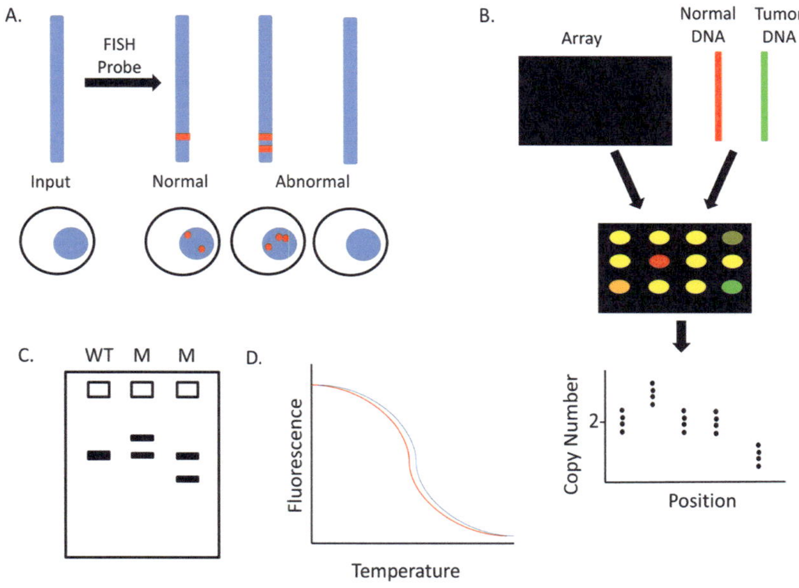

Figure 1. Techniques for measuring gross changes in chromosomes. (A) Fluorescent in situ hybridization (FISH) probes are applied to metaphase spreads or interphase cells. Complementary locations on the target chromosomes are identified as fluorescent spots due to the binding of the probe. Anything other than one locus on each of the sister chromosomes, represented by one fluorescent spot, is abnormal. This is shown at the chromosomal (top panel) and cellular (bottom panel) levels. (B) Array-comparative genomic hybridization binds fluorescently dyed and fragmented genomic DNA to immobilized probes. As tumor and normal DNA are dyed different colors, when both are applied to the array, it will be visualized as yellow if there are equal quantities of DNA from each source. Overrepresentation of green or red indicates overrepresentation of the corresponding DNA source. The fluorescence is then plotted as a graph of copy number *versus* chromosome position. (C) The single-strand conformation polymorphism utilizes the fact that wild-type (WT) and mutant (M) DNA strands will adopt different conformations due to differing intramolecular forces. This will lead them to migrate at different rates during polyacrylamide gel electrophoresis. If a sample of tumor DNA contains a band that migrates at a different rate than a control sample, it is indicative of a mutation. A "normal" band is also expected from the tumor sample due to the likely heterogeneity of the sample. (D) As mutations will alter the forces holding complementary strands of DNA together, a melting curve analysis measures the fluorescence emitted by DNA with increasing temperature. Since the DNA dye only fluoresces when bound to double-stranded DNA, as the DNA denatures the fluorescence decreases.

In lung cancer, FISH is the current FDA-approved gold standard method for detecting translocations involving the ALK gene. ALK translocations were the second driver mutation described in NSCLC [16]. ALK partners in the translocation can vary, but the most frequently involved is the EML4 gene. The FISH test based on the Vysis ALK Break-Apart FISH Probe by Abbott detects the translocation of ALK, but does not identify the fusion partner. This test consists of two probes that bind on either side of the common 2p23 break point. In the absence of a translocation, the probes will be seen as adjacent or overlapping. After a translation, the probes will be visualized with distinct separation. The test results are not always clear cut, and there is a large gray zone area of inconclusive results which can be influenced by subjective judgment. The test is thus highly dependent on optimal sample quality and experienced medical technologist staff.

With appropriate setup, FISH can be used for detection of other less frequent translocations or copy number changes in lung cancer. The technique has a fast TAT and is widely used. The largest drawback of FISH is throughput. Generally, one sample/set of probes is used per slide, making analysis of multiple samples/targets labor intensive.

3.1.3. Comparative genomic hybridization

The sensitivity of karyotyping and FISH is limited by the magnification of the microscope since the results are visualized by the human eye. Comparative genomic hybridization (CGH) is an extension of karyotyping that utilizes fluorescent dyes and microscopy to improve the ability to detect smaller changes in chromosome structure. In this method, chromosomal material from the tumor is dyed with a fluorescent dye, such as red, while chromosomal material from a normal sample is labeled with a different fluorophore, such as green. The two samples are combined, denatured, and allowed to hybridize to a reference metaphase spread in classical CGH. Differential fluorescence (i.e., greater red than green) indicates more or less of that chromosomal segment in the tumor.

This technique has now evolved into an array-based assay. Array-CGH utilizes the same principles, except the labeled input DNA is fragmented and hybridized to an array consisting of small probes rather than a metaphase spread. Where FISH hybridizes fluorescent probes to immobilized chromosomes, array-CGH hybridizes fluorescent genomic DNA to immobilized probes. If the target locus is neither under- or over-represented in the tumor sample, there will be equal numbers of normal and tumor fragments binding to the designated location on the array, and the equal mixture of red and green fluorescence will yield a yellow light. An imbalance of the target DNA in the tumor will lead to a shift in the observed fluorescence to red or green (**Figure 1B**).

While a novel technique, array-CGH has a number of limitations that have prevented it from widespread use in cancer diagnostics. The fundamental principles of the assay allow it to only detect quantitative differences in the amount of the target sequence. Chromosomal abnormalities that involve only the rearrangement of DNA, such as translocations and inversions, cannot be detected. Additionally, the presence of non-tumor cells in the tumor sample will dilute the mutation signal with normal background making the method less sensitive. For this reason, array-CGH is commonly used in oncologic hematology for chronic lymphocytic leukemia (CLL) [17], where a highly pure tumor sample can be obtained, but is rarely used in solid tumors such as lung cancer, which are generally very heterogeneous. Array-CGH is slowly being phased out of the cancer field entirely due to the emergence of next-generation sequencing (NGS), which is discussed in-depth below. The long TAT of NGS currently requires some samples to be analyzed with array-CGH instead, but that will surely improve as the technology evolves. Outside of oncology, array-CGH is routinely used for postnatal diagnostics where a homogeneous sample is readily available [18].

3.2. Analysis of sequence mutations

3.2.1. Sequence mutation screening

Prior to analyzing samples for specific mutations, it is possible to screen samples for the presence of mutations using a qualitative assay yielding a yes or no answer. This is particularly useful when carrying out a large sequencing study as it allows the targeted use of more labor intensive and expensive techniques for only those samples most likely to contain the targeted mutation. These methods can be efficiently scaled to high throughput assays and are based on the chemical and physical principles of DNA structure.

The conformation of single-stranded DNA is a direct function of its nucleotide sequence; therefore, mutant and wild-type DNA adopt different conformations that result in differing migration rates in polyacrylamide gel electrophoresis which can be detected using the single-strand conformation polymorphism technique (**Figure 1C**). Similarly, denaturing high pressure liquid chromatography hybridizes potentially mutant DNA to wild-type DNA. Subsequent ion pair, reverse phase chromatography, can then detect heterodimers as additional peaks due to differences in retention time [19]. Another common technique is melting curve analysis. Changes in sequence will alter the forces holding the double-stranded DNA together, resulting in differences in the temperature required to denature various loci [20]. By staining DNA with intercalating dyes that fluoresce only when bound to double-stranded DNA, the loss of this signal can be monitored with increasing temperature, generating a graph of fluorescence *versus* temperature (**Figure 1D**). While unique fingerprints are sometimes seen for specific mutations, analysis generally consists of simply looking for the presence of any differences compared to the wild-type DNA. If they are identified, other methods may be used to find the exact mutation present.

3.2.2. Allele-specific PCR

Techniques for analyzing single nucleotide mutations can be divided into those that give a direct yes/no readout as to the presence of a specific mutation and those that provide the exact DNA sequence, allowing the user to examine it for various mutations. Allele-specific PCR is an example of the first type of assay. The original allele-specific PCR utilized the fact that Taq polymerase is inefficient when there is a mismatch at the 3′ end of a primer hybridized to the target DNA. Therefore, if the primer is designed such that the final nucleotide will line up exactly with the genomic nucleotide in question, and its sequence is complimentary to the suspected mutation, a much larger quantity of PCR product will be yielded by a sample that contains the target mutation than by a sample that does not (**Figure 2A**). Output can be quantitated in a number of ways including electrophoresis or a follow-up round of qPCR. Due to the exponential nature of PCR, this method is very sensitive, allowing for the detection of mutations in a sample diluted by a large number of normal cells.

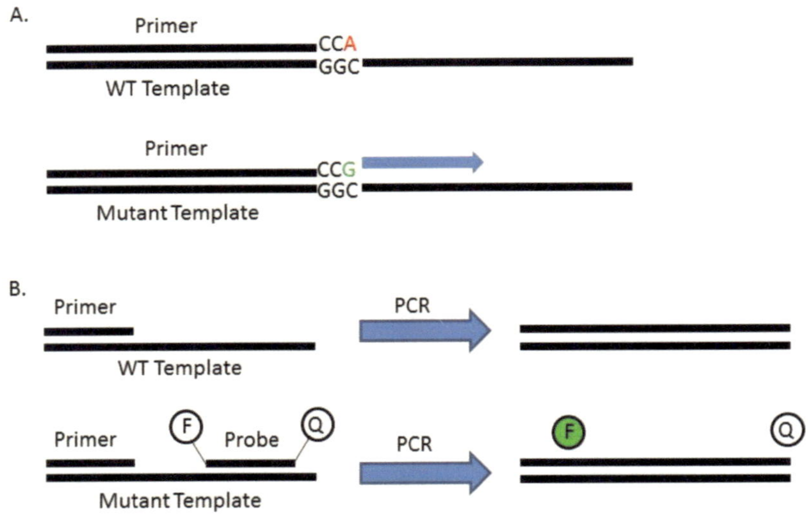

Figure 2. Allele-specific PCR (A) In the original assay, a primer with a 3′ end that aligns perfectly with the nucleotide in question is designed such that it is complementary to the mutant allele and has a mismatch with the wild-type allele. During PCR, elongation will only occur if the mutant allele is present. (B) The TaqMan approach to allele-specific PCR utilizes a probe that will bind only to the mutant allele. The probe contains both fluorescent (F) and quencher (Q) epitopes and does not fluoresce when it is intact. A mutually complementary primer is used to initiate elongation upstream of the probe in both wild-type and mutant alleles. If the elongation encounters the probe, it will release the fluorescent moiety, emitting a detectable signal.

Since its introduction, this method has been simplified, allowing the user to quantitate during the initial PCR step. This is typified by the TaqMan probe system from ThermoFisher Scientific. In this technique, a probe that is complimentary to a mutant, but not wild-type, allele contains a fluorochrome reporter attached to its 5′ end and a quencher moiety on the 3′ end that prevents a fluorescent signal from the reporter being detected. An unlabeled primer upstream of the targeted sequence is used to initiate PCR. As the DNA polymerase elongates the strand starting from the primer, it degrades the oligonucleotide backbone of the TaqMan probe. The fluorochrome reporter emits fluorescence which can now be detected due to this spatial separation from the quencher [21] (**Figure 2B**). This method is highly efficient as it is one step, can easily be done in a 386-well format with multiple probes and samples, and can be automated, resulting in a fast TAT. The assay itself requires only a qPCR instrument, and the reagents are relatively inexpensive. This ease and low cost have resulted in many labs creating their own laboratory-developed tests using this technology, and there are a number of FDA-approved kits available for purchase. As the TaqMan probe assay requires a large amount of genomic DNA per reaction, the number of different probes tested or other diagnostic procedures possible for the sample may be limited.

Having the lowest limit of detection and highest specificity, the Therascreen system from Qiagen combines both of the above methods. A mutation-specific primer is used to amplify the mutated region, and then a Scorpion probe, containing fluorescent and quencher moieties, again binds to this same site. As elongation occurs, the epitopes are separated, and fluorescence occurs. FDA-approved Therascreen kits are available for both EGFR and KRAS genes. However, these assays look only at a limited number of mutations. The EGFR assay can detect 5 point mutations, exon 19 deletions, and exon 20 insertions; the KRAS kit can detect 7 point mutations. The largest flaw of these allele-specific PCR assays is their propensity for false-negatives due to large mutations. The primers and probes are designed to detect single nucleotide mutations and anything greater than that will cause a mismatch and prevent hybridization. A 1% rate of false negatives has been reported for the FDA-approved Therascreen KRAS assay [22]. These assays are promoted as companion assays for therapeutics, such as the BRAF assay from Roche, which is the companion diagnostic assay for therapy with BRAF inhibitor vemurafenib. The test only detects the c.1799T>A p.V600E mutation, though up to 20% of BRAF mutations are non-V600E mutations [23].

3.2.3. Sanger sequencing

The first widely used sequencing method, Sanger sequencing employs PCR in the presence of unlabeled nucleotides and labeled (i.e., radio- or fluorescent labels) chain terminating nucleotides [24]. Since each form of nucleotide (A, T, C, G) is differentially labeled, incorporation of chain terminating nucleotides stops the elongation step and labels the product, indicating the identity of the final nucleotide added (**Figure 3A**). The sample is then subjected to electrophoresis, either gel or capillary, which separates the amplicons by size, allowing the sequence to be read from smallest to largest simply by the label present.

3.2.4. Pyrosequencing

Where Sanger sequencing uses chain termination followed by electrophoresis, pyrosequencing uses a real-time process of sequencing by synthesis [25]. Here, the four possible nucleotides are added and removed sequentially. When the proper nucleotide is added, elongation occurs, releasing pyrophosphate that is converted to light through bioluminescence (**Figure 3B**). The template DNA is immobilized through binding to a biotinylated primer bound to sepharose beads. The technique provides semiquantitative data in regard to prevalence of the mutant allele in the sample [26]. As each template strand is elongated to completion, smaller sample quantities are needed, generally only requiring 10 ng of DNA. For a number of reasons, read lengths obtained with pyrosequencing are not as long as those from Sanger sequencing, generally being well below one hundred bases [27]. This prevents its use for sequencing large-scale mutations. Due to the fact that the technique requires a pre-PCR step and manual analysis of the results, it is time intensive. However, the method is routinely used clinically, both as laboratory-developed tests [28] and commercial kits [29] for analysis of a number of forms of cancer, including lung cancer. Its much lower limit of detection of 5–10% sets it apart from Sanger sequencing and makes it an optimal assay to confirm NGS variants occurring at low variant allele frequency.

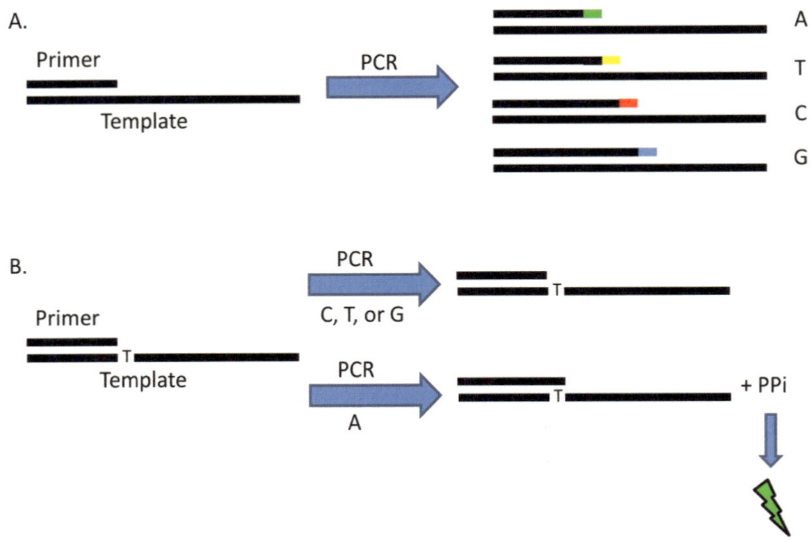

Figure 3. Sequencing technologies. (A) Sanger sequencing consists of PCR of template DNA in the presence of standard and fluorescently labeled chain terminating nucleotides. If a chain terminating nucleotide is incorporated into the strand, it is permanently labeled with a tag that identifies the final nucleotide added. Following PCR, fragments are separated by size, and the sequence is read from smallest to largest strand. (B) Pyrosequencing utilizes a sequencing-by-synthesis approach during PCR. Nucleotides (A, T, C, G) are added sequentially and then removed. When the correct nucleotide is added, elongation occurs, and pyrophosphate is released, resulting in a luciferase reaction and the emission of light.

3.2.5. Next-generation sequencing

If one focuses on detection of only small mutations in a limited number of genes, single-analyte assays will deliver reliable and informative results. However, running mutation assays aiming to capture mutations in all 15 driver mutation-prone genes requires a multianalyte assay, which is why the current direction of the sequencing field is to multiplex. While different technologies that would all be considered next-generation sequencing (NGS) utilize very different sequencing methods, the similarity is that they are able to sequence incredibly large numbers of DNA strands at the same time. This massively parallel sequencing is capable of providing millions or billions of short reads. This ability lends NGS to a wide range of applications including untargeted sequencing of entire genomes, exomes, or transcriptomes, as well as targeted sequencing of large numbers of cancer mutation locations at the same time. The NGS instrument market space is currently occupied by four competitors utilizing slightly different approaches. By far, the largest player is currently Illumina, who offers a wide range of instruments ranging, among others, from the miniSeq to the HiSeq X Ten, the latter of which is capable of producing up to six billion reads. A small range instrument, the MiSeqDx, is FDA approved for *in vitro* diagnostic use. These instruments use chemistry that is a million-wise multiplexed variant of Sanger sequencing with clonal amplification and sequencing by synthesis chemistry. The color of the signal detected when a nucleotide is added indicates the identity of the base added and thus the sequence. Currently, the only other company with a significant market share is ThermoFisher with their Ion Torrent instruments. Similar to traditional pyrosequencing, the Ion Torrent technology sequentially adds and removes nucleotides looking for elongation. Instead of converting pyrophosphate to fluorescence, Ion Torrent measures small-scale changes in pH caused by the release of H^+ during the polymerization of nucleotides [30]. Similarly, their Ion PGM™ Dx System is FDA approved. While both Pacific Biosciences and Qiagen have offerings for NGS, they are not currently widely used. The Pacific Biosciences instruments suffer from low throughput and high cost, while Qiagen only recently entered the market.

3.2.5.1. Clinical NGS workflow

Most NGS runs are conducted on either genomic DNA or mRNA. While formalin-fixed and paraffin-embedded tumor blocks contain suitable quality genomic DNA, the quality of mRNA obtained from these samples will be variable and yield unsatisfactory results in up to 15% of cases. Fresh tissue is required to ensure high-quality mRNA for RNASeq experiments. Prior to beginning the workup, the tumor cell content of the sample must be determined. This requires an experienced and knowledgeable set of eyes. Between 5 and 20% tumor cell content is generally sufficient for NGS [31]. After isolation, DNA is sheared to produce uniform fragments which then undergo multiplex PCR or are hybridized to immobilized probes. The labor required for NGS is dependent on the level of automation available in the lab carrying out the sequencing. Illumina requires 1–2 days of workup, while Ion Torrent requires up to 3 days, although the Ion Torrent instrument has shorter run times. This means that individual labs need to identify their rate-limiting step in order to choose the instrument that will provide the highest throughput and shortest TAT.

3.2.5.2. Targeted sequencing

While NGS has great potential, its cost and massive data generation currently limit its clinical use to targeted sequencing of mutation hotspots rather than genome, exome, or transcriptome sequencing. Disease-specific gene panels are routinely used. The genes are chosen based on their immediate impact on patient care, either due to their use in determining prognosis or in selecting the proper treatment regimen. Sequencing of genes beyond the minimum is determined on a case-by-case basis according to the capability and throughput capacity of the laboratory as well as insurance coverage of the patient. Library preparation kits for NGS generally fall into two categories: those that use PCR amplification or hybridization probes. The first class is typified by Illumina's TruSeq Amplicon Cancer Panel, the Ion AmpliSeq panel from Ion Torrent, and HaloPlex kits from Agilent. The second group contains kits available from sequencing instrument manufactures and also from Agilent, Roche, and Integrated DNA Technologies, along with other third parties. Direct hybridization gives more reliable quantitative data since the possibility of bias introduced by the pre-PCR step is eliminated. These reagents can include probes for intronic regions rearranged in translocations which are detectable in this way [32], though larger rearrangements may lead to poor hybridization and false negatives [33] or misleading copy number data. The internal tandem duplications in the *FLT3* gene in acute myeloid leukemia [34] are an excellent example of mutations that require a special reagent and bioinformatics approach. Generally, with adequate expertise, wet lab and bioinformatics support labs are capable of developing their own lab-developed assays as evidenced by cancer panels developed by Foundation Medicine (Foundation One Assay) [35], Memorial Sloan Kettering (Integrated Mutation Profiling of Actionable Cancer Targets) [36, 37], and many others.

3.2.5.3. *Whole exome sequencing*

While assays for sequencing the entire exome are available, they are not widely used in the clinical setting. As each run is capable of producing a set number of reads, sequencing a greater number of loci reduces the number of reads for each locus. Mutations in a highly heterogeneous sample may not be detected. Exome sequencing may identify rare or previously unidentified mutations, though clinicians would likely not have the knowledge on how to use that information to better care for their patient, so it would have no impact on patient care. Therefore, large-scale exome sequencing has found a better home in the research laboratory than the clinical lab setting.

3.2.5.4. *Bioinformatics*

Perhaps the largest hurdle to the adoption of NGS is data analysis. When an instrument is providing billions of reads, it can be a challenge not only to store the data, but also to utilize them. Instrument manufacturers have greatly improved their software offerings, making it easier to view the data. However, the challenge still remains of how to use the data. With so much information at your fingertips, how do you best utilize it to better care for the patient? Without a meaningful approach, substantial time may be devoted to analyzing irrelevant data. The significance of identified mutations must be denoted, and their impact on treatment must be delineated. A number of companies have begun offering services that would annotate a mutation report with clinically relevant content, including N-of-One, Genome Oncology, and PireanDx. Once the report is generated, commonly outdated electronic medical records systems often make the sharing of the results difficult. Due to file incompatibilities, highly complex documents are all too often printed, scanned, and uploaded as PDF documents. This has prompted data to be stored in third-party systems that greatly enhance the user experience [37].

3.2.5.5. *Reimbursement and government regulation*

In addition to the difficult science, the advancement of NGS in the United States has been hampered by reduced reimbursement rates for molecular pathology testing. Reimbursement is now only available for the test itself, not the interpretation of the results. Additionally, the testing classification has been greatly simplified, failing to differentiate between similar tests that may have very disparate costs while not being redundant [38]. Diagnostic procedures that are conducted in clinical laboratories are regulated by the federal Clinical Laboratory Improvement Amendments (CLIA) that were established in the 1970s. These regulations are administered by federal agencies and by the states, which require laboratories to be properly licensed. Additionally, the College of American Pathologists [39], Association for Molecular Pathology [40], and the American College of Medical Genetics [41] all help to draft technique-specific regulations and offer certification programs of their own and require proficiency testing.

To date, most NGS tests have been developed by individual laboratories, over which the Food and Drug Administration (FDA) has no explicit regulatory oversight. The FDA has warned that NGS technologies, as with older technologies, will be subject to FDA regulation if they advance toward marketable *in vitro* diagnostic status, over which the FDA exerts considerable control. This is generally established on a case-by-case basis. Regulation by all of these bodies is complicated by the fact that NGS is continually evolving and improving. Guidelines must either be routinely revisited or generalized such that their interpretation may change to match the current technology. A fine line must be walked in order to protect the patients for whom the assays are being used, while at the same time not stifling the development of a technology that promises to usher in the era of personalized medicine.

4. Emerging technologies

4.1. Single-analyte vs multianalyte assays

While NGS will likely become the dominant technique for evaluating mutations in cancer moving forward, the other methods discussed here are hardly headed toward imminent obsolescence. Clinical labs must focus not only on the future, but also providing the best diagnostics for current patients. Today's limitations of NGS, including substantial labor requirements and a long TAT, mean that single-analyte methods are still widely used. While NGS may be able to provide a greater quantity of data and increased sample throughput, it has not been found to be qualitatively better than other technologies including allele-specific PCR and Sanger sequencing, among others, with all providing around 96% agreement [42, 43].

4.2. Liquid biopsy

Direct testing of tumor biopsies is preferred; however, circulating tumor DNA may be used to test for mutations after a lung adenocarcinoma diagnosis through direct biopsy has been established. For solid tumors, mutation detection has traditionally required a direct biopsy. In recent years, research has been conducted on the presence of circulating tumor cells, excreted miRNAs, and even tumor genomic DNA floating freely in the bloodstream. The ease of obtaining a blood sample makes sequencing these samples an appealing future technique not only for tumor characterization, but also screening and evaluation of therapeutic efficacy during treatment. The ratio of mutant DNA to normal DNA or tumor to normal cells collected is often very low and seems to be partially dependent on the tumor type, being detectable in greater than 75% of patients with breast, colorectal, and hepatocellular cancers, among others, but in less than half of patients with cancer of the brain, kidney, or prostate [44, 45]. Circulating tumor cells were detected in 78% of small-cell lung cancer patients [46], and both circulating DNA [47] and tumor cells [48] have been successfully used to screen for EGFR mutations in lung cancer. These technologies have not progressed to the point of widespread clinical use and are currently at the research stage. They are more thoroughly reviewed in Ref. [49].

4.3. Future sequencing technologies

Even with NGS technologies still not up to full speed, even better techniques are already being developed. A number of these sequencing instruments are able to decipher the sequence of single, existing DNA strands directly, rather than being based on PCR synthesis [50]. Perhaps showing the most promise, Oxford nanopore technologies has developed a new instrument, the MinION. By passing individual strands through nanopores containing ionic currents, the instrument is able to detect minute changes in current that differ depending on which nucleotide is passing by. The device is small enough to easily hold in the palm of the hand. It is capable of 60 kb read lengths, with 16,000 reads per run [51, 52]. While the portability and capabilities offer amazing promise, the accuracy is currently not sufficient for clinical use. It is gaining significant traction in the research space, however [53].

5. Conclusions

Clinical mutation testing in lung cancer is driven by the available therapies. Currently, there is only a limited armoire of targeted therapy options available which can be employed. If there is not a drug targeting a specific mutated gene available, the fact that the gene shows a mutation is not very meaningful. EGFR-targeted therapeutics may not be used without the presence of EGFR mutations. If the tumor continues to progress after treatment with an EGFR inhibitor, the presence of a resistance-conferring EGFR T790M mutation must be determined prior to giving a third-generation EGFR inhibitor to overcome the resistance. Similarly, ALK inhibitors are only to be given to patients showing ALK rearrangements; however, if treatment fails, there is no need to re-evaluate mutational status. ROS1 inhibitors receive a similar recommendation, while BRAF, RET, ERBB2, KRAS, and MET screenings are only recommended if included as a larger panel or if EGFR, ALK, and ROS1 tests come back negative.

Physicians and laboratories currently have a large number of techniques at their disposal for the interrogation of mutations present in lung cancer. The tests to be performed can be tailored to each patient based on a number of factors including type and number of data points needed, TAT, cost, and availability of quality biopsy material. The absolutely minimal mutation workup includes detection of SNVs and indels in EGFR by Sanger sequencing, pyrosequencing, allele-specific PCR or any other method, and detection of ALK translocations by FISH. However, NGS has the potential to replace many, if not all, of these techniques, but must first continue to improve. Its use in the clinic is currently limited by the fact that it is still quite expensive and has a relatively long TAT, and the results require special skills and reference databases in order to be fully utilized. In the future, it is the hope that every lung cancer patient may have their entire tumor genome sequenced cheaply and efficiently, allowing an in-depth understanding of all mutations driving the tumor and providing information to tailor the best possible treatment for that patient.

Author details

Stephan C. Jahn and Petr Starostik*

*Address all correspondence to: starostik@pathology.ufl.edu

Department of Pathology, Immunology, and Laboratory Medicine, University of Florida College of Medicine, Gainesville, FL, USA

References

[1] Boveri T (2008) Concerning the origin of malignant tumours by Theodor Boveri. Translated and annotated by Henry Harris. J Cell Sci 121(Suppl 1): 1–84.

[2] Cancer Genome Atlas Research Network (2013) Genomic and epigenomic landscapes of adult de novo acute myeloid leukemia. N Engl J Med 368: 2059–2074.

[3] Stratton MR, Campbell PJ, Futreal PA (2009) The cancer genome. Nature 458: 719–724.

[4] Johnson BE, Kris MG, Berry LD, Kwiatkowski DJ, Iafrate AJ, et al. (2013) A multicenter effort to identify driver mutations and employ targeted therapy in patients with lung adenocarcinomas: The Lung Cancer Mutation Consortium (LCMC). ASCO Annual Meeting Proceedings 31: 8019.

[5] Network NCC NCCN Clinical Practice Guidelines in Oncology. Non-Small Cell Lung Cancer (Version 4.2016).

[6] Cancer Genome Atlas Research Network (2014) Comprehensive molecular profiling of lung adenocarcinoma. Nature 511: 543–550.

[7] Tan D, Lynch HT (2013) Principles of Molecular Diagnostics and Personalized Cancer Medicine. Wolters Kluwer Health/Lippincott Williams & Wilkins.

[8] Patel JN, Ersek JL, Kim ES (2015) Lung cancer biomarkers, targeted therapies and clinical assays. Transl Lung Cancer Res 4: 503–514.

[9] Pao W, Miller V, Zakowski M, Doherty J, Politi K, et al. (2004) EGF receptor gene mutations are common in lung cancers from "never smokers" and are associated with sensitivity of tumors to gefitinib and erlotinib. Proc Natl Acad Sci USA 101: 13306–13311.

[10] Lynch TJ, Bell DW, Sordella R, Gurubhagavatula S, Okimoto RA, et al. (2004) Activating mutations in the epidermal growth factor receptor underlying responsiveness of non-small-cell lung cancer to gefitinib. N Engl J Med 350: 2129–2139.

[11] Yu HA, Arcila ME, Rekhtman N, Sima CS, Zakowski MF, et al. (2013) Analysis of tumor specimens at the time of acquired resistance to EGFR-TKI therapy in 155 patients with EGFR-mutant lung cancers. Clin Cancer Res 19: 2240–2247.

[12] Wang J, Wang B, Chu H, Yao Y (2016) Intrinsic resistance to EGFR tyrosine kinase inhibitors in advanced non-small-cell lung cancer with activating EGFR mutations. Onco Targets Ther 9: 3711–3726.

[13] Rodenhuis S, Slebos RJ (1990) The ras oncogenes in human lung cancer. Am Rev Respir Dis 142: S27–30.

[14] Mascaux C, Iannino N, Martin B, Paesmans M, Berghmans T, et al. (2005) The role of RAS oncogene in survival of patients with lung cancer: a systematic review of the literature with meta-analysis. Br J Cancer 92: 131–139.

[15] D'Angelo SP, Janjigian YY, Ahye N, Riely GJ, Chaft JE, et al. (2012) Distinct clinical course of EGFR-mutant resected lung cancers: results of testing of 1118 surgical specimens and effects of adjuvant gefitinib and erlotinib. J Thorac Oncol 7: 1815–1822.

[16] Soda M, Choi YL, Enomoto M, Takada S, Yamashita Y, et al. (2007) Identification of the transforming EML4-ALK fusion gene in non-small-cell lung cancer. Nature 448: 561–566.

[17] Alsolami R, Knight SJ, Schuh A (2013) Clinical application of targeted and genome-wide technologies: can we predict treatment responses in chronic lymphocytic leukemia? Per Med 10: 361–376.

[18] Miller DT, Adam MP, Aradhya S, Biesecker LG, Brothman AR, et al. (2010) Consensus statement: chromosomal microarray is a first-tier clinical diagnostic test for individuals with developmental disabilities or congenital anomalies. Am J Hum Genet 86: 749–764.

[19] OD'Donovan MC, Oefner PJ, Roberts SC, Austin J, Hoogendoorn B, et al. (1998) Blind analysis of denaturing high-performance liquid chromatography as a tool for mutation detection. Genomics 52: 44–49.

[20] Ririe KM, Rasmussen RP, Wittwer CT (1997) Product differentiation by analysis of DNA melting curves during the polymerase chain reaction. Anal Biochem 245: 154–160.

[21] De la Vega FM, Lazaruk KD, Rhodes MD, Wenz MH (2005) Assessment of two flexible and compatible SNP genotyping platforms: TaqMan SNP Genotyping Assays and the SNPlex Genotyping System. Mutat Res 573: 111–135.

[22] Tol J, Dijkstra JR, Vink-Borger ME, Nagtegaal ID, Punt CJ, et al. (2010) High sensitivity of both sequencing and real-time PCR analysis of KRAS mutations in colorectal cancer tissue. J Cell Mol Med 14: 2122–2131.

[23] Millington GW (2013) Mutations of the BRAF gene in human cancer, by Davies et al. (Nature 2002; 417: 949–54). Clin Exp Dermatol 38: 222–223.

[24] Sanger F, Coulson AR (1975) A rapid method for determining sequences in DNA by primed synthesis with DNA polymerase. J Mol Biol 94: 441–448.

[25] Ronaghi M, Uhlen M, Nyren P (1998) A sequencing method based on real-time pyrophosphate. Science 281: 363, 365.

[26] Kringen MK (2015) Analysis of Copy Number Variation by Pyrosequencing(R) Using Paralogous Sequences. Methods Mol Biol 1315: 115–121.

[27] Mashayekhi F, Ronaghi M (2007) Analysis of read length limiting factors in pyrosequencing chemistry. Anal Biochem 363: 275–287.

[28] Poehlmann A, Kuester D, Meyer F, Lippert H, Roessner A, et al. (2007) K-ras mutation detection in colorectal cancer using the pyrosequencing technique. Pathol Res Pract 203: 489–497.

[29] Sundstrom M, Edlund K, Lindell M, Glimelius B, Birgisson H, et al. (2010) KRAS analysis in colorectal carcinoma: analytical aspects of pyrosequencing and allele-specific PCR in clinical practice. BMC Cancer 10: 660.

[30] Boland JF, Chung CC, Roberson D, Mitchell J, Zhang X, et al. (2013) The new sequencer on the block: comparison of Life Technology's Proton sequencer to an Illumina HiSeq for whole-exome sequencing. Hum Genet 132: 1153–1163.

[31] Tsongalis GJ, Peterson JD, de Abreu FB, Tunkey CD, Gallagher TL, et al. (2014) Routine use of the Ion Torrent AmpliSeq Cancer Hotspot Panel for identification of clinically actionable somatic mutations. Clin Chem Lab Med 52: 707–714.

[32] Asan, Xu Y, Jiang H, Tyler-Smith C, Xue Y, et al. (2011) Comprehensive comparison of three commercial human whole-exome capture platforms. Genome Biol 12: R95.

[33] Sboner A, Elemento O (2016) A primer on precision medicine informatics. Brief Bioinform 17: 145–153.

[34] Rustagi N, Hampton OA, Li J, Xi L, Gibbs RA, et al. (2016) ITD assembler: an algorithm for internal tandem duplication discovery from short-read sequencing data. BMC Bioinformatics 17: 188.

[35] Frampton GM, Fichtenholtz A, Otto GA, Wang K, Downing SR, et al. (2013) Development and validation of a clinical cancer genomic profiling test based on massively parallel DNA sequencing. Nat Biotechnol 31: 1023–1031.

[36] Cheng DT, Mitchell TN, Zehir A, Shah RH, Benayed R, et al. (2015) Memorial Sloan Kettering-Integrated Mutation Profiling of Actionable Cancer Targets (MSK-IMPACT): a hybridization capture-based next-generation sequencing clinical assay for solid tumor molecular oncology. J Mol Diagn 17: 251–264.

[37] Hyman DM, Solit DB, Arcila ME, Cheng DT, Sabbatini P, et al. (2015) Precision medicine at Memorial Sloan Kettering Cancer Center: clinical next-generation sequencing enabling next-generation targeted therapy trials. Drug Discov Today 20: 1422–1428.

[38] Ahlman JB, Connelly J, Crosslin R, Dimovski B, Espronceda M, et al. (2015) Current Procedural Terminology 2016. Chicago: American Medical Association.

[39] Aziz N, Zhao Q, Bry L, Driscoll DK, Funke B, et al. (2015) College of American Pathologists' laboratory standards for next-generation sequencing clinical tests. Arch Pathol Lab Med 139: 481–493.

[40] Schrijver I, Aziz N, Farkas DH, Furtado M, Gonzalez AF, et al. (2012) Opportunities and challenges associated with clinical diagnostic genome sequencing: a report of the Association for Molecular Pathology. J Mol Diagn 14: 525–540.

[41] Rehm HL, Bale SJ, Bayrak-Toydemir P, Berg JS, Brown KK, et al. (2013) ACMG clinical laboratory standards for next-generation sequencing. Genet Med 15: 733–747.

[42] Malapelle U, Sgariglia R, De Stefano A, Bellevicine C, Vigliar E, et al. (2015) KRAS mutant allele-specific imbalance (MASI) assessment in routine samples of patients with metastatic colorectal cancer. J Clin Pathol 68: 265–269.

[43] Tsiatis AC, Norris-Kirby A, Rich RG, Hafez MJ, Gocke CD, et al. (2010) Comparison of Sanger sequencing, pyrosequencing, and melting curve analysis for the detection of KRAS mutations: diagnostic and clinical implications. J Mol Diagn 12: 425–432.

[44] Bettegowda C, Sausen M, Leary RJ, Kinde I, Wang Y, et al. (2014) Detection of circulating tumor DNA in early- and late-stage human malignancies. Sci Transl Med 6: 224ra224.

[45] Leon SA, Shapiro B, Sklaroff DM, Yaros MJ (1977) Free DNA in the serum of cancer patients and the effect of therapy. Cancer Res 37: 646–650.

[46] Punnoose EA, Atwal S, Liu W, Raja R, Fine BM, et al. (2012) Evaluation of circulating tumor cells and circulating tumor DNA in non-small cell lung cancer: association with clinical endpoints in a phase II clinical trial of pertuzumab and erlotinib. Clin Cancer Res 18: 2391–2401.

[47] Luo J, Shen L, Zheng D (2014) Diagnostic value of circulating free DNA for the detection of EGFR mutation status in NSCLC: a systematic review and meta-analysis. Sci Rep 4: 6269.

[48] Maheswaran S, Sequist LV, Nagrath S, Ulkus L, Brannigan B, et al. (2008) Detection of mutations in EGFR in circulating lung-cancer cells. N Engl J Med 359: 366–377.

[49] Speicher MR, Pantel K (2014) Tumor signatures in the blood. Nat Biotechnol 32: 441–443.

[50] Thompson JF, Milos PM (2011) The properties and applications of single-molecule DNA sequencing. Genome Biol 12: 217.

[51] Jain M, Fiddes IT, Miga KH, Olsen HE, Paten B, et al. (2015) Improved data analysis for the MinION nanopore sequencer. Nat Methods 12: 351–356.

[52] Ip CL, Loose M, Tyson JR, de Cesare M, Brown BL, et al. (2015) MinION Analysis and Reference Consortium: Phase 1 data release and analysis. F1000Res 4: 1075.

[53] Laver T, Harrison J, OD'Neill PA, Moore K, Farbos A, et al. (2015) Assessing the performance of the Oxford Nanopore Technologies MinION. Biomol Detect Quantif 3: 1–8.

Chapter 6

Sphingolipid in Lung Cancer Pathogenesis and Therapy

Erhard Bieberich and Guanghu Wang

Additional information is available at the end of the chapter

http://dx.doi.org/10.5772/66359

Abstract

Recent genomic research has ranked sphingolipid metabolism as the top dysregulated pathways in lung cancer, demonstrating that these lipids and their metabolic enzymes play key roles in lung cancer pathogenesis. Hence, sphingolipid metabolism has become a forefront in lung cancer research. However, the function of the diverse sphingolipids and their metabolic enzymes and the underlying mechanism in lung cancer are still unclear. In this chapter, we will focus on ceramide and sphingosine-1-phosphate (S1P), the best characterized sphingolipids so far, to summarize the most recent studies and highlight the essential role of sphingolipids in lung cancer pathology, diagnosis, and treatment.

Keywords: lung cancer, NSCLC, sphingolipid, ceramide, sphingosine, sphingosine-1-phosphate (S1P), Spns2

1. Introduction

Lung (pulmonary) cancer is the leading cause of cancer-related death in the United States and worldwide. Its two major types are non–small cell lung cancer (NSCLC) and small-cell lung cancer, among which NSCLC is the most common form accounting for 85–90% of newly diagnosed cases [1, 2]. NSCLC can be further categorized into three major subtypes: large-cell lung cancer, squamous cell carcinoma, and adenocarcinoma.

Most lung cancer is diagnosed at a late stage; thus, chemotherapy is the most common approach for management [3]. However, the effectiveness of conventional chemotherapy for lung cancer has reached its plateau [3]. Multiple genes and signaling pathways have been associated with NSCLC, including the epidermal growth factor receptor (EGFR) family, mitogen-activated protein kinase (MAPK), mesenchymal-epithelial transition factor (c-MET), phosphatidylinositide 3-kinases (PI3K)-Protein Kinase B (PKB/Akt)-mammalian target of rapamycin (mTOR), and vascular endothelial growth factor (VEGF) pathways [1, 2, 4]. Precision therapies have been designed to use inhibitors of these pathways such as gefitinib for EGFR mutations [5]. However, these drugs work for certain patients/for a while and the patients develop drug resistance, and the tumor develops to more aggressive metastatic cancer [2, 6].

Sphingolipid metabolism is among the pathways that show the highest abundance of dysregulation in lung cancer [7]. Yet the function of sphingolipids and underlying mechanism in lung cancer are still not clear, due in part to a lack of suitable in vivo models [8, 9]. Bioactive sphingolipids, including ceramide, ceramide-1-phosphate, sphingosine, and sphingosine-1-phosphate (S1P), regulate a wide range of cell signaling pathways that control cell proliferation, apoptosis, senescence, angiogenesis, and migration, key components of cancer pathology and progression. The roles of sphingolipids in general tumorigenesis have been reviewed extensively, and the readers are encouraged to resort to these resources [10–13]. In this chapter, we will focus on ceramide and S1P to discuss the essential functions of sphingolipids in lung cancer pathology, diagnosis, and treatment. Many enzymes in the sphingolipid metabolism are closely related to lung tumorigenesis. For the ease of discussion, we will first briefly introduce the sphingolipid metabolism pathways.

2. Sphingolipid metabolism

Sphingolipids are acyl derivatives of the amino alcohols sphingosine and dihydrosphingosine. They encompass sphingosine, ceramide, and ceramide derivatives such as ceramide-1-phosphate, S1P, sphingomyelin, and glycosphingolipids (**Figure 1**). These lipids are synthesized

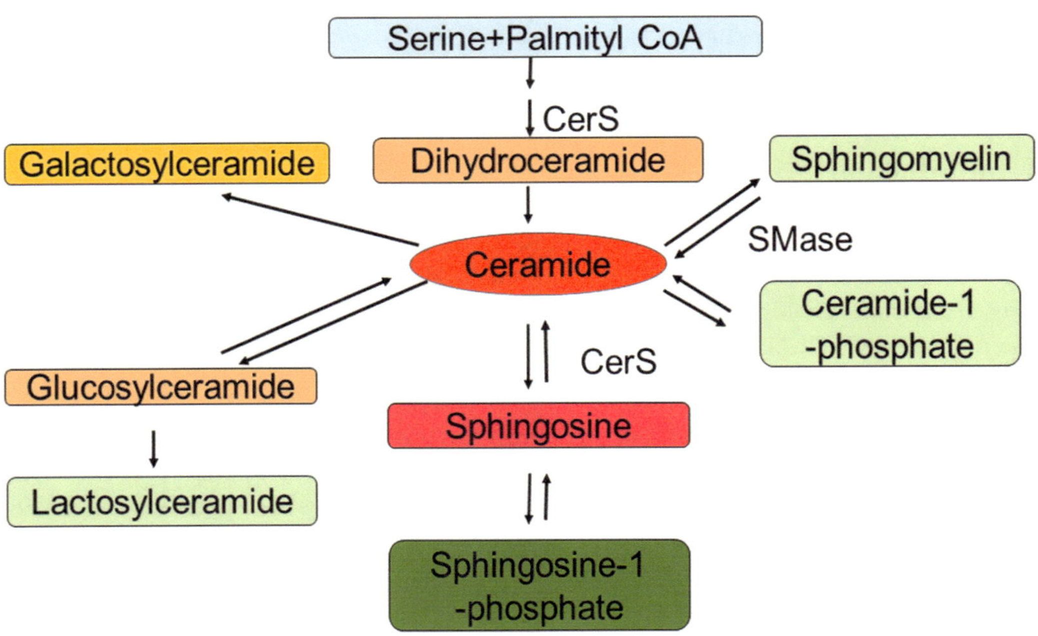

Figure 1. Schematics of ceramide synthesis.

in an interconnected network of enzymes, which is centered on ceramide (**Figure 1**). There are three pathways that produce ceramide, de novo, sphingomyelin cycle, and the salvage pathways [14–16]. In the de novo pathway, ceramide synthesis is initiated by serine palmitoyltransferase which condenses serine and palmitate to form ketosphinganine, followed by reduction of the ketone group to dihydrosphingosine. Dihydrosphingosine is then acylated by ceramide synthase (CerS) to generate dihydroceramides. A desaturation step, which is catalyzed by dihydroceramide desaturase, completes ceramide biosynthesis [14, 16]. In addition, ceramide can be generated by the salvage pathway in which CerS uses sphingosine as an acyl acceptor (**Figure 1**) [14, 16]. In a third pathway, ceramide is generated from sphingomyelin by sphingomyelinase (SMase) (**Figure 1**). The CerS enzymes, which currently encompass six enzymes (CerS1–6, also known as Lass1–6), and neutral SMase2 (nSMase2) are particularly interesting in lung cancer which will be discussed more in detail later. CerS enzymes use different chain lengths of acyl-CoAs and generate ceramide of varying lengths ranging from C14 to C32, while nSmase2 catalyzes sphingomyelin to generate ceramide.

S1P is synthesized intracellularly from sphingosine by the sphingosine kinases SphK1 and SphK2 (**Figure 2**). SphK1 is mainly cytoplasmic and can acutely translocate to the plasma membrane, whereas SphK2 is present predominately in the nucleus but also can be found in the cytoplasm [17]. Once formed, S1P is tightly regulated by three pathways to maintain intracellular homeostasis (**Figure 2**). Firstly, S1P is recycled to ceramide through CerS after dephosphorylation by S1P-specific ER phosphatases, S1P phosphatases 1 (SPP1) and S1P phosphatases 2 (SPP2) [18, 19], or lipid phosphatases. Secondly, S1P can be irreversibly

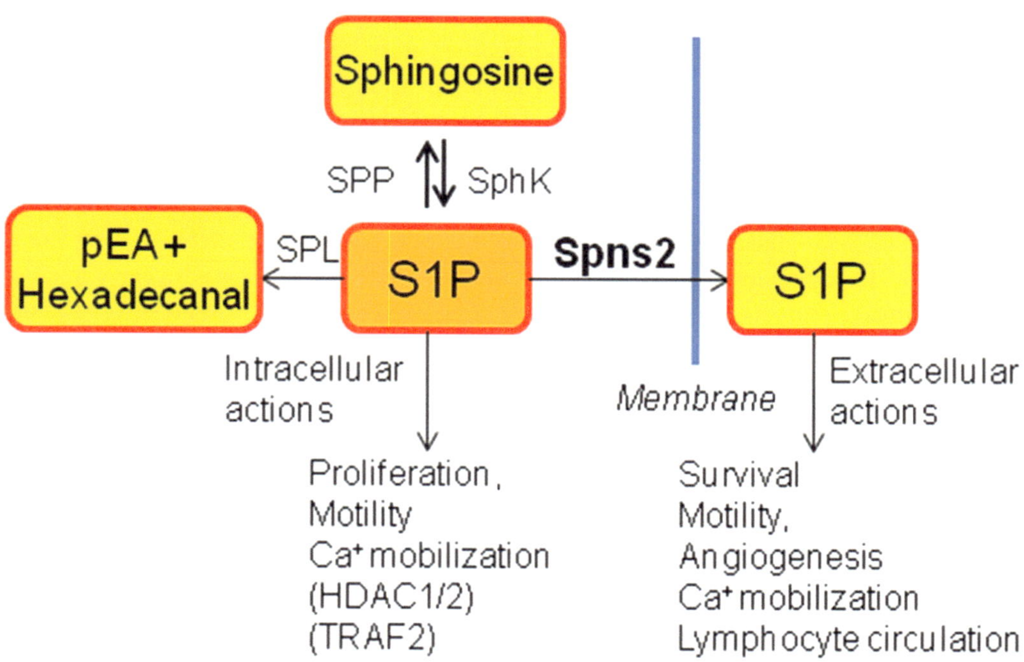

Figure 2. Schematics of S1P metabolism and function.

degraded by S1P lyase (SPL) into phosphoethanolamine (PEA) and hexadecenal [20]. In the third pathway, S1P is released to the extracellular space through transporter proteins, a process that is highly efficient in blood cells and endothelial cells [21, 22]. Several ATP-binding cassette (ABC) transporters are reported to transport S1P in blood cells. However, this notion is still being debated because knockout of the corresponding ABC transporters does not alter serum S1P level. A specific S1P transporter, Spns2, is responsible for S1P secretion in endothelial cells [23–26]. Spns2 gene deficiency in zebrafish and mice leads to significantly reduced extracellular S1P level and impaired egress of lymphocytes and migration of cardiomyocyte precursors [23–25, 27].

3. Ceramide in lung cancer

3.1. Ceramide and related enzymes in lung cancer pathology

Ceramide is generally believed to induce cell death and senescence. However, recent evidence has demonstrated that the roles of ceramide are concentration, cell context, and subcellular localization specific [8, 9, 28–30]. For example, C16 ceramide is shown to favor cancer cell proliferation and promote metastasis in lung cancer patients with CerS6 elevation [28, 29, 31–33]. On the other hand, C18 ceramide mediates cell death [28, 29, 31, 32]. These results emphasize the significance of concentration and cellular context in ceramide-mediated lung cancer cell death.

Most recently, CerS6, the enzyme that catalyzes C16:0 ceramide, was found to be overexpressed in advanced NSCLC patients and inversely correlated with clinical outcome [33]. C16:0 ceramide promotes NSCLC cell migration in vitro through formation of a RAC1-positive lamellipodia/ruffling structure in cells that escape C16 ceramide-induced apoptosis [33]. This notion is supported by data showing that CerS6 knockdown alters the ceramide profile, leading to decreased cell migration/invasion, reduced RAC1-positive lamellipodia formation in vitro, and attenuated lung metastasis in transplanted NSCLC cells in vivo [33].

Ceramide has been linked to cigarette smoking, the number one risk factor for lung cancer [8, 9, 34, 35]. Higher ceramide levels are reported in emphysema patients who are smokers, a subpopulation of patients greatly susceptible to lung cancer [34]. Just like ionizing radiation and chemotherapy drugs, cigarette smoking induces ceramide production which is mediated by nSMase2, an enzyme that hydrolyzes sphingomyelin to ceramide (**Figure 1**) [35]. Further evidence shows that during cigarette smoking, EGFR is favorably co-localized in ceramide-enriched regions of the plasma membrane, suggesting that nSMase2/ceramide plays a role in the aberrant EGFR activation, leading to augmented tumorigenic signaling and drug resistance [36]. Increased ceramide also triggers multidrug-resistant gene expression and synthesis of the pro-survival S1P and cell surface glycosphingolipids Gb3, which provide additional mechanisms for acquired drug resistance [8, 28, 37–39].

3.2. Ceramide as potential lung cancer treatment strategy and monitoring

Ceramide and related signaling is a promising target for lung cancer therapy. Based on the discovery that CerS6 is overexpressed in NSCLC, a combined treatment with

1-α-dimyristoylphosphatidylcholine (DMPC) liposome and the glucosylceramide synthase inhibitor *d*-threo-1-pheny-2-decanoylamino-3-morpholino-1-propanol (D-PDMP) is used to induce cell apoptosis [33]. The combined treatment induced cell death in association with C16 ceramide accumulation and promoted cancer cell apoptosis and tumor regression in murine models.

Based on the observation that the C18 ceramide level is reduced and I2PP2A overexpressed in lung tumors, a study took advantage of FTY-720, an US Food and Drug Administration (FDA)-approved multiple sclerosis drug, which is a sphingosine analog of myriocin [40]. FTY-720 mimics C18 ceramide and binds to I2PP2A, leading to PP2A reactivation, lung cancer cell death, and tumor suppression in vivo [41].

To overcome the cisplatin resistance caused by the increased cell surface glycosphingolipid Gb3, the glucosylceramide synthase inhibitor DL-threo-1-phenyl-2-palmitoylamino-3-morpholino-1-propanol (PPMP) has been tested. PPMP treatment substantially sensitizes cells to cisplatin cytotoxicity [39]. These data suggest that therapies targeting glucosylceramide synthase activity or Gb3 receptors may ameliorate acquired cisplatin drug resistance in lung cancer cells.

An additional exciting advance is that ceramide is a potential indicator of positive response after radiation therapy. Early biomarkers of lung tumor response are urgently needed to distinguish between responders and nonresponders to radiotherapy. A recent study shows that the plasma levels of total ceramide and four main subspecies are significantly higher in objective responders than in nonresponders of lung oligometastases [42]. In patients with increased total plasma ceramide levels, almost complete tumor control is achieved after 1 year, whereas the tumors continue to grow in half of the patients with lower ceramide levels [42]. This is intriguing since plasma ceramide is easily measurable and would enable early segregation of nonresponders so that additional more effective treatment options can be applied.

4. S1P and related signaling in lung cancer

Our understanding of the function of S1P and its signaling in lung cancer pathology is rather limited and fragmented when compared to other cancer types. SphK1, a major enzyme that generates S1P, was found to be overexpressed in lung patient samples [43]. The SphK/S1P pathway was shown to mediate the E2-induced transactivation of EGFR, which is associated with carcinogenesis in lung cancer cells [44]. It has also been reported that expression of the oncogenic K-Ras leads to plasma membrane localization of SphK1 and increased S1P level [45].

In a longitudinal study of 100 cases, plasma S1P level was found to be greater in lung cancer patients, implying that the level of extracellular S1P might contribute to the etiology of lung cancer or be a biomarker [46]. On the other hand, intracellular S1P was found to be increased in lung cancer cells going through epithelial mesenchymal transition, suggesting that intracellular S1P contributes to pathological epithelial mesenchymal transition, which is essential for lung cancer metastasis [47].

Consistent with this, knocking down the S1P transporter Spns2 enhanced migration in NSCLC cells partly due to increased intracellular S1P [26]. Pharmacological inhibition of S1P synthesis in Spns2 knockdown cells abolished the augmented cell migration mediated by Spns2 knockdown, indicating that intracellular S1P plays a key role in migration. Cell signaling studies indicated that Spns2 knockdown increased GSK-3β and Stat3-mediated pro-migration pathways [26]. More importantly, genetic studies showed that the Spns2 mRNA level was reduced in advanced lung cancer patients as quantified by using a small-scale Quantitative PCR (qPCR) array [26]. These data show that Spns2 plays key roles in regulating S1P homeostasis and the cellular functions in NSCLC cells and that Spns2 downregulation is a potential risk factor for lung cancer metastasis and drug resistance [26].

4.1. Targeting S1P for potential lung cancer therapy

S1P functions to enhance survival, proliferation, and angiogenesis; thus, removal of extracellular S1P and the use of SphK inhibitors to reduce S1P biosynthesis are major approaches for lung cancer therapy targeting S1P [48–50].

To remove S1P, an antibody was developed to physically sequester extracellular S1P. In animal models, the S1P-specific monoclonal antibody reduced lung tumor growth [51]. Sequestering extracellular S1P by using this antibody also attenuates lung metastasis of tumor cells from multiple other organs [50, 52].

Although SphK1 is elevated in lung cancer patients suggesting a potentially important role for this enzyme in lung tumor cell proliferation and survival [43, 53], results with novel, highly potent, and selective inhibitors to SphK1 in tumor cells did not affect their growth in vitro or in vivo, suggesting that tumor SphK1 may not be an efficacious therapeutic target for cancer [54, 55]. Hence, inhibitors of SphK2 are developed and tested for inducing lung cancer cell death, among which ABC294640 is a first-in-class drug [56]. One recent study demonstrates that ABC294640 suppressed growth of primary and A549 human lung cancer cells but sparing SphK2-low lung epithelial cells [56]. Inhibition of SphK2 by ABC294640 increased ceramide and decreased S1P levels, leading to lung cancer cell apoptosis. Another study shows that ABC294640 sensitized NSCLC cells to cell death induced by TNF-related apoptosis-inducing ligand (TRAIL) [56]. Compared with TRAIL alone, the combination therapy enhanced the apoptosis induced by TRAIL, and knockdown of SphK2 by siRNA presented a similar effect [57].

5. Concluding remarks

Exciting advances have been made regarding the roles of ceramide and its signaling in lung cancer in the past few years. Excess ceramide clearly has a critical function in inducing cell death in lung cancer cells, although those that escape this verdict are more prone to metastasis, as one important study shows [33]. Further increasing ceramide levels in these cells using combined drug treatment successfully induced apoptosis and reduced tumor size in vitro and in vivo [33]. This kinetic response opens new avenues to treat lung cancer by using ceramide-based therapies, the efficiency of which depends on the successful fine-tuning of ceramide metabolism, by using ceramide-inducing drugs such as fenretinide, and D-PDMP. Another exciting approach is to use ceramide mimics and short-chain ceramide or to increase the sensitizer proteins of ceramide, such as I2PP2A and Par-4, which are found to be reduced in lung cancer patients [41, 58, 59].

In terms of targeting S1P in lung cancer, aside from the antibody, using SphK2 inhibitors and its combination with SphK1 inhibitors seem to be promising approaches that merit further discovery [60]. In addition, agents such as transporter Spns2 [26] have shed new insights into the biology of S1P signaling. Such mechanistic insights have revealed additional control points for potential lung cancer therapeutic intervention. Even though receptor modulators have become the mainstream of current drug discovery [61], only one drug that targets the SphK/S1P axis (FTY-720, Fingolimod) is approved by FDA. And, the precise function of FTY-720 is very complicated and context/concentration dependent [41].

One important way that lung cancer cells overcome ceramide-induced cell death and senescence is to generate S1P, the pro-survival sphingolipid. Therefore, compounds that prevent S1P conversion from ceramide or further metabolize S1P to other derivatives which potentially sensitize cells to chemotherapy-induced tumor cell death are becoming an important approach for treating patients with lung cancer [62, 63].

In summary, growing evidence suggests that targeting sphingolipid metabolism is essential in improving lung cancer therapy and overcoming drug resistance. Due to the complexity and ubiquity of the sphingolipid metabolism and signaling, it is likely that a combined therapy employing conventional or novel targeted drugs and strategies based on chemical compounds or genetic approaches to modulate ceramide and S1P metabolism can be more beneficial than monotherapy. However, some important caveats should be considered in order to allow the development of more specific drug targets and inhibitors, in particular, the complexity of biological events that involve sphingolipids and the redundancy of the functions of the different enzymes.

Acknowledgements

This study was supported by grants NIH R01AG034389, R01NS095215, and NSF1121579 to E.B. and American Lung Association RG-351596 to GW. We are also grateful to the institutional support by the Department of Neuroscience and Regenerative Medicine (chair Dr. Lin Mei), Medical College of Georgia at Augusta University.

Abbreviations

S1P	Sphingosine-1-phosphate
CerS	Ceramide synthase
SMase	Sphingomyelinase
nSMase2	Neutral sphingomyelinase2
SphK	Sphingosine kinase
SPP1 and SPP2	S1P phosphatases 1 and 2

SPL	S1P lyase
PEA	Phosphoethanolamine
NSCLC	Non–small cell lung cancer
DMPC	Dimyristoylphosphatidylcholine
TRAIL	TNF-related apoptosis-inducing ligand

Author details

Erhard Bieberich and Guanghu Wang*

*Address all correspondence to: gwang@augusta.edu

Department of Neuroscience and Regenerative Medicine, Medical College of Georgia at Augusta University, Augusta, GA, U.S.A

References

[1] Heist, R.S., L.V. Sequist, and J.A. Engelman, Genetic changes in squamous cell lung cancer: a review. J Thorac Oncol, 2012. **7**(5): pp. 924–33.

[2] Herbst, R.S., J.V. Heymach, and S.M. Lippman, Lung cancer. N Engl J Med, 2008. **359**(13): pp. 1367–80.

[3] Custodio, A., M. Mendez, and M. Provencio, Targeted therapies for advanced non-small-cell lung cancer: current status and future implications. Cancer Treat Rev, 2012. **38**(1): pp. 36–53.

[4] West, L., et al., A novel classification of lung cancer into molecular subtypes. PLoS One, 2012. **7**(2): p. e31906.

[5] Shepherd, F.A., et al., Erlotinib in previously treated non-small-cell lung cancer. N Engl J Med, 2005. **353**(2): pp. 123–32.

[6] American Cancer Society. Cancer Facts & Figures 2012. Atlanta: American Cancer Society; 2012.

[7] Chen, Y., et al., Biomarker identification and pathway analysis by serum metabolomics of lung cancer. Biomed Res Int, 2015. **2015**: p. 183624.

[8] Goldkorn, T., S. Chung, and S. Filosto, Lung cancer and lung injury: the dual role of ceramide. Handb Exp Pharmacol, 2013. **216**: pp. 93–113.

[9] Goldkorn, T., S. Filosto, and S. Chung, Lung injury and lung cancer caused by cigarette smoke-induced oxidative stress: molecular mechanisms and therapeutic opportunities involving the ceramide-generating machinery and epidermal growth factor receptor. Antioxid Redox Signal, 2014. **21**(15): pp. 2149–74.

[10] Spiegel, S., et al., Roles of sphingosine-1-phosphate in cell growth, differentiation, and death. Biochemistry (Mosc), 1998. **63**(1): pp. 69–73.

[11] Huang, Y.L., W.P. Huang, and H. Lee, Roles of sphingosine 1-phosphate on tumorigenesis. World J Biol Chem, 2011. **2**(2): pp. 25–34.

[12] Giussani, P., et al., Sphingolipids: key regulators of apoptosis and pivotal players in cancer drug resistance. Int J Mol Sci, 2014. **15**(3): pp. 4356–92.

[13] Furuya, H., Y. Shimizu, and T. Kawamori, Sphingolipids in cancer. Cancer Metastasis Rev, 2011. **30**(3–4): pp. 567–76.

[14] Bieberich, E., There is more to a lipid than just being a fat: sphingolipid-guided differentiation of oligodendroglial lineage from embryonic stem cells. Neurochem Res, 2011. **36**(9): pp. 1601–11.

[15] Rahmaniyan, M., et al., Identification of dihydroceramide desaturase as a direct in vitro target for fenretinide. J Biol Chem, 2011. **286**(28): pp. 24754–64.

[16] Hannun, Y.A. and L.M. Obeid, Principles of bioactive lipid signalling: lessons from sphingolipids. Nat Rev Mol Cell Biol, 2008. **9**(2): pp. 139–50.

[17] Igarashi, N., et al., Sphingosine kinase 2 is a nuclear protein and inhibits DNA synthesis. J Biol Chem, 2003. **278**(47): pp. 46832–9.

[18] Ogawa, C., et al., Identification and characterization of a novel human sphingosine-1-phosphate phosphohydrolase, hSPP2. J Biol Chem, 2003. **278**(2): pp. 1268–72.

[19] Le Stunff, H., et al., Recycling of sphingosine is regulated by the concerted actions of sphingosine-1-phosphate phosphohydrolase 1 and sphingosine kinase 2. J Biol Chem, 2007. **282**(47): pp. 34372–80.

[20] Zhou, J. and J.D. Saba, Identification of the first mammalian sphingosine phosphate lyase gene and its functional expression in yeast. Biochem Biophys Res Commun, 1998. **242**(3): pp. 502–7.

[21] Pappu, R., et al., Promotion of lymphocyte egress into blood and lymph by distinct sources of sphingosine-1-phosphate. Science, 2007. **316**(5822): pp. 295–8.

[22] Venkataraman, K., et al., Vascular endothelium as a contributor of plasma sphingosine 1-phosphate. Circ Res, 2008. **102**(6): pp. 669–76.

[23] Kawahara, A., et al., The sphingolipid transporter spns2 functions in migration of zebrafish myocardial precursors. Science, 2009. **323**(5913): pp. 524–7.

[24] Nagahashi, M., et al., Spns2, a transporter of phosphorylated sphingoid bases, regulates their blood and lymph levels and the lymphatic network. FASEB J, 2013. Mar;27(3):1001-11. doi: 10.1096/fj.12-219618. Epub 2012 Nov 24.

[25] Fukuhara, S., et al., The sphingosine-1-phosphate transporter Spns2 expressed on endothelial cells regulates lymphocyte trafficking in mice. J Clin Invest, 2012. **122**(4): pp. 1416–26.

[26] Bradley, E., et al., Critical role of spns2, a sphingosine-1-phosphate transporter, in lung cancer cell survival and migration. PLoS One, 2014. Oct 20;**9**(10):e110119. doi: 10.1371/journal.pone.0110119. eCollection 2014.

[27] Nijnik, A., et al., The role of sphingosine-1-phosphate transporter Spns2 in immune system function. J Immunol, 2012. **189**(1): pp. 102–11.

[28] Ogretmen, B., Sphingolipids in cancer: regulation of pathogenesis and therapy. FEBS Lett, 2006. **580**(23): pp. 5467–76.

[29] Saddoughi, S.A. and B. Ogretmen, Diverse functions of ceramide in cancer cell death and proliferation. Adv Cancer Res, 2013. **117**: pp. 37–58.

[30] Morad, S.A. and M.C. Cabot, Ceramide-orchestrated signalling in cancer cells. Nat Rev Cancer, 2013. **13**(1): pp. 51–65.

[31] Ogretmen, B. and Y.A. Hannun, Biologically active sphingolipids in cancer pathogenesis and treatment. Nat Rev Cancer, 2004. **4**(8): pp. 604–16.

[32] Ponnusamy, S., et al., Sphingolipids and cancer: ceramide and sphingosine-1-phosphate in the regulation of cell death and drug resistance. Future Oncol, 2010. **6**(10): pp. 1603–24.

[33] Suzuki, M., et al., Targeting ceramide synthase 6-dependent metastasis-prone phenotype in lung cancer cells. J Clin Invest, 2016. **126**(1): pp. 254–65.

[34] Petrache, I., et al., Ceramide upregulation causes pulmonary cell apoptosis and emphysema-like disease in mice. Nat Med, 2005. **11**(5): pp. 491–8.

[35] Levy, M., et al., Neutral sphingomyelinase 2 is activated by cigarette smoke to augment ceramide-induced apoptosis in lung cell death. Am J Physiol Lung Cell Mol Physiol, 2009. **297**(1): pp. L125–33.

[36] D'Angelo, S.P., et al., Incidence of EGFR exon 19 deletions and L858R in tumor specimens from men and cigarette smokers with lung adenocarcinomas. J Clin Oncol, 2011. **29**(15): pp. 2066–70.

[37] Cole, S.P., et al., Overexpression of a transporter gene in a multidrug-resistant human lung cancer cell line. Science, 1992. **258**(5088): pp. 1650–4.

[38] Galluzzi, L., et al., Molecular mechanisms of cisplatin resistance. Oncogene, 2012. **31**(15): pp. 1869–83.

[39] Tyler, A., et al., Targeting glucosylceramide synthase induction of cell surface globotriaosylceramide (Gb3) in acquired cisplatin-resistance of lung cancer and malignant pleural mesothelioma cells. Exp Cell Res, 2015. **336**(1): pp. 23–32.

[40] Cohen, J.A., et al., Oral fingolimod or intramuscular interferon for relapsing multiple sclerosis. N Engl J Med, 2010. **362**(5): pp. 402–15.

[41] Saddoughi, S.A., et al., Sphingosine analogue drug FTY720 targets I2PP2A/SET and mediates lung tumour suppression via activation of PP2A-RIPK1-dependent necroptosis. EMBO Mol Med, 2013. **5**(1): pp. 105–21.

[42] Dubois, N., et al., Plasma ceramide, a real-time predictive marker of pulmonary and hepatic metastases response to stereotactic body radiation therapy combined with irinotecan. Radiother Oncol, 2016. **119**(2): pp. 229–35.

[43] Johnson, K.R., et al., Immunohistochemical distribution of sphingosine kinase 1 in normal and tumor lung tissue. J Histochem Cytochem, 2005. **53**(9): pp. 1159–66.

[44] Sukocheva, O., et al., Estrogen transactivates EGFR via the sphingosine 1-phosphate receptor Edg-3: the role of sphingosine kinase-1. J Cell Biol, 2006. **173**(2): pp. 301–10.

[45] Gault, C.R., et al., Oncogenic K-Ras regulates bioactive sphingolipids in a sphingosine kinase 1-dependent manner. J Biol Chem, 2012. **287**(38): pp. 31794–803.

[46] Alberg, A.J., et al., Plasma sphingolipids as markers of future lung cancer risk: a population-based, nested case–control study. Cancer Epidemiol Biomarkers Prev, 2013.

[47] Meshcheryakova, A., et al., Exploring the role of sphingolipid machinery during the epithelial to mesenchymal transition program using an integrative approach. Oncotarget, 2016. **7**(16): pp. 22295–323.

[48] Pyne, N.J. and S. Pyne, Sphingosine 1-phosphate and cancer. Nat Rev Cancer, 2010. **10**(7): pp. 489–503.

[49] Pyne, N.J., et al., Sphingosine 1-phosphate signalling in cancer. Biochem Soc Trans, 2012. **40**(1): pp. 94–100.

[50] Proia, R.L. and T. Hla, Emerging biology of sphingosine-1-phosphate: its role in pathogenesis and therapy. J Clin Invest, 2015. **125**(4): pp. 1379–87.

[51] Visentin, B., et al., Validation of an anti-sphingosine-1-phosphate antibody as a potential therapeutic in reducing growth, invasion, and angiogenesis in multiple tumor lineages. Cancer Cell, 2006. **9**(3): pp. 225–38.

[52] Ponnusamy, S., et al., Communication between host organism and cancer cells is transduced by systemic sphingosine kinase 1/sphingosine 1-phosphate signalling to regulate tumour metastasis. EMBO Mol Med, 2012. **4**(8): pp. 761–75.

[53] Heffernan-Stroud, L.A. and L.M. Obeid, Sphingosine kinase 1 in cancer. Adv Cancer Res, 2013. **117**: pp. 201–35.

[54] Schnute, M.E., et al., Modulation of cellular S1P levels with a novel, potent and specific inhibitor of sphingosine kinase-1. Biochem J, 2012. **444**(1): pp. 79–88.

[55] Kharel, Y., et al., Sphingosine kinase type 1 inhibition reveals rapid turnover of circulating sphingosine 1-phosphate. Biochem J, 2011. **440**(3): pp. 345–53.

[56] Guan, S., et al., Inhibition of ceramide glucosylation sensitizes lung cancer cells to ABC294640, a first-in-class small molecule SphK2 inhibitor. Biochem Biophys Res Commun, 2016. **476**(4): pp. 230–6.

[57] Yang, J., et al., ABC294640, a sphingosine kinase 2 inhibitor, enhances the antitumor effects of TRAIL in non-small cell lung cancer. Cancer Biol Ther, 2015. **16**(8): pp. 1194–204.

[58] Joshi, J., et al., Par-4 inhibits Akt and suppresses Ras-induced lung tumorigenesis. EMBO J, 2008. **27**(16): pp. 2181–93.

[59] Bieberich, E., et al., Selective apoptosis of pluripotent mouse and human stem cells by novel ceramide analogues prevents teratoma formation and enriches for neural precursors in ES cell-derived neural transplants. J Cell Biol, 2004. **167**(4): pp. 723–34.

[60] Tran, H.B., et al., Cigarette smoke inhibits efferocytosis via deregulation of sphingosine kinase signaling: reversal with exogenous S1P and the S1P analogue FTY720. J Leukoc Biol, 2016. **100**(1): pp. 195–202.

[61] Kunkel, G.T., et al., Targeting the sphingosine-1-phosphate axis in cancer, inflammation and beyond. Nat Rev Drug Discov, 2013. **12**(9): pp. 688–702.

[62] Maceyka, M., et al., Sphingosine-1-phosphate signaling and its role in disease. Trends Cell Biol, 2012. **22**(1): pp. 50–60.

[63] Shirahama, T., et al., In vitro and in vivo induction of apoptosis by sphingosine and N, N-dimethylsphingosine in human epidermoid carcinoma KB-3-1 and its multidrug-resistant cells. Clin Cancer Res, 1997. **3**(2): pp. 257–64.

Chapter 7

Prognostic and Predictive Value of PD-L1 in Patients with Lung Cancer

Mirjana Rajer

Additional information is available at the end of the chapter

http://dx.doi.org/10.5772/66757

Abstract

Improved understanding of the molecular mechanisms has led to identification of checkpoint signalling and development of checkpoint inhibitors in the treatment of many cancers, including lung cancer. To be able to select the patients who benefit most from checkpoint inhibitors, predictive biomarkers are needed. Currently, the only predictive biomarker that has been approved in clinical use is PD-L1, the ligand of the inhibitory T-cell checkpoint PD-1. The use of PD-L1 as a predictive biomarker is confounded by multiple unresolved issues, from testing issues (e.g., cut-off values for positivity) to clinical use (e.g., the response to anti–PD-1 and anti–PD-L1 antibodies in patients without any expression of PD-L1). Even more open questions exist in the evaluation of PD-L1 as a prognostic biomarker. In the future, we expect that an improved understanding of immune system, tumor microenvironment, mechanism of action of immunotherapeutic drugs, and PD-L1 testing methods will elucidate the value of PD-L1 as a prognostic and predictive biomarker in detail.

Keywords: immunotherapy, PD-L1, prognostic factor, predictive factor, lung cancer

1. Introduction

Immunotherapy represents an important step forward in the management of patients with lung cancer. Careful selection of patients, who benefit most from any new treatment including immunotherapy, is essential. To be able to select the patients, prognostic and predictive markers are needed. Prognostic biomarkers provide information about the patient's overall cancer outcome, regardless of the therapy. Predictive biomarkers give information about the effect of a therapeutic intervention [1–3].

PD-1 is a T cell immune checkpoint involved in dampening autoimmunity in the peripheral effector phase of T-cell activation, leading to immune tolerance of cells expressing its ligands PD-L1 and PD-L2. Activation of PD-1–PD-L1 leads to peripheral immunological tolerance in T cells. Multiple solid tumors (melanoma, RCC, and lung cancer) express PD-L1 to generate immunosuppressive tumor microenvironment and avoid destruction of their cells by T lymphocytes. In healthy tissues, PD-1 is thought to limit the activity of antigen-specific T cells to prevent collateral tissue damage during infection. In cancer, the PD-1 pathway can be exploited by some tumor cells to inactivate T cells [4].

The importance of the PD-L1 together with the development of drugs that inhibit its action suggest a candidate for a prognostic and/or predictive biomarker: PD-L1 expression in tumor or inflammatory cells. The (few) trials that evaluated PD-L1 as a prognostic biomarker yielded inconclusive results. Some of them showed that patients with PD-L1 or PD-1 positive expression have significantly shorter overall survival, while in others, no correlation between biomarker expression and outcome was seen. Many questions remain open even when considering PD-L1 as a predictive biomarker, for example, what cut-off percentage of expression can be considered as positive or can PD-L1 testing be performed only on fresh or archival tissues also. Above all, the most important question whether PD-L1 can really be considered as a predictive biomarker still has to be answered. In the lack of definitive answers, currently researchers propose other biomarkers as supplemental (e.g., pre-existing CD8+ T, cytokines, ...) [4].

In this chapter, the value of PD-L1 as a prognostic and predictive biomarker will be presented together with all open questions and possible answers.

2. Change in the insight of lung cancer

Lung cancer was first described a century ago, and since then every year, around 1.6 million of new cases are diagnosed [4]. Nonsmall cell lung cancer (NSCLC) remains the main cause of death due to cancer worldwide. About 60% of lung cancers are diagnosed at Stage IV, and these patients have a very poor prognosis, since 5-year survival is only 1–4% [5]. New treatments, developed in the last years, lead to improved survival in the different groups of NSCLC patients with advanced disease. Patients who benefit most are those with adenocarcinomas and specific mutations, such as EGFR activating mutations and ALK translocations. A median survival of 20 months has been reached with EGFR tyrosine kinase inhibitors (EGFR-TKI), which can be considered a milestone in the treatment of advanced lung cancer. Despite promising results, many patients with advanced lung cancer still have a poor prognosis. Patients with squamous carcinomas, patients with adenocarcinomas not harboring specific mutations, and patients with small cell lung cancers still have a poor prognosis, with survival often less than a year. To be able to improve survival in lung cancer in general, the next step should be to focus on the treatment of those patients. Immunotherapy nowadays seems a step forward in reaching this goal [1].

Changes in lung cancer have became evident in recent years. A strong connection between lung cancer and smoking is supposed to be one of the main reasons [4]. Main changes observed are the increase of adenocarcinomas at the expense of squamous tumors and a change in the position of cancers. Previously centrally located, they now arise mainly at the periphery of the lung. Possible explanations are changes in the smoking patterns. Nicotine is known to be one of the most addictive substances in the world. To be able to get enough nicotine with new sorts of cigarettes (light and ultra light low-nicotine, and low-tar), smokers have to inhale deeper and for a longer time. This leads to the change of locations of tumors, since the smoke now enters deeply in the lungs and stays there for a longer time [6–8]. The increased incidence of adenocarcinomas is also suspected to be related to new forms of cigarettes and a higher amount of nitrosamines in them. Nitrosamines are known to cause adenocarcinomas in experimental animal models, and it is supposed that the same carcinogenic process occurs also in smokers [4, 9].

In recent years, changes at the "macroscopic level" are supplemented by the insight in the microscopic world of the lung cancer such as discovery of EGFR mutations and more and more important knowledge about complex immunologic interactions between tumors and the host environment [1].

3. Immune system and cancer

When cells transform to be malignant, activation of innate and adaptive immune responses occurs. The purpose of this activation is control of early cancer growth by elimination of cancer cells. Cancer cells have different genetic and epigenetic alterations leading to an expression of different antigens that can be recognized and eliminated by the immune system [10].

The process starts at the cancer site, where tumor cells disintegrate and tumor antigens become available to the immune system. Antigen presenting cells (APC) uptake these antigens and under maturation, signals, activate, and migrate to the lymph nodes or tertiary lymphoid structures [11]. Maturation signals are necessary, since without them immune tolerance rather than activation occurs. Examples of maturation signals are intracellular proteins, heat-shock proteins, DNA, ATP, uric acid, etc. Activated APCs migrate to lymph nodes, where they present as antigens in the context of mayor histocompatibility complex Classes I and II molecules to the T lymphocytes. Antigen-specific CD 4 and CD 8 T lymphocytes recognize the antigens and become activated. Costimulatory and coinhibitory signals are essential for this activation to regulate and balance a proper immunological response. CD 28 complex represents a costimulatory signal and acts together with other stimulatory and inhibitory signals on T lymphocytes. They regulate T-cell activation, differentiation, survival, and effector function. Examples of costimulatory receptors are GITR, OX 40, CD 30, and CD 40, while coinhibitory signals, beside LAG, TIM, BTLA, VISTA, etc., include also CTLA-4 and PD-1 with its ligand PD-L1 currently implemented as important targets of cancer immunotherapy. After activation, T lymphocytes migrate to the tumors trough and the systemic vasculature by following a chemokine gradient. T cells then go through the process of extravasation, migrate into the tumor, and recognize the tumor targets that lead finally to tumor cell destruction [11]. Lymphocytic infiltration of tumors is frequently observed in a variety of human cancers and in numerous trials tumor-infiltrating lymphocytes have been correlated with a more favorable prognosis [10].

When tumors develop, tumor cells acquire several mutations that lead to tumor "immortality." The results of these mutations are abnormal proteins on the cell surface that can be recognized by the immune system. A higher number of mutations, commonly called mutation burden, is connected to higher immunogenicity of tumors. NSCLC and melanomas are cancers with the highest burden among several solid tumors and because of that they are believed to be good targets for immunotherapy [1]. The problem of immune recognition and cancer is that cancers have the ability to evade the immune system, and this is one of the hallmarks of cancer [5]. Several mechanisms of immune evasion exist, but one of the most important is that tumor-infiltrating lymphocytes become inactivated by the effect of PD-L1 expression on tumor cells [10, 12].

4. Why do we need prognostic and predictive biomarkers

Prognostic and predictive biomarkers have become important in recent years with the development of new highly selective therapies. A prognostic biomarker offers insight into the possible natural evolvement of the disease and most likely outcome like duration of survival of the patients. It is not related to treatment, but rather to tumor biology. It helps physicians and patients to predict the course of the disease [1, 13–15]. Before a marker is labelled predictive, the effect of a marker as a prognostic marker must be taken into account [16].

A predictive biomarker, on the other hand, predicts the effect of the treatment that should be different in patients with the biomarker compared to those without it [1, 7]. In lung cancer, examples of predictive biomarkers include the presence of EGFR-activating mutations and response to EGFR-TKIs. Predictive biomarkers are important in treatment decisions because they can improve the treatment effectiveness and at the same time, reduce costs and potential harm to the patients by avoiding treatment when the biomarker is not present [1]. In a trial presented by Lopes *et al.*, the use of biomarkers to select proper patients in clinical trials resulted in a sixfold increase in clinical trial success [17].

Regarding immunotherapy, the median duration of response, once the response is achieved, is often longer than response to classical chemotherapy and even some targeted agents. However, response rates in nonselected populations are still low; they are achieved in only 15–20% of the patients. This fact, together with the high expenses of immunotherapy, leads to the necessity of finding reliable predictive biomarkers to identify which patients are most likely to benefit from it [16].

5. PD-L1 as a prognostic and predictive biomarker

Programmed cell death protein 1 (PD-1) is a cell surface protein that has two ligands PD-L1 and PD-L2. PD-1 and PD-L1 negatively regulate immune responses. The PD-1/PD-L1 pathway mediates one of the mechanisms of cancer "escape" from the immune system. Cancer microenvironment induces PD-L1 expression on tumor cells that results in inhibition of the immune response, permitting cancer growth, progression, and metastases [5, 18].

http://dx.doi.org/10.5772/66757

PD-L1 expression has been studied widely in different trials as a prognostic and predictive biomarker. Poor responses and high expression of PD-L1 have been found in several cancers including melanoma, breast, bladder, ovary, pancreas, kidney, esophagus, and hematologic malignancies [1, 18, 19]. Results are not constant; some authors report no correlation or even improved survival of patients with tumors highly expressing PD-L1 [18, 20].

Regarding expression of PD-L1 as a prognostic biomarker in lung cancer, several contradictive data have been published. Many authors suggest that high expression is connected to better prognosis, while others found just the opposite [19]. Cha *et al*. evaluated the prognostic significance of PD-L1 expression in 323 surgically resected lung adenocarcinomas Stages I–III. PD-L1 expression in tumor cells was positive in 60 of the cases (18.6%). PD-L1 positivity was more frequent in male patients ($p = 0.001$), tumors greater than 3 cm ($p = 0.03$), higher-stage tumors ($p < 0.001$), solid, predominant tumors ($p < 0.001$), and EGFR wild-type tumors ($p = 0.022$). Higher expression (over 50%) was more prevalent in former or current smokers compared to nonsmokers ($p = 0.026$) and was associated with more pack-years of smoking ($p = 0.016$) [19]. Survival analysis was performed on 316 patients who underwent complete surgical resection (Stages I–IIIA disease). Poor, recurrence-free, and overall survival in patients with high PD-L1 expression assessed with univariate analysis were reported (both $p < 0.001$), exact median PFS and overall survival (OS) were not reported in numbers (e.g., months). Authors conclude that high PD-L1 expression is associated with poor prognosis of patients [19].

Aguiar *et al*. recently published a meta-analysis aiming to answer the question about PD-L1 as a predictive biomarker. The analysis included 13 studies with 1979 patients who were treated with checkpoint inhibitors. Five different checkpoint inhibitors were used: nivolumab in six trials, atezolizumab in three trials, pembrolizumab in one trial, MEDI4736 in two, and avelumab in one trial. The most frequent histology was nonsquamous NSCLC (67%). Majority of the patients were previously treated (84%), male (58%), current or previous smokers (64%), and with ECOG performance status 1 (62%). All included trials reported overall response rate (ORR). The ORR in 652 PD-L1–positive patients was 29%, and 13% among 915 PD-L1–negative patients. Difference was statistically significant (relative risk (RR) 2.08, 95% confidence interval (CI) 1.49–2.91, $p < 0.01$). The ORR increased proportionally with increase in PD-L1 expression, regardless of tumor histology or line of treatment (Pearson's correlation $r = 0.43$). Regarding PFS, authors evaluated 24 weeks PFS rate. Data were available for 767 patients. In PD-L1–positive patients 24 weeks PFS was 35% (358 patients), while in 409 PD-L1–negative patients, it was 26% (RR 0.79, 95% CI 0.71–0.89, $p < 0.01$). One-year overall survival (OS) was reported in nine trials with 1396 patients. OS did not differ between the PD-L1–positive and PD-L1–negative groups. Among the 617 positive patients the rate was 28%, while among 779 PD-L1–negative, it was 27% (RR 0, 96, 95% CI 0.87–1.06, $p = 0.39$). Authors also evaluated the response to immune checkpoint inhibitors compared to docetaxel in PD-L1 negative patients (PD-L1 expression below 1%). Two Phase III and one Phase II trials compared nivolumab or atezolizumab with docetaxel in the second-line setting. Among the 407 PD-L1–negative patients, ORR was 12% in both arms (RR 1, 95% CI 0.59–1.7, $p = 1$). PFS was also similar between the two arms (hazard ratio (HR) 0.98, $p = 0.93$ for PFS). Regarding OS even if not statistically significant, there was even a trend toward better survival among patients receiving checkpoint inhibitors (HR 0.83, $p = 0.12$). Authors conclude that even if tumor PD-L1 expression is related to improved survival and better outcome of patients with advanced NSCLC, PD-L1 currently cannot be considered as a biomarker for selection of patients who benefit from immune checkpoint inhibitors treatment since many PD-L1–negative patients also benefit from them, and the response is not inferior to the response to chemotherapy [1].

Other authors like Schmidt *et al.* also evaluated prognostic and predictive values of PD-L1 expression. Three hundred and twenty-one curatively resected NSCLC patients who had available tumor material and clinical data from the Thoracic Departments in Ostrcapepeln, Germany, were included. Median age of patients was 66 years and all NSCLC histology included, except NSCLC non-other specified. Cut-off for positivity was ≥5% of tumor cells PD-L1–positive. Twenty-four percent of cells expressed PD-L1 in NSCLC samples. For the whole group, PD-L1 expression was not the prognostic factor for OS ($p = 0.256$). The better survival in the patients with PD-L1–positive tumors compared to patients with no PD-L1 expression was observed only in some subgroups: squamous histology (HR 0.45, 95% CI 0.25–0.83, $p = 0.005$), patients that received adjuvant therapy (HR 0.35, CI 0.14–0.86, $p = 0.01$), had positive lymph nodes reviled by surgery (HR 0.47, CI 0.26–0.85, $p = 0.005$), and had greater tumor size (HR 0.55, CI 0.36–0.84, $p = 0.004$. According to the authors, these findings suggest that PD-L1 expression might be prognostic in these subgroups of patients, but because of the small sample size, firm conclusions cannot be done [21].

Cooper retrospectively analyzed 681 Australian patients who underwent surgical resection for Stages I–III NSCLC between 1990 and 2008 for PD-L1 expression. Tumors with ≥50% of the cells showing positive membrane staining were considered to have high expression of PD-L1. Several clinicopathological factors were compared regarding PD-L1 expression. Associations were encountered comparing patient's age, tumor size, and grade. High PD-L1 expression was associated with younger patient's age ($p = 0.07$). Median age in the "younger" group was 67 and "older" group 69 years. High PD-L1 expression was statistically significantly higher in bigger tumors (median size 45 mm vs. 40 mm, $p = 0.02$) and tumors with higher histological grade ($p < 0.01$). Even if not statistically significant, squamous and large cell tumors had more "high" expression compared with adenocarcinomas (8.1 and 12.5 vs. 5.1% of samples, $p = 0.13$). High PD-L1 expression was not associated with factors such as gender, tumor size, stage, nodal involvement, EGFR, k-ras, or ALK mutations. Authors also compared patients' outcome between the two PD-L1 groups. Patients with high expression had longer median survival compared to patients with low (113.2 months vs. 85.5 months, $p = 0.023$). High PD-L1 as the prognostic factor for better survival was confirmed in Cox model (HR 0.59, 95% CI 0.4–0.8, $p > 0.01$). Even if high PD-L1 expression was a prognostic factor in this trial, authors conclude that the evidence was still not firm enough to claim its prognostic value, and they state that any prognostic significance relates not on single marker of immune signals, but to the overall balance of the host-tumor immune response [22].

6. Immune checkpoint inhibitors in lung cancer and PD-L1 as predictive biomarker

The aim of cancer immunotherapies is to change the adoptive immune system toward tumor rejection. One of the possible approaches is immune checkpoint blockade, which aims to relieve inhibition of immune checkpoints [5, 23]. NSCLC was considered to be an immunotherapy nonresponsive tumor type, when the earliest clinical trials with interleukins, vaccines, and interferon failed to show clinical benefit. More recently, good treatment responses and improved overall survival have been observed with the use of immune checkpoint inhibitors. Patients that respond to these treatments have durable responses that are usually longer than responses to chemotherapy or targeted therapies. However, some drawbacks exist in nonselected patients' response and can be seen only in 15–20% of the patients, and the cost of these drugs is extremely high [12, 16].

Currently, two checkpoint inhibitors (PD-L1 inhibitors) pembrolizumab and nivolumab are being used in everyday clinical practice, but it is supposed that soon others such as atezolizumab, durvalumab, and avalumab will enter into everyday clinical use [24]. Quick development of new immunotherapeutic drugs is not followed by proper development in optimal biomarkers for patient selection. In clinical trials, anti–PD-1 and anti–PD-L1 antibodies produce 20% of response in nonselected population [25]. This can be well seen in the interpretation of clinical trials with nivolumab and pembrolizumab. General conclusions from nivolumab trials is that patient selections should not be done on the PD-L1 expression, while pembrolizumab trials suggest the opposite [16].

6.1. Nivolumab

CheckMate 017, a Phase III trial, compared treatment with docetaxel in one arm and nivolumab in second arm in patients with Stage IIIB or Stage IV squamous NSCLC that progressed on the first-line therapy with platinum-containing regimen. From October 2012–December 2013, 272 eligible patients were included. Patients were randomized to receive either nivolumab at dose 3 mg/kg or docetaxel 75 mg/m^2 every 3 weeks. The primary endpoint was OS. Median age was 63, most were men (76%), had ECOG performance status score 1 (76%), and were current or former smokers (92%). The nivolumab group had longer overall survival (9.2 vs. 6 months, HR 0.59, $p < 0.001$) and longer progression-free survival (3.5 vs. 2.8 months, HR = 0.62, $p < 0.001$). Response was 20% in nivolumab and 9% in docetaxel arm ($p = 0.008$). PD-L1 expression was assessed retrospectively in 83% (225 of 272) of the patients who underwent randomization. Patients were categorized as positive if the expression was 1, 5, or 10%. No differences in overall survival was found between different expression groups in patients that received nivolumab or docetaxel regardless of the percentage (%) of positivity (>1% HR 0.96, CI 0.45–1.05; >5% HR 0.53, CI 0.3–0.89; >10% HR 0.70, CI 0.47–1.01). Authors concluded that the expression of PD-L1 was not a prognostic or a predictive factor for treatment with nivolumab [16, 26].

CheckMate 057 was a second Phase III trial comparing nivolumab with docetaxel for patients with previously treated nonsquamous NSCLC Stage IIIB or Stage IV that progressed on previous therapy. From November 2012 to December 2013, 582 patients were randomized to receive either 3 mg/kg of nivolumab every 3 weeks or docetaxel 75 mg/m^2 every 3 weeks. Patients treated with nivolumab had longer overall survival (12.2 vs. 9.4 months, HR 0.73, $p = 0.002$) and a higher response rate (19% vs. 12%, $p = 0{,}02$) compared to patients receiving docetaxel. Differences in PFS were not established (2.3 months for nivolumab vs. 4.2 for docetaxel, HR 0.92, CI 0.77–1.11, $p = 0.39$). PD-L1 expression was evaluated in the same way as in CheckMate 017 with cut-offs at 1, 5, and 10%. PD-L1 testing was performed in 78% (455 of 582) of the patients. Objective response rate was 9% (CI 5–16) in patients with less than 1% PD-L1 expression, 36% (CI 26–46) in patients with >5%, and 37 (CI 7–48) in patients with more than 10% expression. Similarly, differences were seen in OS, with patients who have expression more than 5% (median OS 19.4 months), having longer survival with nivolumab treatment compared to patients with expression less than 1% (median OS 10.5 months) ($p < 0.01$). The study showed a predictive association between PD-L1 expression and benefit from anti–PD-1 treatment. Although the benefit of nivolumab was observed in the overall population, the magnitude of benefit across all the efficacy endpoints appeared to be greater among patients whose tumors expressed PD-L1 than among those whose tumors did not express PD-L1 [16, 27].

6.2. Pembrolizumab

Keynote 001 was a Phase I trial in which patients received three different schedules of treatment with pembrolizumab (2 mg/kg every 2 weeks, 10 mg/kg every two or every 3 weeks). From May 2012 to February 2014, 495 patients with Stage IIIB or Stage IV of NSCLC were included. ORR with pembrolizumab treatment was 19.4%, and PFS and OS were 3.7 and 12.5 months, respectively. PD-L 1 was assessed and cut-off defined at 50% of tumor cells expression. In defining PD-L1 positivity, authors used received-data-characteristic curves (ROC). Prevalence of PD-L1 positivity (>50%) was 23.2, 1–49, 37.6, and 39.2% less than 1%. Among patients with the score of at least 50%, the progression-free survival was 6.3 (95% CI 2.9–12.5) months, and overall survival was not reached. Progression-free and overall survival were shorter among patients with a proportion score of 1–49% or a score of less than 1% than among those with a score of at least 50%. Median PFS was 6.1 months (CI 4.2-not reached) in positive group and 4 months (CI 2.1–2.4) in <1% group. Median OS was not reached in a positive group and 10.4 (CI 5.8-not reached) in <1% group. Authors conclude that a proportion score of at least 50% may represent a new biomarker for the treatment of nonsmall-cell lung cancer [16, 25].

Keynote 010 was a Phase II/III trial comparing two schedules of pembrolizumab (2 mg/kg every 3 weeks, 10 mg/kg every 3 weeks) with docetaxel 75 mg/m^2 for patients with PD-L1 expression (>1% of tumor cells) that progressed on previous chemotherapy. Between August 2013 and February 2015, 1034 patients were included. Median overall survival was 10.4 months with pembrolizumab 2 mg/kg, 12.7 months with pembrolizumab 10 mg/kg, and 8.5 months with docetaxel. Overall survival was significantly longer for both doses of pembrolizumab vs. docetaxel (pembrolizumab 2 mg/kg vs. docetaxel: HR 0.71, 95% CI 0.58–0.88, $p = 0{\cdot}0008$), and (pembrolizumab 10 mg/kg vs. docetaxel: HR 0.61, 95% CI 0.49–0.75, $p < 0{\cdot}0001$). Median progression-free survival was 3.9 months with pembrolizumab 2 mg/kg, 4.0 months with pembrolizumab 10 mg/kg, and 4.0 months with docetaxel, with no significant difference for pembrolizumab 2 mg/kg or for pembrolizumab 10 mg/kg. As expected, patients with at least 50% of tumor cells expressing PD-L1 had overall survival significantly longer with pembrolizumab 2 mg/kg than with docetaxel (median 14.9 months vs. 8.2 months; HR 0·54, 95% CI 0.38–0.77, $p = 0.0002$), and with pembrolizumab 10 mg/kg than with docetaxel (17.3 months vs. 8.2 months; 0.50, 0.36–0.70; $p < 0.0001$). For this patient population, progression-free survival was also significantly longer with pembrolizumab 2 mg/kg than with docetaxel (median 5.0 months vs. 4.1 months, HR 0.59, 95% CI 0.44–0.78, $p = 0.0001$), and with pembrolizumab 10 mg/kg than with docetaxel (5.2 months vs. 4.1 months, 95%, HR 0.59, 95% CI 0.45–0.78, $p < 0.0001$). This trial confirmed the results of Keynote 001 and added additional data to the assumed predictive value of PD-L1 positivity [16, 28].

6.3. Atezolizumab

PD-L1 expression in trials with atezolizumab is reported somehow differently. First expression is reported in tumor cells (TC) and immune cells infiltrating tumor (IC) separately. Tumors are categorized into four different groups:

- TC3/IC3: at least 10% of cells expressing PD-L1.
- TC2/IC2: at least 5% of cells expressing PD-L1.
- TC1/IC1: at least 1% of cells expressing PD-L1.
- TC0/IC0: less than 1% of cells expressing PD-L1.

The association between the response to atezolizumab and PD-L1 expression was first assessed in a Phase I trial of Herbst *et al.* Two hundred and seventy-seven patients with advanced incurable cancer received MPDL-3280A (atezolizumab) intravenously every 3 weeks. Responses (complete and partial responses) were observed in 32 of 175 (18%) with all tumor types including NSCLC, melanoma, renal cell carcinoma, and other tumors (including colorectal cancer, gastric cancer, and head and neck squamous cell carcinoma). Authors found the association between response and the expression of PD-L1. The association of response to atezolizumab treatment and tumor-infiltrating immune cell PD-L1 expression was statistically significant ($p = 0.007$), while the association with tumor cell PD-L1 expression was not ($p = 0.920$) [29].

POPLAR was a Phase II trial comparing treatment with atezolizumab with docetaxel in patients progressing on previous chemotherapy treatments. One hundred forty-four patients between August 2013 and March 2014 randomly received either atezolizumab 1200 mg or docetaxel 75 mg/m^2 once every 3 weeks. Patients on atezolizumab had longer overall survival (12.6 vs. 9.7 months, HR = 0.73, $p = 0.04$), although no differences in response rate or progression-free survival were encountered. Higher PD-L1 expression in TC/IC was associated with improved overall survival (TC3/IC3 HR 0.49, 95% CI 0.22–1.07, $p = 0.068$; TC2/3 or IC2/3 HR 0.54, 95% CI 0.33–0.89. $p = 0.014$, TC1/2/3 or IC1/2/3 HR 0.59, 95%CI 0.40–0.85, $p = 0.005$; TC0 and IC0 HR 1.04. 95% CI 0.62–1.75, $p = 0.871$). Authors believe PD-L1 expression is predictive for atezolizumab's benefits [16, 30].

BIRCH trial was a Phase II trial in which patients with locally advanced or metastatic NSCLC were divided into three cohorts. All the patients received atezolizumab at the dose of 1200 mg every 3 weeks. Patients were included if they had TC2–3/IC 2-3 PD-L1 expression. One hundred thirty-nine patients in Cohort I received atezolizumab as first-line treatment, 267 patients in Cohort II as second, and 253 in Cohort III as third or more line of treatment. Higher PD-L1 expression was associated with higher response rate in all cohorts.

Name of the trial (phase)	Compound	PD-L1 expression and OS (HR compared to control arm or months)	PD-L1 expression and PFS (HR compared to control arm or months)	PD-L1 expression and RR (%)
Checkmate 017 (Phase 3)	Nivolumab versus docetaxel	<1% (0.58) ≥1% (0.69) <5% (0.70) ≥5% (0.53) <10% (0.70) ≥10% (0.50)	<1% (0.66) ≥1% (0.67) <5% (0.75) ≥5% (0.54) <10% (0.70) ≥10% (0.58)	<1% (17) ≥1% (17) <5% (15) ≥5% (21) <10% (16) ≥10% (19)
Checkmate 057 (Phase III)	Nivolumab versus docetaxel	<1% (0.90) ≥1% (0.59) <5% (1.01) ≥5% (0.43) <10% (1.00) ≥10% (0.40)	<1% (1.19) ≥1% (0.70) <5% (1.31) ≥5% (0.54) <10% (1.24) ≥10% (0.52)	<1% (9) ≥1% (31) <5% (10) ≥5% (36) <10% (11) ≥10% (37)
Keynote 001 (Phase I)	Pembrolizumab	<1% 10.4 months 1–49% 10.6 months ≥50% not repoted	<1% 4.0 months 1–49% 4.1 months ≥50% 6.4 months	<1% (10.7) 1–49% (16.5) ≥50% (45.2)
Keynote 010 (Phase III)	Pembrolizumab 2 mg/kg versus docetaxel	>1% (0.71) ≥50% (0.54)	>1% (0.88) ≥50% (0.59)	>1% (18) ≥50% (30)
Keynote 010 (Phase III)	Pembrolizumab 10 mg/kg versus docetaxel	>1% (0.61) ≥50% (0.50)	>1% (0.79) ≥50% (0.59)	>1% (18) ≥50% (29)
Atezolizumab (Phase I)	Atezolizumab	TC0–2/IC0–2 16 months TC3/IC3 18 months	TC0–2/IC0–2 4 months TC3/IC3 4 months	TC0–2/IC0–2 (16) TC3/IC3 (48)
POPLAR (Phase 2)	Atezolizumab versus docetaxel	TC0/IC (1.04) TC0–2/IC 0–2 (0.59) TC2–3/IC 2–3 (0.54) TC3/IC3 (0.49)	TC0/IC (1.12) TC0–2/IC 0–2 (0.85) TC2–3/IC 2–3 (0.72) TC3/IC3 (0.60)	TC0/IC (8) TC0–2/IC 0–2 (18) TC2–3/IC 2–3 (22) TC3/IC3 (38)
BIRCH (Phase II, Cohort I)	Atezolizumab	TC2–3/IC2–3 (82%)* TC3/IC3 (79%)*	TC2–3/IC2–3 5.5 months TC3/IC3 5.5 months	TC2–3/IC2–3 (19) TC3/IC3 (26)
BIRCH (Phase II, Cohort II)	Atezolizumab	TC2–3/IC2–3 (76%)* TC3/IC3 (80%)*	TC2–3/IC2–3 2.8 months TC3/IC3 4.1 months	TC2–3/IC2–3 (17) TC3/IC3 (24)
BIRCH (Phase II, Cohort III)	Atezolizumab	TC2–3/IC2–3 (71%)* TC3/IC3 (75%)*	TC2–3/IC2–3 2.8 months TC3/IC3 4.2 months	TC2–3/IC2–3 (17) TC3/IC3 (27)
Avelumab (Phase Ib)	Avelumab	>1% (4.6 months) ≤1% (8.9 months)	>1% (5.9 weeks) ≤1% (12.0 weeks)	>1% (10) ≤1% (15)
Durvalumab (Phase I/II)	Durvalumab	<25% not reported ≥25% not reported	<25% not reported ≥25% not reported	<25% (5) ≥25% (27)

*Six-month overall survival.

Table 1. Response to checkpoint inhibitors according to PD-L1 expression.

In Cohort I, ORR was 26% (95% CI 16–39) in patients with TC3/IC2 vs. 19% (95% CI 13–27) in patients with TC2–3/IC 2–3. In Cohort II, ORR was 24% (95% CI 17–32) in patients with TC3/IC2 vs. 17% (95% CI 13–22) in patients with TC2–3/IC 2–3. In Cohort III ORR was 27% (95% CI 19–36) in patients with TC3/IC2 vs. 17% (95% CI 13–23) in patients with TC2–3/IC 2–3. These results also suggest that PD-L1 is a possible biomarker for treatment with atezolizumab [31].

6.4. Avelumab and durvalumab

Patients received avelumab in a Phase Ib trial. The response rate, median progression-free survival, and median overall survival were 13.6%, 11.6 weeks and 8.4 months. PD-L1 cut-off for positivity was 1% of the expression and was associated with higher response rate, longer progression-free, and overall survival [16]. Response rate of 16% was achieved in Phase I/II trial of durvalumab treatment. PD-L1 positivity was defined as an expression of more than 25% of cells and was correlated with higher response rate [16].

Trials with checkpoint inhibitors are summarized in **Table 1**.

7. The problems of PD-L1 as a biomarker

The assessment of PD-L1 tumor expression is currently a controversial issue with more open questions than known facts. PD-L1 expression is a dynamic rather than static process that varies according to different tumor and host factors (15–30). Several data show that anti–PD-L1 drugs are more effective in patients whose tumors express PD-L1, but responses in the population of patients without the expression lead to the conclusion that these patients also benefit from this treatment. How to select right patients for anti–PD-L1 treatment remains an open question in these circumstances [5].

7.1. Tests

Currently, several different monoclonal antibodies for testing PD-L1 positivity exist. In a meta-analysis of Aguiar *et al.* among 13 included trials, 5 different antibodies were used (DAKO 28-8, DAKO 22C3, VENTANA SP 142, and two nonspecified), and 3 different threshold values for immunohistochemical positivity selected (1, 5, and 50%). Authors conclude that standardized approach to PD-L1 status assessment is lacking [1]. For the details of Aguiar's meta-analysis, please see the Section 5 of this chapter.

Today several differences exist between tests:

1. Every test uses it own antibody.
2. Some tests evaluate the percentage of tumor cells stained, while others evaluate not only tumor cells but also tumor infiltrating immune cells.
3. Cut-off points and scoring systems differ between tests.
4. Different staining techniques (manual vs. automated).

All these differences make the comparison between results of different tests difficult if not impossible [16, 23].

7.2. Positivity and response to treatment

The threshold of immunohistochemical PD-L1 expression positivity is not well established today. Thresholds of 1, 5, or 50% of positive cells are being used in different trials. It is estimated that any expression of PD-L1 can be found in 45–50% of NSCLC biopsies [18]. In a trial of Cha *et al.*, the threshold of 5% showed the most significant *p* value regarding overall survival predictions [19]. For details of Cha *et al.* trial, please see the Section 5 of this chapter. Even if considered positive (regardless of the positivity cut-off), not all patients respond to the treatment with immunotherapy. Response is seen only in 15–45% of "positive" patients and on the other end, many "negative" patients also respond [16].

7.3. Concordance

Checkpoint inhibitors recently demonstrated efficacy in the treatments of metastatic NSCLC that are being used more and more in clinical trials and everyday clinical practice. Despite their benefits, the association of responses with a predictive biomarker PD-L1 remains uncertain. Today, several PD-L1 IHC tests exist, and concordance between them is not very clear. Sheffield *et al.* compared multiple methods of testing. Tissue microarrays of matched primary and metastatic NSCLCs were used to compare four different PD-L1 IHC techniques. Tissues from 80 patients were included. Multiple IHC methodologies showed a high rate of agreement (Kappa = 0.67). Concordance between PD-L1 positivity among different tests (antibodies) was from 73.4 to 76%. Determination of which test is the best one is challenging due to the lack of a reference standard [32].

Significant discordance between the PD-L1 status of primary tumors and metastases was observed. PD-L1 status of primary and metastatic tumors was discordant in 17 (22%) cases. Because of the variability of the biomarker, also changes in positivity during immunotherapy treatment have been studied. Discordance between primary tumor and metastatic sites is supposed to be because of the intratumoral heterogeneity and sampling bias [32]. Variability seems to be even more substantial, since immunohistochemical status changes during treatment in 12–35% of the patients [16].

7.4. Tissue

Keynote 001 trial revealed another unanswered issue in the PD-L1 expression testing. Deterioration in the PD-L1 expression in archival tissue samples that had been sectioned 6 months or more before testing was encountered. Researches decided to evaluate only the samples taken in the 6-months period before testing. Of the 1143 screened patients, only 824 had eligible tumor samples. Why this deterioration in expression occurs, and how to treat patients with pembrolizumab that do not have tissue available for testing are another of the two questions to be solved [25].

7.5. Open questions

To be able to continue the story of the PD-L1 as a predictive biomarker, these open questions will have to be answered [33]:

1. Is a predictive biomarker in immunotherapy necessary?
2. Is localization of the biomarker important (expression of PD-L1 in tumor and/or tumor-infiltrating lymphocytes)?
3. What is/are the optimal detection test/tests?
4. Does PD-L1 expression change over time (after different treatments such as chemotherapy and irradiation) and space (primary tumor vs. metastases)?

8. Conclusion

Immune checkpoint inhibitors are new and very promising treatment options in patients with several solid malignancies including lung cancer. For an optimal selection of patients who benefit most, predictive biomarkers are needed. PD-L1 has been suggested as a potential biomarker, but due to many open questions, today, it is not considered the only reliable immunotherapy biomarker since responses can be encountered even in patients considered PD-L1 negative. A possible solution to this issue is finding new and maybe more reliable predictive biomarkers that will for sure evolve in the next years of immunotherapy treatment development.

Author details

Mirjana Rajer

Address all correspondence to: mrajer@onko-i.si

Institute of Oncology Ljubljana, Ljubljana, Slovenia

References

[1] Aguiar, P.N., Jr., et al., The role of PD-L1 expression as a predictive biomarker in advanced non-small-cell lung cancer: a network meta-analysis. Immunotherapy, 2016. **8**(4): pp. 479–488.

[2] Homet Moreno, B. and Ribas, A., Anti-programmed cell death protein-1/ligand-1 therapy in different cancers. Br J Cancer, 2015. **112**(9): pp. 1421–1427.

[3] McDermott, D.F. and Atkins, M.B., PD-1 as a potential target in cancer therapy. Cancer Med, 2013. **2**(5): pp. 662–673.

[4] Domagala-Kulawik, J., The role of the immune system in non-small cell lung carcinoma and potential for therapeutic intervention. Transl Lung Cancer Res, 2015. **4**(2): pp. 177–190.

[5] Aguiar, P.N., Jr., et al., A pooled analysis of nivolumab for the treatment of advanced non-small-cell lung cancer and the role of PD-L1 as a predictive biomarker. Immunotherapy, 2016. **8**(9): pp. 1011–1019.

[6] Janssen-Heijnen, M.L. and Coebergh, J.W., Trends in incidence and prognosis of the histological subtypes of lung cancer in North America, Australia, New Zealand and Europe. Lung Cancer, 2001. **31**(2–3): pp. 123–137.

[7] Janssen-Heijnen, M.L. and Coebergh, J.W., The changing epidemiology of lung cancer in Europe. Lung Cancer, 2003. **41**(3): pp. 245–258.

[8] Charloux, A., et al., The increasing incidence of lung adenocarcinoma: reality or artefact? A review of the epidemiology of lung adenocarcinoma. Int J Epidemiol, 1997. **26**(1): pp. 14–23.

[9] Burns, D.M., Changing rates of adenocarcinoma of the lung. Chem Res Toxicol, 2014. **27**(8): pp. 1330–1335.

[10] Santarpia, M., et al., Programmed cell death protein-1/programmed cell death ligand-1 pathway inhibition and predictive biomarkers: understanding transforming growth factor-beta role. Transl Lung Cancer Res, 2015. **4**(6): pp. 728–742.

[11] Zamarin, D. and Postow, M.A., Immune checkpoint modulation: rational design of combination strategies. Pharmacol Ther, 2015. **150**: pp. 23–32.

[12] Chakravarti, N. and Prieto, V.G., Predictive factors of activity of anti-programmed death-1/programmed death ligand-1 drugs: immunohistochemistry analysis. Transl Lung Cancer Res, 2015. **4**(6): pp. 743–751.

[13] Ballman, K.V., Biomarker: predictive or prognostic?. J Clin Oncol, 2015. **33**(33): pp. 3968–3971.

[14] Chan, J.Y., Choudhury, Y., and Tan, M.H., Predictive molecular biomarkers to guide clinical decision making in kidney cancer: current progress and future challenges. Expert Rev Mol Diagn, 2015. **15**(5): pp. 631–646.

[15] Burotto, M., et al., Biomarkers in early-stage non-small-cell lung cancer: current concepts and future directions. J Thorac Oncol, 2014. **9**(11): pp. 1609–1617.

[16] Shukuya, T. and Carbone, D.P., Predictive markers for the efficacy of Anti-PD-1/PD-L1 antibodies in lung cancer. J Thorac Oncol, 2016. **11**(7): pp. 976–988.

[17] Falconi, A., Lopes, G., and Parker, J.L., Biomarkers and receptor targeted therapies reduce clinical trial risk in non-small-cell lung cancer. J Thorac Oncol, 2014. **9**(2): pp. 163–169.

[18] D'Incecco, A., et al., PD-1 and PD-L1 expression in molecularly selected non-small-cell lung cancer patients. Br J Cancer, 2015. **112**(1): pp. 95–102.

[19] Cha, Y.J., et al., Clinicopathological and prognostic significance of programmed cell death ligand-1 expression in lung adenocarcinoma and its relationship with p53 status. Lung Cancer, 2016. **97**: pp. 73–80.

[20] Baxevanis, C.N., et al., Immune biomarkers: how well do they serve prognosis in human cancers?. Expert Rev Mol Diagn, 2015. **15**(1): pp. 49–59.

[21] Schmidt, L.H., et al., PD-1 and PD-L1 expression in NSCLC indicate a favorable prognosis in defined subgroups. PLoS One, 2015. **10**(8): p. e0136023.

[22] Cooper, W.A., et al., PD-L1 expression is a favorable prognostic factor in early stage non-small cell carcinoma. Lung Cancer, 2015. **89**(2): pp. 181–188.

[23] Chae, Y.K., et al., Biomarkers for PD-1/PD-L1 blockade therapy in non-small-cell lung cancer: is PD-L1 expression a good marker for patient selection?. Clin Lung Cancer, 2016. **17**(5): pp. 350–361.

[24] Grigg, C. and Rizvi, N.A., PD-L1 biomarker testing for non-small cell lung cancer: truth or fiction?. J Immunother Cancer, 2016. **4**: p. 48.

[25] Garon, E.B., et al., Pembrolizumab for the treatment of non-small-cell lung cancer. N Engl J Med, 2015. **372**(21): pp. 2018–2028.

[26] Brahmer, J., et al., Nivolumab versus docetaxel in advanced squamous-cell non-small-cell lung cancer. N Engl J Med, 2015. **373**(2): pp. 123–135.

[27] Borghaei, H., et al., Nivolumab versus docetaxel in advanced nonsquamous non-small-cell lung cancer. N Engl J Med, 2015. **373**(17): pp. 1627–1639.

[28] Herbst, R.S., et al., Pembrolizumab versus docetaxel for previously treated, PD-L1-positive, advanced non-small-cell lung cancer (KEYNOTE-010): a randomised controlled trial. Lancet, 2016. **387**(10027): pp. 1540–1550.

[29] Herbst, R.S., et al., Predictive correlates of response to the anti-PD-L1 antibody MPDL3280A in cancer patients. Nature, 2014. **515**(7528): pp. 563–567.

[30] Fehrenbacher, L., et al., Atezolizumab versus docetaxel for patients with previously treated non-small-cell lung cancer (POPLAR): a multicentre, open-label, phase 2 randomised controlled trial. Lancet, 2016. **387**(10030): pp. 1837–1846.

[31] Besse, B., et al., 16LBA phase II, single-arm trial (BIRCH) of atezolizumab as first-line or subsequent therapy for locally advanced or metastatic PD-L1-selected non-small cell lung cancer (NSCLC). Eur J Cancer, 2015. **51**: pp. S717–S718.

[32] Sheffield, B.S., et al., Investigation of PD-L1 biomarker testing methods for PD-1 axis inhibition in non-squamous non-small cell lung cancer. J Histochem Cytochem, 2016. **64**(10): 587–600.

[33] Sundar, R., et al., Immunotherapy in the treatment of non-small cell lung cancer. Lung Cancer, 2014. **85**(2): pp. 101–109.

Chapter 8

Checkpoint Inhibitors in Nonsmall Cell Lung Cancer

Karen G. Zeman, Joseph E. Zeman,
Christina E. Brzezniak and Corey A. Carter

Additional information is available at the end of the chapter

http://dx.doi.org/10.5772/64611

Abstract

Lung cancer remains the leading cause of cancer-related deaths worldwide. The majority of NSCLC patients present with advanced stage disease. Lung cancer was once thought of as a low antigenicity cancer unlikely to benefit from immunotherapy, but has recently been found to have a high level of antigenicity. Moreover, a large body of research now exists to support both the safety and efficacy of immunotherapy in advanced stage NSCLC. The checkpoint inhibitors nivolumab, pembrolizumab, and atezolizumab are now approved by the U.S. Federal Drug Administration for second-line treatment in advanced stage NSCLC. In addition to being efficacious, checkpoint inhibitors have a superior safety profile compared to previous standard of care, chemotherapy. Further trials are needed to investigate the checkpoint inhibitors' role in combination treatment, first-line treatment, and early stage disease.

Keywords: PD-1, PD-L1, checkpoint inhibitors, NSCLC, nivolumab, pembrolizumab, atezolizumab, mutational load, PD-L1 expression, immunotherapy

1. Introduction

Lung cancer is the second most common cancer in both men and women; approximately 14% of all new cancers diagnosed are lung cancer. Lung cancer is the leading cause of cancer death among both men and women; one in four cancer deaths in the Unites States is due to lung cancer and worldwide it accounts for 1.59 million deaths annually [1, 2]. The survival rates for nonsmall cell lung cancer (NSCLC) remain low with 49% of Stage IA patients, 14% of Stage IIIA, and 1% of Stage IV patients alive at 5 years. The majority of NSCLC patients present with advanced stage disease [3]. Despite years of research in treatment strategies for NSCLC, few significant improvements on outcomes with available cytotoxic chemotherapy have been made. In addition, a large portion of patients with advanced disease are not treated with aggressive cytotoxic therapy due to performance status or other comorbidities [4]. Major inroads have been made for patients with targetable driver mutations who make up a minority of NSCLC patients but for the vast majority of patients further innovative treatments are needed. In the last half decade, there has been an explosion of evidence demonstrating lung cancer's antigenicity and clinical response to immune therapy.

2. Lung cancer and the immune system

One of the primary functions of our immune system is the ability to detect and destroy abnormal cells, which includes malignant cells. In lymphoid tissue, T cells are activated by the antigen presenting cells (APCs) carrying antigen from the tumor. T cells are then activated by the APCs and migrate to the peripheral tissues where they search and destroy antigen-expressing tumor cells. The human immune system maintains regulatory mechanisms to prevent autoimmunity or more specifically the immune system from attacking self.

In lymphatic tissue, expression of cytotoxic T-lymphocyte-associated antigen 4 (CTLA-4) negatively regulates the early stages of T-cell activation by competing with the T-cell costimulatory receptor CD28 for binding with CD80 and CD86 expressed on the APC (**Figure 1**) [3, 5]. Antibody blockade of CTLA-4 has been shown to increase antitumor immunity in clinical settings, and this has been well described in the melanoma therapy [6, 7].

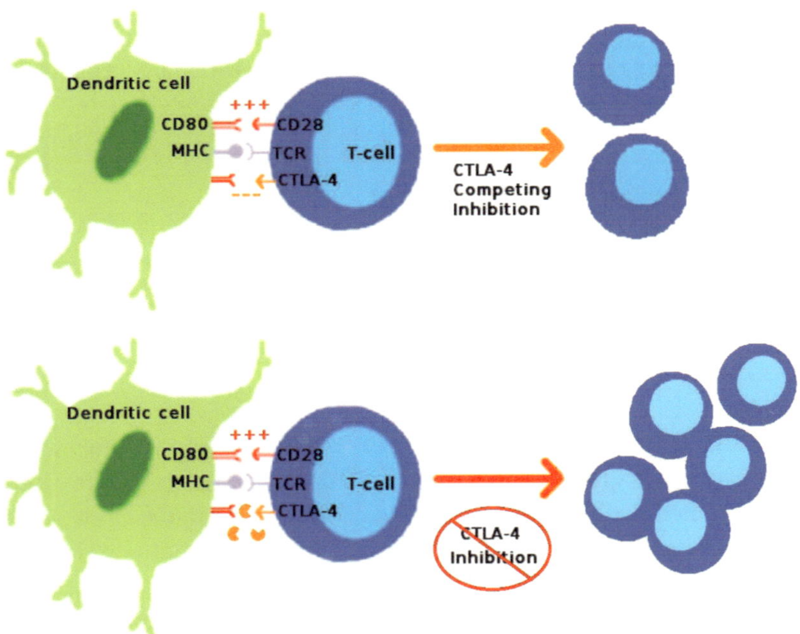

Figure 1. Immune system activation and inhibition in the lymphoid tissue. MHC, major histocompatibility complex; CTLA-4, cytotoxic T-lymphocyte-associated antigen 4; TCR, T-cell receptor.

In the peripheral tissues, the adaptive immune system is negatively regulated in part through binding of the programmed cell death protein 1 (PD-1) expressed on activated T cells with the

http://dx.doi.org/10.5772/64611

programmed death ligand 1 (PD-L1) and/or programmed death ligand 2 (PD-L2). Tumor cells can evade the immune response through upregulation of expression of PD-L1, resulting in decreased T-cell response and immune resistance (**Figure 2**). PD-1 and PD-L1 inhibitors can take the breaks off the T-cell activity in peripheral tissues by blocking PD-1 binding to PD-L1.

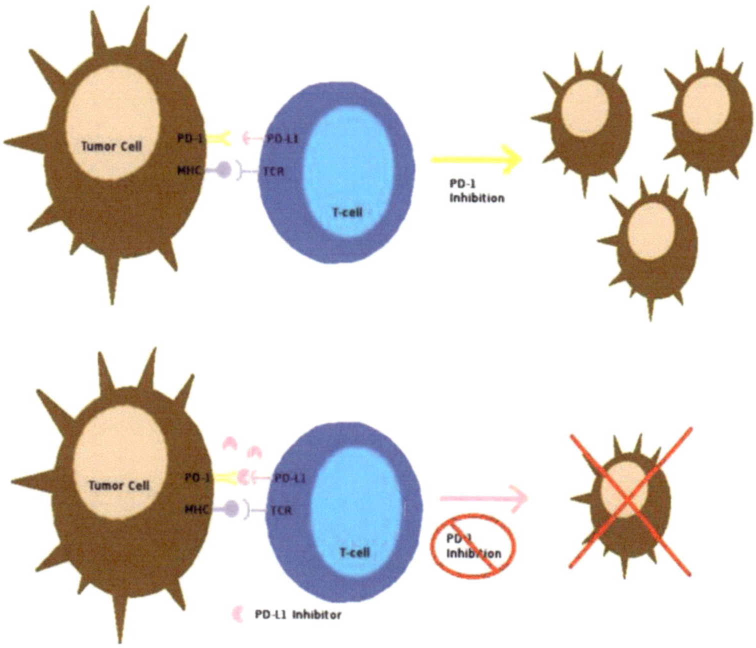

Figure 2. Immune system activation and inhibition in the peripheral tissue. MHC, major histocompatibility complex; TCR, T-cell receptor; PD-1, programmed cell death protein 1; PD-L1, programmed death ligand.

It has been a previously accepted belief that lung tumors have a very low antigenicity and approaching lung cancer with immunotherapy would have little hope of causing any significant benefit. However, through thoughtful translational research, immunotherapy is now being seen as promising therapeutic agents with a significant potential to affect NSCLC. Smokers' tumors are now understood to have some of the most complex and extensive genetic mutations seen in solid malignancies, and consequentially they have some of the highest antigenicity [8, 9].

In 2015, the benefits of checkpoint inhibition in the treatment of NSCLC went from theoretical to breaking news with new agents such as pembrolizumab, nivolumab, and atezolizumab receiving breakthrough drug designation and later approval by the U.S. Federal Drug Administration (FDA) for treatment of advanced stage NSCLC in the second-line setting after progression on or after platinum containing chemotherapy [10–12]. In the case of pembrolizumab, treatment was indicated only for patients with tumors expressing PD-L1 greater than 50% by the Dako assay. Nivolumab was approved without the need for PD-L1 testing. Here is a review of the key trials that brought immunotherapy into standard of care treatment for NSCLC. Summarization of key clinical trials in checkpoint inhibition is presented in **Table 1**.

Clinical trial	Phase trial	Line of treatment	Histology	Patients	Treatment regimen	OS (months)	PFS (months)	Median DOR (months)
CheckMate 063	2	Third	Squamous	117	Nivolumab 3 mg/kg every 2 weeks	8.2	1.9	NR
CheckMate 017	3	Second line	Squamous	272	Nivolumab 3 mg/kg every 2 weeks Docetaxel 75 mg/m^2 every 3 weeks	9.2 6.0	3.5 2.8	NR 8.4
CheckMate 057	3	Second line	Nonsquamous	582	Nivolumab 3 mg/kg every 2 weeks Docetaxel 75 mg/m^2 every 3 weeks	12.2 9.4	2.3 4.2	17.6 5.6
Keynote-001	1	First to fifth	All histologies	495	Pembrolizumab efficacy reported for all doses	12.0	3.7	12.5
Keynote-010	2/3	Second line	All histologies	1034	Pembrolizumab 2 mg/kg every 3 weeks Pembrolizumab 10 mg/kg every 3 weeks Docetaxel 75 mg/m2 every 3 weeks	10.4 12.7 8.5	5.0 5.2 4.1	NR NR 6.0
CheckMate 012 Gettinger et al.	1	First line	All histologies	52	Nivolumab 3 mg/kg every 2 weeks	19.4	3.6	NR
CheckMate 012 Rizvi et al.	1	First line	All histologies	56	Nivolumab 10 mg/kg + gemcitabine-cisplatin (squamous) Nivolumab 10 mg/kg + pemetrexed-cisplatin (nonsquamous) Nivolumab 5 mg/kg +paclitaxel-carboplatin (all histologies) Nivolumab 10 mg/kg + paclitaxel-carboplatin (all histologies)	11.6 19.2 NR 14.9	5.7 6.8 7.1 4.8	10.3 5.8 19.6 5.5

http://dx.doi.org/10.5772/64611

Clinical trial	Phase trial	Line of treatment	Histology	Patients	Treatment regimen	OS (months)	PFS (months)	Median DOR (months)
CheckMate 012 Hellman et al.	1	First line	All histologies	148	Nivolumab 3 mg/kg every 2 weeks + Ipilimumab 1 mg/kg every 12 weeks Nivolumab 3 mg/kg every 2 weeks + Ipilimumab 1 mg/kg every 6 weeks Nivolumab 3 mg/kg every 2 weeks	n/a	8.1 3.9 3.6	NR NR NR
POPLAR	2	Second line	All histologies	287	Atezolizumab 1200 mg every 3 weeks Docetaxel 75 mg/m2 every 3 weeks	12.6 9.7	2.7 3	NR 7.8

OS, overall survival; PFS, progression-free survival; DOR, duration of response; NR, not reached; n/a, not available.

Table 1. Summary of key checkpoint inhibitor trials efficacy data.

3. Key trials in checkpoint inhibition therapy of NSCLC

3.1. Checkpoint inhibitor trials: pembrolizumab second line and beyond

3.1.1. Keynote-001

Keynote-001 was a phase I study assessing safety and efficacy of treatment with pembrolizumab of advanced NSCLC [13]. The primary objectives were to investigate safety, side effect profile, and efficacy of pembrolizumab. Treatment-related adverse events were 70.9% and grade 3 or higher severe adverse events were 9.5%. With regards to efficacy, overall response rate was 19.4%: 18% in previously treated patients and 24.8% in treatment naïve patients. There was no significant difference noted between treatment dose and dose interval. Current smokers had an increased response rate at 22.3% and never smokers had a 10.3% response rate. Median duration of response was 12.5 months and median progression-free survival was 3.7 months with an overall median survival of 12 months. Additionally, the study sought to evaluate PD-L1 as a biomarker and evaluated tissue obtained within 6 months of treatment for PD-L1 expression. They concluded that a percentage of 50% PD-L1 tumor cell expression was associated with a higher response rate and longer progression-free survival (PFS) and overall survival (OS).

Keynote-001 was a phase I study that established safety and efficacy of pembrolizumab in heavily treated patients with NSCLC. Furthermore, it used the DAKO PD-L1 expression assay with 22C3 antibody clone for patient selection to solidify this as the chosen PD-L1 assay [13].

3.1.2. Keynote-010

Keynote-010 was a randomized phase II/III study assessing pembrolizumab versus docetaxel in PD-L1 positive advanced NSCLC [14]. Eligible patients had advanced NSCLC that had progressed despite two or more cycles of platinum doublet chemotherapy or appropriate tyrosine kinase inhibitor (TKI) therapy, a fresh tumor sample showing PD-L1 expression of at least 1% was required. The primary endpoints were overall survival and progression-free survival both in the total population and in patients with PD-L1 expression ≥50%. Secondary endpoints were safety/toxicity, response rate, and duration of response.

In patients with a PD-L1 tumor proportion score of 50% or greater, median overall survival was 14.9 months for pembrolizumab 2 mg/kg, 17.3 months for pembrolizumab 10 mg/kg, and 8.2 months for the docetaxel group. In the total population, median overall survival was 10.4 months for pembrolizumab 2 mg/kg, 12.7 months for pembrolizumab 10 mg/kg, and 8.5 months for the docetaxel group. Pembrolizumab demonstrated improvement in progression-free survival in patients with tumor proportion score of ≥50% but progression-free survival was not significantly different in the total population. Neither pembrolizumab dosage reached the median duration of response for patients with tumor proportion score of ≥50% or all patients. The docetaxel group duration of response was 8 months in the tumor proportion score of ≥50% or all patients and 6 months in all patients.

With regards to toxicity, treatment-related adverse events were 13% for pembrolizumab 2 mg/kg, 16% for pembrolizumab 10 mg/kg, and 35% for docetaxel. Severe adverse events, grade 3 or higher, were reported as 63% for pembrolizumab 2 mg/kg, 66% for pembrolizumab 10 mg/kg, and 81% for docetaxel.

Based on these two landmark clinical trials, pembrolizumab was approved by the FDA for metastatic NSCLC in patients with PD-L1 expressing tumors who have progression on platinum doublet chemotherapy and tyrosine kinase inhibitor therapy for EGFR or ALK mutant tumors [12–14].

3.2. Checkpoint inhibitor trials: nivolumab second line and beyond

3.2.1. CheckMate 017

Previous phase I and II studies, CheckMate 003 and CheckMate 063, respectively, demonstrated both safety and efficacy of nivolumab in heavily pretreated NSCLC patients. CheckMate 003 defined treatment dose at 3 mg/kg every 2 weeks. CheckMate 063 demonstrated efficacy endpoints of OS of 8.2 months and overall response rate (ORR) of 14.5% with an adverse event rate of 74% with 17% grade 3–4 [15, 16].

Checkmate 017 was a phase 3, randomized, study investigating nivolumab as compared to docetaxel in the second-line setting for treatment of advanced squamous cell NSCLC in 272 patients [17]. Eligible patients had advanced squamous cell NSCLC and progression after one prior platinum containing regimen, prior treatment with EGFR TKI therapy was allowed. The primary endpoint was overall survival. Secondary endpoints were ORR, PFS, patient-reported outcomes, efficacy by PD-L1 expression, and safety.

The median overall survival was 9.2 months in the nivolumab group, which is significantly higher compared to 6 months in the docetaxel treatment group. The ORR was 20% with nivolumab and 9% with docetaxel. The median duration of response was not reached in the nivolumab treatment group (2.9–20.5+ months) compared to the docetaxel treatment group 8.4 months (1.4–15.2). The median PFS for nivolumab and docetaxel treatment groups was 3.5 and 2.8 months, respectively. PD-L1 expression in this study was neither predictive nor prognostic of any efficacy endpoints.

With regards to toxicity, treatment-related adverse events were less frequent in the nivolumab treatment group. The nivolumab and docetaxel treatment groups demonstrated 58% and 86% of patients with any adverse event (AE), respectively. Furthermore, only 7% of the nivolumab treatment group demonstrated grade 3 or 4 events and no grade 5 events. Docetaxel had a 55% grade 3 or 4 event rate and 2% of patients had events of grade 5. Docetaxel demonstrated higher rates of treatment-related serious adverse events mainly attributable to hematologic toxic events and infections.

This study demonstrated improved overall survival and safety profile with nivolumab treatment over standard of care second-line therapy in squamous-cell NSCLC. Additionally, PD-L1 expression was not found to be predictive or prognostic of any efficacy endpoints.

3.2.2. CheckMate 057

Checkmate 057 expanded on the results of checkmate 017 and evaluated nivolumab versus docetaxel in advanced nonsquamous NSCLC. This study was a randomized phase 3 trial specifically looking at nivolumab versus docetaxel in the second-line setting for nonsquamous histology NSCLC [18]. A total of 582 patients with advanced nonsquamous cell NSCLC, progression after one prior platinum containing regimen, prior treatment with EGFR TKI therapy were enrolled. Patients were treated until disease progression or discontinuation of treatment due to toxic side effects or other reasons. The primary endpoint was overall survival. Secondary endpoints included safety, confirmed objective response, PFS, patient-reported outcomes, and efficacy by PD-L1 expression.

With regards to efficacy, the median overall survival was 12.2 months in the nivolumab group and was significantly higher compared to 9.4 months in the docetaxel treatment group. The ORR was 19% with nivolumab and 12% with docetaxel. The median duration of response in the nivolumab treatment group was 17.2 months compared to the docetaxel treatment group 5.6 months. The median PFS was for nivolumab and docetaxel treatment groups were 2.3 and 4.2 months, respectively.

Treatment-related adverse events were less frequent in the nivolumab treatment group. The nivolumab and docetaxel treatment groups demonstrated 69% and 88% of patients with any AE. Furthermore, only 10% of the nivolumab treatment group demonstrated grade 3 or 4 events compared to docetaxel, which had a 54% grade 3 or 4 event rate. Docetaxel demonstrated higher rates of treatment-related serious adverse events as seen in prior study.

PD-L1 expression demonstrated a strong predictive association between increased PD-L1 expression and clinical outcomes. Improved clinical outcomes was noted in this study but the magnitude of improvement across all efficacy endpoints was greater with tumors expressing PD-L1 compared to those who did not. Patients whose tumors expressed PD-L1 demonstrated a nearly doubled median overall survival compared to docetaxel. Patients whose tumors did not demonstrate PD-L1 expression, defined as <1%, demonstrated similar overall survival. This finding differed compared to Checkmate 017 where PD-L1 expression was not predictive or prognostic for all comers.

This study demonstrated improved overall survival and safety profile with nivolumab treatment over standard of care second-line therapy in nonsquamous cell NSCLC. It also found no significant difference in overall survival in patients whose tumors did not express PD-L1 although safety profile and durability of response remain compelling arguments of the use of checkpoint inhibitors over chemotherapy.

These two studies resulted in the FDA approving nivolumab for the treatment of NSCLC in both squamous and nonsquamous after progression on a platinum containing doublet and TKI if applicable [11]. Nivolumab's approval and indication are not contingent on PD-L1 expression. This difference has greatly impacted medical oncology's use of both drugs as pembrolizumab requires the tissue be assessed for PD-L1 expression with varying costs and the availability of testing available in addition to the wait time for testing results, whereas nivolumab is approved regardless of expression level.

3.3. Checkpoint inhibitor clinical trials of nivolumab first line

3.3.1. CheckMate 012: nivolumab as monotherapy in first-line advanced NSCLC

The purpose of Checkmate 012 was to determine if in a phase I, multicohort study, there was clinical benefit of nivolumab as monotherapy or combined with current standard therapies in first-line advanced NSCLC [19]. Eligibility criteria for this study was Stage IIIB or IV NSCLC of any histology who had no prior chemotherapy for advanced disease. Prior adjuvant or neoadjuvant chemotherapy was allowed. Additionally, prior radiotherapy or TKI therapy was permitted if completed at least 2 weeks before treatment on study. Patients were treated with nivolumab until disease progression, discontinuation due to toxicity, withdrawal of consent, or loss to follow up. The primary objective of this study was to investigate safety and tolerability of nivolumab monotherapy. Secondary study objectives were ORR and PFS with OS included as an exploratory efficacy endpoint.

The study found an ORR of 23% with four patients with ongoing complete responses. Stable disease was seen in 27% of patients with a median DOR was not reached, range 4.2–25.8 months+, and 75% was achieved by the first tumor assessment at week 11. Median OS was 19.4 months, 16.8 months for squamous and not reached for nonsquamous histology. Median PFS was 3.6 months. The primary endpoint was to assess safety and tolerability, and the study demonstrated a 71% AE rate and 19% of grade 3 and 4 with treatment-related adverse events led to discontinuation in 12% of patients.

Additionally, Checkmate 012 investigated several variables for correlation with clinical response to include PD-L1 expression, KRAS, and EGFR mutation status. Tumors specimens were evaluable in 88% of the patients for PD-L1 expression, finding 70% of patients had ≥1% and 30% <1%. Clinical activity was observed regardless of PD-L1 expression across all expression levels although higher response rates correlated with higher expression levels. Confirmed ORR was 28 and 14% in tumors with ≥1% or <1%. This study did not demonstrate a relationship between PFS and OS and baseline PD-L1 expression. ORRs and disease control rates were higher among patients with a history of smoking. Additionally, median PFS was longer in current smokers compared to former smokers although the study was not powered to assess this. Median PFS was lower for patients with EGFR-mutant tumors vs. EGFR-wild-type. In contrast, median PFS was longer in KRAS mutant tumors compared to wild-type.

This study demonstrated good tolerance compared to standard first-line therapy in addition to demonstrating promising DOR and survival. It is important to note that this trial was not randomized, had a selected patient population with good performance status, and no standard of care comparison arm. Of note, four patients had durable complete clinical responses which are unlikely in chemotherapy treatment of NSCLC. Two phase III clinical trials will further assist answering the question is nivolumab monotherapy superior to current standard of care or is indicated first line in a select patient population? CheckMate 026, NCT02041533, is investigating nivolumab in the first-line setting compared to standard of care therapy, platinum doublet chemotherapy, in advanced NSCLC patients with PD-L1 expressing tumors [20]. CheckMate 227, NCT02477826, is a multiarm study comparing nivolumab vs. nivolumab+ipilimumab vs. standard of care therapy platinum doublet chemotherapy ± nivolumab [21].

Checkmate 012 established safety and efficacy of nivolumab monotherapy in the first-line setting of NSCLC. There are ongoing clinical trials comparing nivolumab to standard of care and in combination.

3.3.2. CheckMate 012: nivolumab in combination with platinum-based doublet

Another cohort of Checkpoint 012 was released studying nivolumab in combination with platinum-based doublet chemotherapy for first-line treatment of advanced NSCLC. Patients were assigned by histology to receive nivolumab 10 mg/kg plus gemcitabine-cisplatin (squamous) or pemetrexed-cisplatin (nonsquamous) or nivolumab 5 or 10 mg/k plus paclitaxel-carboplatin (all histologies) followed by nivolumab monotherapy [22]. In this study, nivolumab was administered every 3 weeks to coincide with chemotherapy administration. Eligibility criteria included patients with newly diagnosed advanced NSCLC with no prior treatment. The primary objective of this study was to assess safety and tolerability of immunotherapy and platinum doublet chemotherapy. Secondary objective was antitumor activity measured by PFS and ORR. A total of 56 patients were enrolled in this study.

For patients treated with 10 mg/kg nivolumab plus platinum based chemotherapy adverse events of any grade occurred at 93% and grade 3 or 4 occurred in 50%. In the overall population, 95% of patients experienced any grade adverse event and 45% of patients experienced graded 3 or 4 treatment-related events. Median PFS time ranging from 4.8 to 7.1 months and median OS in the 10 mg/kg nivolumab plus platinum-based chemotherapy ranged from 11.6 to 19.2 but was not reached in the nivolumab 5 mg/kg plus paclitaxel/carboplatin arm. PD-L1 expression was able to be quantified for 79% of patients in the study, no association was found between PD-L1 expression and PFS or OS. No difference in ORR or PFS was noted between histologies although median DOR was longer in the squamous histology subset. Median OS was longer with nonsquamous versus squamous NSCLC.

Treatment-related adverse events resulted in 21% of patients discontinuing the clinical trial. No treatment related deaths were reported in this study.

Based on these results, it is not clear if there is an OS benefit to combination therapy of nivolumab plus platinum-based chemotherapy. There was an increase in adverse events although no patient-related deaths were reported with combination therapy.

3.3.3. CheckMate 012: safety and efficacy of first-line nivolumab and ipilimumab in advanced NSCLC

CheckMate 012 recently presented an abstract at ASCO 2016 on another cohort-investigating nivolumab and ipilimumab in advanced NSCLC in their phase I clinical trial [23]. This study extrapolated from efficacy in nivolumab and ipilimumab combination therapy in melanoma and monotherapy efficacy and safety in NSCLC. The trial enrolled 148 patients with all NSCLC histologies and distributed patients between four cohorts varying in nivolumab and ipilimumab drug dosing. Primary endpoints investigated were safety and secondary endpoints were ORR and PFS. Exploratory endpoints included overall survival and efficacy by tumor PD-L1 expression. The primary endpoint demonstrated adverse events in 69–77% of patients across cohorts and 28–35% grade 3–4 toxicities. Treatment-related adverse events resulting in discontinuation of therapy was reported at 10% similar to nivolumab monotherapy trials. Efficacy endpoints, ORR, and PFS were improved at the higher dosing of nivolumab 3 mg/kg compared to 1 mg/kg. Recommended dosing for further testing is nivolumab 3 mg/kg q2 weeks and ipilimumab 1 mg/kg q6 weeks. PD-L1 expression corresponded with higher efficacy response rates.

This data helped to establish safety of dual complimentary checkpoint inhibition although final publication is pending. CheckMate 227 trial, NCT02477826, will further evaluate dual checkpoint inhibition with nivolumab 3 mg/kg and ipilimumab 1 mg/kg compared to standard of care therapy [21].

3.4. Checkpoint inhibitor clinical trials of pembrolizumab first line

3.4.1. KEYNOTE 024

KEYNOTE 024 was an open-lab phase 3 randomized controlled trial investigating pembrolizumab versus platinum-based doublet chemotherapy in first-line setting. Inclusion criteria included patients with stage IV NSCLC, no sensitizing EGFR mutations or ALK translocations, no previous chemotherapy for metastatic disease, and PD-L1 expression of 50% of greater. The patients were assigned either pembrolizumab 200 mg every 3 weeks for 35 cycles or the investigators choice of one of five platinum-based chemotherapy regimens for 4–6 cycles. The primary endpoint was progression-free survival. Secondary endpoints include overall survival, objective response rate, and safety. A total of 305 patients were enrolled in this study [24].

The estimated percentage of patients alive at 6 months was 80.2% in the pembrolizumab group and 72.4% in the chemotherapy group. The ORR was 44.8% with pembrolizumab and 27.8% in the chemotherapy group. The median duration of response was not reached in the pembrolizumab treatment group (1.9 to 14.5+ months) compared to the chemotherapy treatment group of 6.3 months (2.1–12.6). The median PFS for pembrolizumab and docetaxel treatment groups was 10.3 and 6.0 months, respectively.

The pembrolizumab and chemotherapy treatment groups demonstrated 73.4% and 90% of patients with any adverse event (AE), respectively. The pembrolizumab treatment group demonstrated 26.6% of patients with grade 3 or 4 events and no grade 5 events. The chemotherapy arm had twice the incidence of grade 3, 4, or 5 events at 53.3%.

This trial was a landmark for demonstrating superiority of checkpoint inhibition therapy with pembrolizumab over that of standard of care platinum-based chemotherapy. An important feature is that this population was selected for patients with at least 50% PD-L1 expression. Also of recurring significance, checkpoint inhibition therapy was better tolerated with less overall adverse events and significantly decreased severe adverse events.

3.5. Checkpoint inhibitor clinical trials with PD-L1 inhibitors

3.5.1. POPLAR study

POPLAR was an open label phase 2 randomized controlled trial investigation of atezolizumab vs. docetaxel in 287 patients with advanced NSCLC with progression on platinum-based therapies [25]. Atezolizumab is currently the only approved anti-PD-L1 inhibitor approved by the U.S. FDA for the second-line treatment of bladder cancer. It is not approved for the treatment of lung cancer. The primary endpoint for the POPLAR trial was overall survival and secondary endpoints were ORR, PFS, and DOR. Of note, in addition to testing PD-L1 expression on tumor cells it also investigated PD-L1 expression on tumor-infiltrating lymphocytes.

Atezolizumab demonstrated a trend toward improvement in overall survival of 12.6 months compared to the 9.7 months with docetaxel. PFS was similar between groups, 2.7 months with atezolizumab vs. 3.0 months with docetaxel. Median DOR for atezolizumab and docetaxel respectively was 14.3 months compared with 7.2 months. The survival benefit with atezolizumab correlated with increasing PD-L1 expression on tumor cells and tumor infiltrating cells. Survival in patients with minimal PD-L1 expression was similar to that of the docetaxel treatment group.

Treatment-related adverse events were less frequent in the atezolizumab treatment group. The atezolizumab and docetaxel treatment groups demonstrated 67% and 88% of patients with any AE. Atezolizumab treatment group demonstrated a 40% grade 3 or 4 events rate and docetaxel had a 53% grade 3 or 4 event rate. Docetaxel demonstrated higher rates of treatment-related serious adverse events as previously demonstrated in PD-1 checkpoint inhibitor second-line trials.

POPLAR was the first study of a PD-L1 checkpoint inhibitor in a randomized clinical trial of patients with previously treated NSCLC. Atezolizumab showed a superior overall survival compared with docetaxel in patients with advanced NSCLC similar to those findings in CheckMate 017 and 057. A trend toward increased efficacy was appreciated with increased PD-L1 tumor expression. Patients with the lowest PD-L1 expression group demonstrated similar overall survival to the docetaxel treatment group.

At the European Society for Medical Oncology Conference held on October 2016, the OAK, NCT02008227, phase 3 randomized clinical trial comparing atezolizumab to docetaxel in locally advanced disease or metastatic NSCLC who have failed platinum therapy was presented. OAK demonstrated increased overall survival with atezolizumab, 13.8 months, vs. docetaxel, 9.6 months [26]. On October 18, 2016, the FDA approved atezolizumab for the treatment of patients with metastatic NSCLC in the second-line setting based on the findings of the POPLAR and OAK clinical trials [10].

http://dx.doi.org/10.5772/64611

4. Adverse events in checkpoint inhibition

Checkpoint inhibitors confer a unique toxicity profile compared to chemotherapy as a result of activation of the patient's immune system. Immune-related adverse events (irAEs) are a direct result of immune system's stimulation resulting in both activation against tumor and against self. irAEs include but are not limited to colitis, pneumonitis, hepatitis, dermatitis, neuropathies, nephritis, and endocrinopathies [4, 27]. Of note, these irAEs were first appreciated with a different checkpoint inhibitor, ipilimumab, designed to affect CTLA-4. Additionally, irAEs from anti-PD-1 and anti-PD-L1 treatment occur at a lower rate than from anti-CTLA-4 [28].

Ipilimumab's side effect profile is well studied in the treatment of melanoma. Gastrointestinal and dermatologic immune-mediated toxicities were the most common. Moreover, they frequently appear in predictable time courses with dermatologic toxicities typically appearing in the first 2 weeks of therapy and gastrointestinal manifestations emerging after week 6 of therapy. Endocrinopathies are typically seen after longer duration of therapy although it is important to note that toxicities can occur at any time and even after cessation of therapy [29].

Anti-PD-1 and anti-PD-L1 treatment as mentioned above has a superior side effect profile compared to CTLA-4 inhibitions. The most common irAEs are rash, diarrhea, and colitis. These typically present at grade 1 or 2 and do not require discontinuation of therapy. Endocrinopathies include hypothyroidism as the most common, thyroiditis, hyperthyroidism, hypophysitis, and adrenal insufficiency [4, 13, 16]. Pneumonitis is a rare irAE but can be life threatening and occurs more often in lung cancer patients [3, 28].

PD-L1 inhibition was previously theorized to result in fewer irAEs as a result of targeting the tumor cell ligand and sparing PD-L2 which is more prevalent in healthy tissue, notably lung cells. Unfortunately, the POPLAR study did not demonstrate reduced irAE with PD-L1 inhibition compared to other trials that reported adverse event rates of PD-1 inhibitors [25].

The first and foremost purpose of checkpoint inhibitors is to determine efficacy either in monotherapy or in a combination regimen. One common thread in the clinical trials reviewed and markedly apparent in clinical trials comparing checkpoint inhibitors to docetaxel is that in subpopulations with the lowest rate of response to checkpoint inhibitors treatment efficacy is similar but adverse events are reduced compared to chemotherapy as well as grade 3 or 4 severe adverse events (**Table 2**) [18]. Therefore, if in the case of CheckMate 017, CheckMate 057, and POPLAR, we review the results for patients with minimal PD-L1 expression, EGFR mutants, and never smokers and observe similar efficacy but reduced adverse events. This argues in favor of checkpoint inhibition therapy secondary to its improved safety profile [17, 18, 25].

Treatment of grade 3 or 4 irAE typically requires discontinuation of therapy and systemic immunosuppression with high dose corticosteroids as the first-line therapy. Immune modulators such as infliximab can be used for patients that are steroid refractory. Grade 1 and 2 toxicities can be managed with supportive care alone and may not require discontinuation of checkpoint inhibition [30].

Clinical trial	Line of treatment	Treatment	All adverse events (AE) %	Grade 3 or 4 AE %
CheckMate 017	3	Nivolumab 3 mg/kg every 2 weeks Docetaxel 75 mg/m2 every 3 weeks	58 86	7 55
CheckMate 057	3	Nivolumab 3 mg/kg every 2 weeks Docetaxel 75 mg/m2 every 3 weeks	69 88	10 54
Keynote-010	2/3	Pembrolizumab 2 mg/kg every 3 weeks Pembrolizumab 10 mg/kg every 3 weeks Docetaxel 75 mg/m2 every 3 weeks	63 66 81	13* 16* 35*
POPLAR	2	Atezolizumab 1200 mg every 3 weeks Docetaxel 75 mg/m2 every 3 weeks	67 88	40 53

AE, adverse events.

*Annotates data including grade 3, 4, and 5.

Table 2. Summary of adverse events in trials for checkpoint therapy in second line setting compared to docetaxel therapy.

5. PD-L1 expression

PD-L1 expression has been looked at extensively to identify patients who will confer benefit from checkpoint inhibitor therapy. Most studies to date have demonstrated increased PD-L1 expression as a positive prognostic indicator of response but there is substantial debate in its appropriateness for patient selection for therapy. In KEYNOTE 001 and KEYNOTE 010, PD-L1 expression was utilized as inclusion criteria for enrollment where patients demonstrating at least 1% expression were eligible for the trial and divided into cohorts of 1–49% expression and ≥50% expression [13, 14]. The FDA-approved pembrolizumab for second-line therapy of advanced NSCLC for PD-L1 expressing patients only, defined as patients with ≥50% PD-L1 expression on tumor cells. In CHECKMATE 017, PD-L1 was neither significantly prognostic nor predictive of efficacy although this study was not powered for this subset analysis [17]. In CHECKMATE 057, PD-L1 expression was strongly correlated with ORR and predictive of OS [18]. POPLAR interestingly investigated both tumor cell and immune cell expression of PD-L1 and found both were prognostic of response to PD-L1 inhibition with significant improvement in OS with increased expression. OS in patient with TC0 and IC0 was consistent with that of the docetaxel treatment group (**Table 3** for comparison of studies) [25].

While several studies have supported the finding of PD-L1 as a prognostic and predictive factor there is debate on how to use this information if at all. First, PD-L1 expression assays have varied across studies to include usage of Dako 28-8, Dako 22C3, Ventana SP142, and Ventana SP263 [31]. Second, the cut-off expression percentage has varied throughout published trials

http://dx.doi.org/10.5772/64611

Clinical trial	Treatment regimen	Phase trial	Histology	PD-L1 expression	PD-L1 assay	ORR PD-L1+ vs. PDL1-	Overall survival
Checkmate 063	Nivolumab	2	Squamous	59% ≥ 1% 33% ≥ 5% 33% ≥ 10%	Dako 28-8	20% vs. 13% 24% vs. 14% 24% vs. 14%	NR
Checkmate 017	Nivolumab vs. docetaxel	3	Squamous	47% ≥ 1% 31% ≥ 5% 27% ≥ 10%	Dako 28-8	17% vs. 17% 21% vs. 15% 19% vs. 16%	HR 0.69 vs. 0.58 HR 0.53 vs. 0.70 HR 0.50 vs. 0.70
Checkmate 057	Nivolumab vs. docetaxel	3	Nonsquamous	53% ≥ 1% 41% ≥ 5% 37% ≥ 10%	Dako 28-8	31% vs. 9% 36% vs. 10% 37% vs. 11%	HR 0.67 vs. 0.56 HR 0.54 vs. 0.75 HR 0.58 vs. 0.70
KEYNOTE-001	Pembrolizumab	1	All	23% < 1% 38% ≥ 1% and < 50 34% ≥ 50%	Dako 22C3	10.7% vs. NR 16.5% vs. NR 45.2% vs. NR	10.4 mo vs. NR 10.6 mo vs. NR NR vs. NR
KEYNOTE-010	Pembrolizumab vs. docetaxel	1	All	43% ≥ 50%	Dako 22C3	30% vs. NR	2 mg/kg: 14.9 mo vs. NR 10 mg/kg: 17.3 mo vs. NR
CheckMate 012 Gettinger et al	Nivolumab	1	All	70% ≥ 1% 57% ≥ 5%	Dako 28-8	28% vs. 14% 31% vs. 15%	1 yr OS: 69% vs. 70% 1 yr OS: 73% vs. 70%
CheckMate 012 Rizvi et al	Nivolumab + PD-CT	1	All	52% ≥ 1%	Dako 28-8	48% vs. 43%	1 yr OS: 70% vs. 76% 20.2 mo vs. 19.2 mo
CheckMate 012 Hellman et al	Nivolumab + ipilimumab	1	All	77% ≥ 1%* 23% ≥ 50%*	Dako 28-8	57% vs. 0% 86% vs. 30%	1 yr OS: 83% vs. NR 1 yr OS: 100% vs. NR
POPLAR	Atezolizumab vs. docetaxel	2	All	32% TC-IC 0 < 1% 68% TC-IC 1/2/3 ≥ 1% 37% TC-IC 2/3 ≥ 5% 16% TC3 ≥ 50% or IC3 ≥ 10%	Ventana SP142	NR	1.04 vs. NR 0.59 vs. NR 0.54 vs. NR 0.49 vs. NR

OS, overall survival; ORR, objective response rate; NR, not reported; PD-1L, programmed cell death-1 ligand; mo, month.
*Annotates reported nivolumab 3 mg/kg q2 week + ipilimumab 1 mg/kg q6 week data only.

Table 3. PD-L1 expression and clinical benefit.

and includes exclusion of a small proportion of responders. Finally, PD-L1's expression is dynamic calling into question the reliability in its use as a biomarker if expression varies by time accessioned, recent treatment, and variability in expression between sites biopsied [31–33]. To answer some of these questions, the "Blueprint Project" was established to formulate the cross-platform standards for PD-L1 positivity [34]. Ultimately, we hope to either validate one assay or demonstrate consistent reliability between assays of PD-L1 expression. As we continue to learn the complex symphony of the tumor microenvironment it is likely PD-L1 expression will be one of many prognostic tests utilized to tailor individual treatment.

6. Genomics and predicting clinical efficacy to checkpoint inhibition

While checkpoint inhibition appears promising at this time, it confers improvement of overall survival in only a minority of patients. Yet, many patients that do respond to checkpoint inhibition demonstrate durable response to therapy making patient selection and identifying predictive and prognostic factors necessary for future clinical decision-making. Despite the numerous studies that have found PD-L1 expression to correspond with disease response, PD-L1 expression is not without its own shortcomings with the most significant being its validity and its negative predictive value. There is a large variability in mutation burden within tumor types ranging from tens to thousands of mutations. This heterogeneity is appreciated in NSCLC secondary to the variability within the disease compared to smokers, nonsmokers, and patients with driver mutations such as EGFR-mutant [35]. In the studies reviewed here, smoking has been found to correspond to clinical efficacy while decreased clinical efficacy was found in checkpoint inhibitor therapy with EGFR-mutant patients and nonsmokers [3]. Significant research is currently underway evaluating molecular determinants of clinical benefit to include evaluating for mutational load, mismatch-repair deficiency, and isolating specific somatic neoepitopes [36, 37]. Rizvi et al. [35] found using whole-exome sequencing of NSCLC patients treated with pembrolizumab that higher nonsynonymous mutation burden in tumors was associated with improved objective response, durable clinical benefit, and PFS. In a recently published genetic analysis of clinical response to anti-CTLA-4 in melanoma tumors, evaluating neoantigens was assessed in patients with clinical response. They found the presence of the neoepitope signature peptides correlated strongly with survival. They also found a correlation with high mutational load. Although this was not statistically significant in their study to support clinical benefit, the mutational load seen in many lung cancer patients make this an interesting topic for future research [36].

7. Conclusion

Lung cancer remains the leading cause of cancer-related mortality worldwide with the majority of NSCLC patients presenting with advanced stage disease. We now have robust literature demonstrating both efficacy and increased safety using checkpoint inhibition compared to standard of care chemotherapy in advanced stage disease. Still, immunotherapy and its efficacy in treatment of NSCLC as well as our understanding of how to best utilize this therapy remains in its infancy. We currently have data to support improved efficacy with advanced stage disease with checkpoint inhibition in the first and second line. CheckMate 026, NCT02041533, is investigating nivolumab in the first-line setting compared to standard of care therapy, platinum doublet chemotherapy, in advanced NSCLC patients with PD-L1 expressing tumors [20]. CheckMate 227, NCT02477826, is a multiarm study comparing nivolumab vs. nivolumab+ipilimumab vs. standard of care therapy platinum doublet chemotherapy ± nivolumab in the first-line setting [21]. KEYNOTE 042, NCT02220894, is an ongoing clinical trials investigating pembrolizumab in the first-line setting in PD-L1 expressing tumors [38, 39]. Atezolizumab is the first FDA-approved PD-L1 inhibitor approved in the second-line setting. As more studies mature, we look to further understand checkpoint inhibition in combination therapy, the sequence of therapy, and defining the appropriate population.

An additional question which remains unanswered is the efficacy of checkpoint inhibitors in early stage disease. Also, which patients benefit the most from checkpoint inhibition is still to be determined. It is generally accepted that patients who are smokers, have squamous histology, high expression of PD-L1, and a high mutational load are more likely to respond to checkpoint inhibition, whereas patients who are nonsmokers, EGFR-mutant, minimal or no PD-L1 expression, and low mutational load are less likely to respond to checkpoint inhibition. Future investigation will help delineate which of these factors can reliably predict response to therapy. The ability for us to define mechanisms by which tumors evade our immune system complemented with our ability to predict response will hold the key to successful incorporation of immunotherapy in a wide population of patients with lung cancer.

Author details

Karen G. Zeman[1]*, Joseph E. Zeman[2], Christina E. Brzezniak[3] and Corey A. Carter[1]

*Address all correspondence to: karengmayr@gmail.com

1 Department of Hematology Oncology, Walter Reed National Military Medical Center, Bethesda, Maryland, USA

2 Department of Pulmonary and Critical Care Medicine, Walter Reed National Military Medical Center, Bethesda, Maryland, USA

3 Thoracic Oncology and Immuno-Oncology, Walter Reed National Military Medical Center, Bethesda, Maryland, USA

The views expressed in this article are those of the author and do not necessarily reflect the official policy or position of the Department of the Navy, Department of Defense, nor the U.S. Government

References

[1] Brambilla E, Travis WD. Lung Cancer. In: World Cancer Report 2014 (Internet). Lyon, France: International Agency for Research and Cancer; 2014. 350-61 p.

[2] American Cancer Society: Global Cancer Facts and Figures (ed 3). Atlanta, GA: American Cancer Society; 2015.

[3] Melosky B, Chu Q, Juergens R, Leighl N, McLeod D, Hirsh V. Pointed progress in second-line advanced non-small-cell lung cancer: the rapidly evolving field of checkpoint inhibition. Journal of Clinical Oncology. 2016;34(14):1676–U235.

[4] Reckamp KL. Advances in immunotherapy for non-small cell lung cancer. Clinical Advances in Hematology & Oncology: H&O. 2015;13(12):847–53.

[5] Lyford-Pike S, Peng SW, Young GD, Taube JM, Westra WH, Akpeng B, et al. Evidence for a Role of the PD-1:PD-L1 pathway in immune resistance of HPV-associated head and neck squamous cell carcinoma. Cancer Research. 2013;73(6):1733–41.

[6] Wolchok JD, Kluger H, Callahan MK, Postow MA, Rizvi NA, Lesokhin AM, et al. Nivolumab plus ipilimumab in advanced melanoma. New England Journal of Medicine. 2013;369(2):122–33.

[7] Hodi FS, O'Day SJ, McDermott DF, Weber RW, Sosman JA, Haanen JB, et al. Improved survival with ipilimumab in patients with metastatic melanoma. New England Journal of Medicine. 2010;363(8):711–23.

[8] Hoser G, Domagala-Kulawik J, Droszcz P, Droszcz W, Kawiak J. Lymphocyte subsets differences in smokers and nonsmokers with primary lung cancer: a flow cytometry analysis of bronchoalveolar lavage fluid cells. Medical Science Monitor: International Medical Journal of Experimental and Clinical Research. 2003;9(8):BR310–15.

[9] Hoser G, Kawiak J, Domagala-Kulawik J, Kopinski P, Droszcz W. Flow cytometric evaluation of lymphocyte subpopulations in BALF of healthy smokers and nonsmokers. Folia Histochemica Et Cytobiologica. 1999;37(1):25–30.

[10] Atezolizumab (TECENTRIQ) (press release). 10/2016.

[11] FDA expands approved use of Opdivo to treat lung cancer (press release). 3/2015 Update.

[12] FDA approves Keytruda for advanced non-small cell lung cancer: First drug approved in lung cancer for patients whose tumors express PD-L1 (press release). 10/2015.

[13] Garon EB, Rizvi NA, Hui RN, Leighl N, Balmanoukian AS, Eder JP, et al. Pembrolizumab for the treatment of non-small-cell lung cancer. New England Journal of Medicine. 2015;372(21):2018–28.

[14] Herbst RS, Baas P, Kim DW, Felip E, Perez-Gracia JL, Han JY, et al. Pembrolizumab versus docetaxel for previously treated, PD-L1-positive, advanced non-small-cell lung cancer (KEYNOTE-010): a randomised controlled trial. Lancet. 2016;387(10027):1540–50.

[15] Gettinger SN, Horn L, Gandhi L, Spigel DR, Antonia SJ, Rizvi NA, et al. Overall survival and long-term safety of nivolumab (Anti-Programmed Death 1 Antibody, BMS-936558, ONO-4538) in patients with previously treated advanced non-small-cell lung cancer. Journal of Clinical Oncology. 2015;33(18):2004–U32.

[16] Rizvi NA, Mazieres J, Planchard D, Stinchcombe TE, Dy GK, Antonia SJ, et al. Activity and safety of nivolumab, an anti-PD-1 immune checkpoint inhibitor, for patients with advanced, refractory squamous non-small-cell lung cancer (CheckMate 063): a phase 2, single-arm trial. Lancet Oncology. 2015;16(3):257–65.

[17] Brahmer J, Reckamp KL, Baas P, Crino L, Eberhardt WEE, Poddubskaya E, et al. Nivolumab versus docetaxel in advanced squamous-cell non-small-cell lung cancer. New England Journal of Medicine. 2015;373(2):123–35.

[18] Borghaei H, Paz-Ares L, Horn L, Spigel DR, Steins M, Ready NE, et al. Nivolumab versus docetaxel in advanced nonsquamous non-small-cell lung cancer. New England Journal of Medicine. 2015;373(17):1627–39.

[19] Gettinger S, Rizvi NA, Chow LQ, Borghaei H, Brahmer J, Ready N, et al. Nivolumab monotherapy for first-line treatment of advanced non-small-cell lung cancer. Journal of Clinical Oncology. 2016;34(25):2980–87.

[20] ClinicalTrials.gov.: An Open-Label, Randomized, Phase 3 Trial of Nivolumab Versus Investigator's Choice Chemotherapy as First-Line Therapy for Stage IV or Recurrent PD-L1+ Non-Small Cell Lung Cancer (CheckMate 026) Updated 9/2016 (Available from: https://clinicaltrials.gov/ct2/show/NCT02041533?term=NCT02041533&rank=1.

[21] ClinicalTrials.gov.: A Trial of Nivolumab, or Nivolumab Plus Ipilimumab, or Nivolumab Plus Platinum-doublet Chemotherapy, Compared to Platinum Doublet Chemotherapy in Patients With Stage IV Non-Small Cell Lung Cancer (NSCLC) (CheckMate 227) Updated 9/2016 (Available from: https://clinicaltrials.gov/ct2/show/NCT02477826?term =NCT02477826&rank=1.

[22] Rizvi NA, Hellmann MD, Brahmer JR, Juergens RA, Borghaei H, Gettinger S, et al. Nivolumab in combination with platinum-based doublet chemotherapy for first-line treatment of advanced non-small-cell lung cancer. Journal of Clinical Oncology. 2016;34(25):2969–79.

[23] Hellmann MD. CheckMate 012: Safety and efficacy of first-line nivolumab and ipilimumab in advanced NSCLC. 2016 ASCO Annual Meeting; Chicago: Journal of Clinical Oncology. 2016. p. Abs 3001.

[24] Reck M, Rodriguez-Abreu D, Robinson AG, Hui R, Csoszi T, Fulop A, et al. Pembrolizumab versus chemotherapy for PD-L1-positive non-small-cell lung cancer. New England Journal of Medicine. 2016; 375(19):1823–1833.

[25] Fehrenbacher L, Spira A, Ballinger M, Kowanetz M, Vansteenkiste J, Mazieres J, et al. Atezolizumab versus docetaxel for patients with previously treated non-small-cell lung cancer (POPLAR): a multicentre, open-label, phase 2 randomised controlled trial. Lancet. 2016;387(10030):1837–46.

[26] ClinicalTrials.gov. A Randomized Phase 3 Study of Atezolizumab (an Engineered Anti-PDL1 Antibody) Compared to Docetaxel in Patients With Locally Advanced or Metastatic Non-Small Cell Lung Cancer Who Have Failed Platinum Therapy - "OAK" Updated 9/2016 (Available from: https://clinicaltrials.gov/ct2/show/NCT02008227?term =NCT02008227&rank=1.

[27] Brahmer JR, Tykodi SS, Chow LQM, Hwu W-J, Topalian SL, Hwu P, et al. Safety and activity of anti-PD-L1 antibody in patients with advanced cancer. New England Journal of Medicine. 2012;366(26):2455–65.

[28] Johnson DB, Rioth MJ, Horn L. Immune checkpoint inhibitors in NSCLC. Current Treatment Options in Oncology. 2014;15(4):658–69.

[29] Weber JS, Kahler KC, Hauschild A. Management of immune-related adverse events and kinetics of response with ipilimumab. Journal of Clinical Oncology. 2012;30(21):2691–7.

[30] Howell M, Lee R, Bowyer S, Fusi A, Lorigan P. Optimal management of immune-related toxicities associated with checkpoint inhibitors in lung cancer. Lung Cancer. 2015;88(2):117–23.

[31] Grigg C, Rizvi NA. PD-L1 biomarker testing for non-small cell lung cancer: truth or fiction? Journal for Immunotherapy of Cancer. 2016;4:48.

[32] Chae YK, Pan A, Davis AA, Raparia K, Mohindra NA, Matsangou M, et al. Biomarkers for PD-1/PD-L1 blockade therapy in non-small-cell lung cancer: is PD-L1 expression a good marker for patient selection? Clinical Lung Cancer. 2016;17(5):350–361.

[33] Sheng J, Fang W, Yu J, Chen N, Zhan J, Ma Y, et al. Expression of programmed death ligand-1 on tumor cells varies pre and post chemotherapy in non-small cell lung cancer. Scientific Reports. 2016;6:20090.

[34] FR H, McElhinny A, Stanforth D, al e. PD-L1 IHC assays for lung cancer: results from phase 1 of the "blueprint PD-L1 assay comparison project." AACR Annual Meeting; New Orleans 2016.

[35] Rizvi NA, Hellmann MD, Snyder A, Kvistborg P, Makarov V, Havel JJ, et al. Mutational landscape determines sensitivity to PD-1 blockade in non-small cell lung cancer. Science. 2015;348(6230):124–8.

[36] Snyder A, Makarov V, Merghoub T, Yuan J, Zaretsky JM, Desrichard A, et al. Genetic basis for clinical response to CTLA-4 blockade in melanoma. New England Journal of Medicine. 2014;371(23):2189–99.

[37] Le DT, Uram JN, Wang H, Bartlett BR, Kemberling H, Eyring AD, et al. PD-1 blockade in tumors with mismatch-repair deficiency. New England Journal of Medicine. 2015;372(26):2509–20.

[38] ClinicalTrials.gov. Study of Pembrolizumab (MK-3475) Compared to Platinum-Based Chemotherapies in Participants With Metastatic Non-Small Cell Lung Cancer (MK-3475-024/KEYNOTE-024) Updated 8/2016 (Available from: https://clinicaltrials.gov/ct2/show/NCT02142738?term=NCT02142738&rank=1.

[39] ClinicalTrials.gov. Study of MK-3475 (Pembrolizumab) Versus Platinum-based Chemotherapy for Participants With PD-L1-positive Advanced or Metastatic Non-small Cell Lung Cancer (MK-3475-042/KEYNOTE-042) Updated 8/2016 (Available from: https://clinicaltrials.gov/ct2/show/NCT02220894?term=NCT02220894&rank=1.

Chapter 9

Repurposing Metformin for Lung Cancer Management

Chuan-Mu Chen, Jiun-Long Wang, Yi-Ting Tsai,
Jie-Hau Jiang and Hsiao-Ling Chen

Additional information is available at the end of the chapter

http://dx.doi.org/10.5772/67160

Abstract

In this article, we introduced the background knowledge of lung cancer management and considered repurposing old drugs to overcome therapy bottleneck. We chose metformin to prove both its antihyperglycemia and antitumor formation effects. Based on the metformin-related AMPK-dependent pathway, we tried to explore the AMPK-independent pathway in inhibition of lung tumorigenesis by metformin. Using preclinical data mining from clinical settings with a literature review, we attempted to clarify the role of metformin in lung cancer management. Additional objective and strong evidence are needed using randomized control studies to verify the benefit of metformin in clinical practice. Furthermore, we proposed two lung cancer animal models and showed the establishment processes thoroughly. We hope that these two lung cancer animal models provide a useful platform for furthering old drug repurposing as well as new drug investigations in the future.

Keywords: lung cancer, metformin, animal model, AMPK pathway, orthotopic injection

1. Introduction

1.1. Background

Lung cancer is known as a major cause of cancer-related mortality worldwide. Newly discovered drugs focus on the issue of improving survival and need vast time and investment. In Ref. [1], it was estimated that it took 13 years and cost of 1.8 billion dollars for one newly developed drug. Additionally, just only one of the 5000 promising antitumor agents had the potential to pass the U.S. Food and Drug Administration (FDA) regulation and obtain final approval. With respect to currently used drugs, it is convenient to quickly access the "repurposing" or "repositioning" effect of converting them into anticancer management. In recent years, more and more studies have involved the antidiabetes drug metformin. Initially, Evans et al. [2] observed that patients with type 2 diabetes mellitus (DM) under metformin treatment had a reduction of cancer incidence. It caused a 23% reduction of risk of any cancer for the metformin group. Though it was an observational study, more and more research and experimental designs followed the path. Bo et al. [3] showed that the cancer incidence of type 2 DM patients with metformin was lower than that compared with other oral antidiabetic (OAD) agents. For pancreatic and colon cancer patients, Currie et al. [4] found that the metformin users among the type 2 DM group had lower cancer incidence. For breast cancer patients, some studies found that metformin was beneficial for neoadjuvant chemotherapy groups [5,6]. Regarding animal models, Algire et al. [7] proved the efficacy of metformin in lung cancer. From the preliminary result of above studies, we could understand the utilization of metformin in different types of cancers, including lung cancer.

1.2. Diabetes mellitus and metformin

Diabetes mellitus is a common metabolic disease, and the associated prevalence is approximately 7–10% [8]. Patients with DM have higher risk of cardiovascular disease, nephropathy (renal function impairment), retinopathy and polyneuropathy (numbness of distal part of four limbs). It is known that hyperglycemia is crucial for the development of many cancers, including breast, liver, colorectal, kidney and lung cancer. Among the diverse ODA agents for type 2 DM, metformin was the common first-line choice worldwide. It is estimated that approximately 120 million patients initially took metformin for controlling blood sugar. Moreover, the safety of metformin is confirmed due to a lower incidence of lactic acidosis compared with other OAD.

Metformin (N′,N′-dimethylbiguanide) belongs to the biguanide class. It possesses hypoglycemic effect by inhibition of gluconeogenesis. Further it could lower insulin resistance, which is very important for cancer growth. From earlier studies, scientists found metformin could activate the adenosine monophosphate-activated protein kinase (AMPK) pathway to negatively regulate the mammalian target of rapamycin (mTOR) pathway with the aid of liver kinase B1 (LKB1) [9,10]. The mTOR pathway helps proliferation for cell viability [11]. Therefore, metformin could demonstrate an antiproliferative effect in cells, even for cancer cells. Based on this implication, metformin showed the potential for an antitumor effect. In addition to the AMPK-dependent pathway, some studies supposed metformin could exert an AMPK-independent pathway in dealing with tumorigenesis [1]. Later, we will focus on the issue of the antitumor effects of metformin in lung cancer.

2. Mechanism of metformin on antitumorigenesis

2.1. The antitumor effect of metformin

2.1.1. Metformin corrects hyperglycemia

Metformin can accumulate within the matrix of mitochondria, and it could exert the inhibition of the complex I of the mitochondrial electron transport chain. Further, reduction of nicotinamide adenine dinucleotide hydride (NADH) oxidation can also cause the reduction of synthesis of adenosine triphosphate (ATP). After the activation of AMP-activated protein kinase (AMPK), it enhances catabolic activity instead of the anabolic process. It initiates transcriptional signal transduction, inhibition of gluconeogenesis, and induction of glucose uptake into muscle cells via glucose transporters (GLUT2) [12]. Moreover, metformin can indirectly cause the induction of insulin receptor expression to facilitate insulin sensitivity and reduce insulin resistance, which is associated with tumor growth [13].

2.1.2. Metformin upregulates AMPK

Metformin can activate AMPK to initiate the downstream signal transduction to affect the transcription of tumor suppressor liver kinase B1 (LKB1) [14]. Once AMPK is activated, it negatively regulates the mTOR pathway by phosphorylation and activation of tuberous sclerosis complex 2 (TSC2) and inhibition of downstream small GTPase (RHEB). The mTOR pathway is crucial for tumor cell survival because mTOR plays a vital role in cell growth, proliferation and protein synthesis. Moreover, the mTOR pathway could be activated via mitogenic responsive phosphoinositide 3-kinase/protein kinase B/AKT (PI3K/PKB/AKT) pathway. When metformin-related AMPK dependent pathway is affected, the inhibition of mTOR signal transduction and reduction of cancer cell proliferation are achieved [15].

2.1.3. AMPK and p53 pathways

It is known that p53 can activate numerous genes to negatively regulate the AKT and mTORC1 pathways, resulting in cancer cell quiescence, senescence and further apoptosis. Thus, once AMPK phosphorylates p53, it could lead to p53-mediated cell cycle arrest in p53-expressing cells and cell apoptosis for cells with mutated p53 [11].

2.1.4. Inflammatory pathway and metformin

For tumorigenesis, chronic inflammation is attributed to tumor growth and development. Once the inflammatory process is stimulated, it causes DNA adduct formation and increases the amount of inflammation biomarkers (such as cytokine/chemokines, immune-related effectors, acute phase proteins, reactive oxygen and nitrogen species, prostaglandins, cyclooxygenase-related factors and transcription factors and growth factors) [16]. Like tumor necrosis factor-alpha (TNF-α), nuclear factor-kappa B (NF-kB) and signal transducer and activator of transcription 3 (STAT3) are important components of the inflammation reaction. Arai et al. elucidated that metformin reduces the process and production of TNF-α in human monocytes [17].

Reactive oxygen species (ROS) play a vital role in the formation of advanced glycation end products to enrich oxidative stress. Metformin can reduce the production of endogenous reactive oxygen species via inhibition of mitochondrial complex I [18].

2.1.5. Cell cycle pathway and metformin

Sahra et al. found that metformin has an antiproliferation effect, which is mediated by G1 cell cycle arrest. In a study with prostate cancer cells, metformin-induced cell cycle arrests by inhibiting the expression of cyclin D1 and retinoblastoma-protein (pRb) [19].

2.1.6. *Angiogenesis and metformin*

For tumor cells growth, vast amounts of nutrition and oxygen are needed. As the tumor enlarges and begins to invade and cause distant metastasis, angiogenesis is the cornerstone. Tumor cells easily develop pro-angiogenic agents once exposed to a hypoxic environment [8]. The vascular endothelial growth factor (VEGF) formation is the key step. The VEGF group is consisted of four members (VEGF-A, B, C and D), and VEGF-A is the most potent. VEGF-A has four isoforms: VEGF-A_{121}, VEGF-A_{165}, VEGF-A_{189} and VEGF-A_{206}. VEGF-A_{165} functions in both the angiogenic process and cell growth. Moreover, the angiogenesis process needs a cofactor (neuropilin; NRP-1) to facilitate the VEGF ligand interaction with the VEGF receptor (VEGF-R2) [16,20]. In our previous lung cancer cell line (A549) experiments, the expression of NRP-1 decreased after the addition of metformin.

2.1.7. *Models of metformin using different cell lines*

In the beginning, anticancer studies were started from cell lines and animal models (commonly using a xenograft model). There are a vast number of antitumor studies with metformin on ovarian cancer, gastric cancer, pancreatic cancer and breast cancer. Some emphasize cell cycle-related proteins (CD1, CDK4 and CDK6) and some focus on microRNA (miR) regulation and signal transduction [21–24]. Moreover, cancer stem cells (CSC) were also found to be involved in the antitumor effect of metformin in both cell lines and xenograft models. The dosage and administration route of metformin were diverse. We provided a brief summary of previous findings of the antitumor effects of metformin on different cell lines in **Table 1** [21, 22, 24, 25].

Cancer cell type	**Ovarian cancer**	**Gastric cancer**	**Breast cancer, prostate cancer, lung cancer**	**Pancreatic cancer**
Lab material	1. Cell line 2. Xenograft model 3. Live tumor analysis	1. Cell line 2. Xenograft 3. miRNA	1. Cell line 2. Xenograft	1. Human pancreatic cancer cells
Mechanism	1. Inhibit tumor proliferation (IHC: Ki-67↓, Cyclin D1↓) 2. pACC↑: downstream target of AMPK (pmTOR↓)	1. Cell cycle–related protein (CD1↓,CDK4↓, CDK6 ↓) 2. Block G0-G1 phase 3. Cell proliferation assay	1. Cancer stem cells (CD44↑, CD24↓)	1. microRNA analysis 2. RT-PCR
Results	1. Inhibits angiogenesis (IHC stain for VEGF, CD-31) 2. Microvessel density: CD-31 3. Inhibits metastasis of ovarian cancer 4. Enhances cytotoxicity of chemotherapy reagents (Cisplatin: colony formation assay)	1. Reduced Cyclin D1 expression	1. Metformin reduces the dosage of chemotherapy (Doxorubicin) 2. Lung cancer cell line (A549)	1. Metformin up-regulates the expression of miR-26a, miR-192 and let-7c. 2. Cell migration 3. Cell proliferation assay 4. Metformin suppresses the oncogene: HMGA1

Cancer cell type	Ovarian cancer	Gastric cancer	Breast cancer, prostate cancer, lung cancer	Pancreatic cancer
Route	Oral feeding metformin in drinking water 200 ml	i.p. injection (intraperitoneal)	Oral intake in drinking water.	1. i.p. (Xenograft) 2. Cell line
Dosage	Reagan-Shaw formula 1. Human: 480 mg/60 kg 2. Mouse: 100 mg/kg	1. 1 mmol/L, 5 mmol/L 10 mmol/L 1 or 2 mg/day, i.p., 5 times/week for 4 weeks	200 μg/mL (15 mg/kg)	1. 1. i.p: 250 mg/kg (100 μL/mouse) 2. 2. Cell line: (0~10 mmol/L)
Reference	[24]	[22]	[21]	[25]

Table 1. The associated antitumor mechanism of metformin on different cancer cells.

2.2. Literature review of the present studies on the issue of metformin in lung cancer

First, we searched the articles on PubMed that included with metformin and lung cancer in the title. From basic, preclinical research (including cell lines and animal studies) to observational studies, we attempt to explain the association of the antitumor mechanism by metformin.

2.2.1. Preclinical studies

2.2.1.1. Metformin and lung cancer cell lines

Initially, Ashinuma et al. investigated the effect of metformin on the inhibition of clonogenicity, cell growth and proliferation using four different lung cancer cell lines [26].

2.2.1.2. Synergistic effect of metformin with chemotherapy reagents

Chemotherapy is widely used for the treatment of advanced lung cancer (stage IIIB and IV). Some studies aim to overcome chemoresistance by the combination of metformin and chemotherapy. The report of Tseng et al. [27] showed metformin mediated the downregulation of p38 mitogen-activated protein kinase-dependent excision repair cross-complementing 1 and decreased DNA repair ability. Additionally, it could further sensitize human lung cancer cells to cisplatin and paclitaxel agents [27,28].

2.2.1.3. Synergistic effect of metformin and tyrosine kinase inhibitors (TKIs)

Tyrosine kinase inhibitors (TKIs) such as gefitinib (Iressa), erlotinib (Tarceva) and afatinib (Giotrif) are now validated as the first-line therapy for advanced lung adenocarcinoma bearing mutant epidermal growth factor receptor (EGFR). Studies designed to evaluate the possible synergistic effect of metformin and TKIs were launched. Morgillo et al. [29] showed that metformin with gefitinib had more obvious antiproliferative and proapoptotic effects in both cell line and animal models (xenograft).

2.2.1.4. Synergistic effect of metformin and TKI in EGFR-TKI–resistant lung cancer cell line

First-line TKIs in lung adenocarcinoma encountered the issue of drug resistance due to the development of EGFR-resistant strains (such as T790M). To overcome this problem, Li et al. [30] proved that metformin could reverse epithelial-to-mesenchymal transition (EMT) and interleukin-6 (IL-6) signaling activation in EGFR-TKI–resistant lung cancer cells. Then, they proved metformin could increase sensitivity for EGFR-resistant strains to TIKs (gefitinib and erlotinib) therapy.

2.2.1.5. Effect of metformin in radiation therapy for lung cancer

Radiation therapy is one therapy modality for lung cancer patients. However, the possible effects when adding metformin to radiation therapy are unknown. Storozhuk et al. showed that metformin may enhance the radiation response of nonsmall cell lung cancer through the ataxia-telangiectasia mutated protein kinase (ATM) and AMPK pathway [31].

2.2.2. Observational studies

2.2.2.1. Population-based studies in Taiwan

In Taiwan, the National Health Insurance Registered Database (NHIRD) is popular for further assessment and discovery of medical issues. Experts attempt to find the association between metformin and lung cancer risk among type 2 DM patients. Lai et al. performed an epidemiological study and found that in patients treated with metformin, compared with the non-metformin (other OAD) group in type 2 DM patients, the reduction of lung cancer risk was approximately 39–45% [32].

2.2.2.2. Population-based studies outside Taiwan

From a retrospective study performed by Tan et al., they defined diabetic nonsmall cell lung cancer (NSCLC) patients receiving chemotherapy as the first-line treatment. Patients were divided into three groups: (A) Chemotherapy + metformin; (B) Chemotherapy + insulin, and (C) Chemotherapy + other OAD. They found that group A had superior median overall survival (OS) compared with the other two groups (20 months vs. 13.1 months vs. 13.0 months, respectively, $P = 0.007$) [33]. Like the NHIRD in Taiwan, the USA has a similar system called the SEER (surveillance, epidemiology and end results) database. Lin et al. collected 750 diabetic patients diagnosed with stage IV NSCLC and showed that the metformin group was associated with a benefit in survival. The hazard ratio (HR) was 0.80 and 95%, and the confidence interval (CI) is 0.71–0.89, respectively [33,34]. A study by Zhu et al. [35] showed metformin was significantly associated with a 16% reduction of lung cancer risk in type 2 DM patients. The relative risk (RR) is 0.84 and 95% CI (confidence interval was 0.73–0.97, $P < 0.05$).

3. Animal models applied to lung cancer studies

Animal models are indispensable for transforming *in vitro* studies into an *in vivo* setting. Subcutaneous xenograft models are commonly used as lung cancer animal models. In this model, lung cancer cell lines are injected subcutaneously to the flank side of nude mice. Different designed reagents are administered, and the response after medical therapy is observed. The tumor is not directly initiated from the original lung tissue. Thus, it is an indirect way to observe the so-called lung tumor formation.

Here, we introduced two lung cancer animal models developed in our laboratory. **Model 1** was transgenic mice with an overexpression of human vascular endothelial growth factor (*hVEGF*)-A_{165}. The model emphasized angiogenesis in the lung cancer formation process. **Model 2** was an *in vivo* image model of orthotopic lung adenocarcinoma formation in mice by using dual fluorescence reporting genes (pCAG-iRFP-2A-Venus). We could track the lung tumor formation and response to therapy more directly. We provide a summary for these two animal models and compare them with the subcutaneous xenograft model as shown in **Table 2**.

Animal models for lung cancer study	Model 1	Model 2	Current model
Mechanism	hVEGF-A165 over-expression transgenic mice	Orthotopic lung xenograft (transpleural injected) dual fluorescence reporter	Subcutaneous xenograft
Species of animal	Transgenic mice (FVB)	Nude mice (BALB/cAnN. Cg-Foxnlnu/CrlNARL)	Nude mice
Lung cancer cell line selected	Not applied	A549	A549
Tumor formation site	Lung	Lung	Trunk or flank area
Tumor formation duration	Approximately 12 months	Approximately 4–6 weeks	Approximately 4–6 weeks
IVIS setting	No	Yes	No
Lung tumor formation	Direct	Direct	Indirect
Reference	[37]	[40]	[21]

Table 2. Comparison of our two types of animal models with the current subcutaneous xenograft model for lung tumor formation.

3.1. Animal model 1: overexpression of human vascular endothelial growth factor (*hVEGF*)-A_{165}-induced lung tumorigenesis in transgenic mice

3.1.1. Background

When a tumor develops, it demands a vast amount of oxygen and nutrition for tumor growth. When a tumor is small in size, approximately 10^5 to 10^6 tumor cells, it depends on the diffusion effect for nutrition transport. As the tumor enlarges, it must overcome hypoxia and develop an angiogenic switch, including proangiogenic and angiogenic factors. Once vasculogenesis and angiogenesis are established, the tumor can invade extensively and cause distant metastasis [36]. Based on this theory, we demonstrate lung tumor formation via the angiogenesis model.

3.1.2. Materials and methods, see Ref. [37]

1. **Create transgenic mice carrying the mccsp-Vegf-A_{165}-sv40 transgenic fusion gene (Figure 1A)**

   - A 1975-bp *mccsp-Vegf-A_{165}*–sv40 transgene was directly microinjected into pronuclear stage FVB mouse embryos and then transferred into the fallopian tube of the recipient females mice.
   - Transgenic mice were mated with littermates or normal FVB mice to produce offspring.
   - The resulting 12-month transgenic offspring were the candidates for performing the lung cancer model.

2. **Gross picture of homozygous transgenic mice compared with wild-type mice (Figure 1B)**

   - Illustration of the whole picture of lung tissues from transgenic mice (homozygous) and wild type mice. We can observe the mass with a bulging appearance of lung tissue, with tumor formation in the transgenic mice (**Figure 1B**, upper panel).

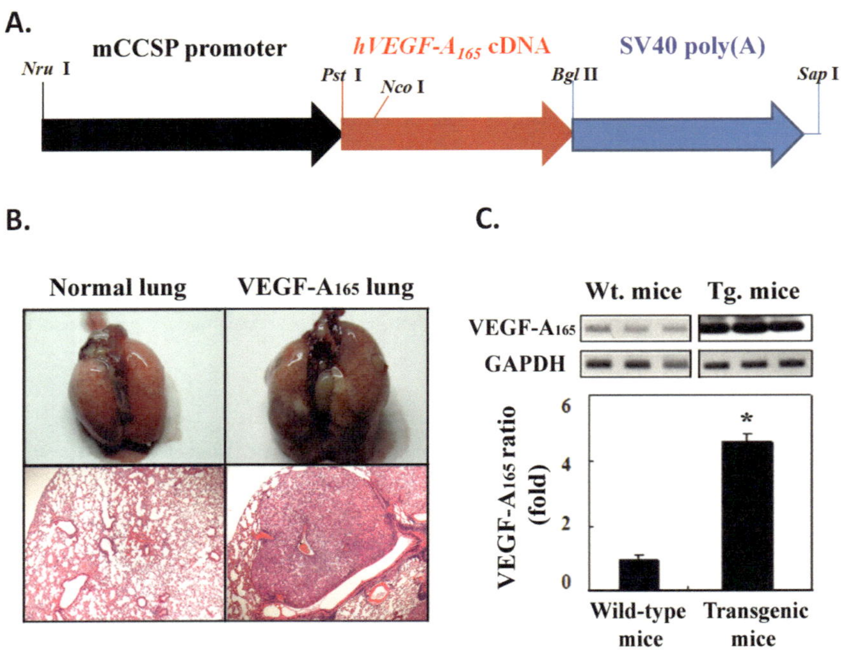

Figure 1. Animal model 1 for overexpressing human vascular endothelial growth factor (*hVEGF*)-A_{165}-induced lung tumorigenesis in transgenic mice. (A) Construction map of *hVEGF*-A_{165} overexpression, which is controlled by mouse Clara cell-specific protein (*mccsp*) promoter. The structure of the transgene is approximately 1975-base pairs in length. (B) The whole exterior (upper panel) and histopathologic sections of the lung tissues (lower panel) in the transgenic mice (right side) and wild-type mice (left side). (**C**) Western blot analysis of the hVEGF-A_{165} protein expression level in the lung tissue of wild type and transgenic mice (upper panel) and the quantification data.

3. **Histopathologic analysis of the lung tissue in transgenic mice and wild-type mice (Figure 1B)**

   - From the lower part of **Figure 1B**, we can easily find the lung tumor formation with bizarre cell shapes and increased nucleus/cytoplasm (N/C) ratios in the lung tissues of transgenic mice. The wild type mice showed no tumor-specific appearance.

4. **Validation of *hVEGF*-A_{165} protein expression of transgenic mice was performed by western blot analysis**

   - In the lung tissue of 12-month transgenic mice, the western blot data proved, there were more than 5-fold higher levels of VEGF expression compared with wild type mice (**Figure 1C**).

3.2. Animal model 2: dual fluorescence reporting genes expressed by an *in vivo* imaging model of orthotopic lung adenocarcinoma in mice

3.2.1. Background

In cancer research, it is important to perform *in vivo* animal experiments to further mimic the effects on human beings. During the study period, it is necessary to record images simultaneously. Real time imaging depends on the *in vivo* image system (IVIS). The creation of good IVIS images is necessary and demands comprehensive consideration. The property of good IVIS images requires an optimal imaging window. For the mammalian tissue study, obtaining deep optical images requires near-infrared (NIR) fluorescent probes. The NIR optical window is around from 650 to 900 nm. Under this optical window, mammalian tissue is considered more transparent to light due to the limited combined absorption of water, melanin and hemoglobin. Moreover, under this spectral region, it could eliminate autofluorescence and have low light scattering [38]. The common used near-infrared fluorescent proteins (iRFP) included iRFP670, iRFP682, iRFP702 and iRFP720 [39]. Based on this concept, we designed a near-infrared fluorescent mice tumor model to further evaluate the IVIS expression during lung tumor formation.

3.2.2. Material and methods, see Ref. [40]

3.2.2.1. Construction of dual fluorescence-expression vector

- The construction map of the pCAG-iRFP-2A-venus transgene is shown (**Figure 2A**).
- Transfection of lung adenocarcinoma cell line (A549) with pCAG-iRFP-2A-venus expression was performed. The iRFP can show red fluorescence. Venus can show green fluorescence. And DAPI (4′,6-diamidino-2-phenylindole) emits blue fluorescence in cell nuclei as a background control (**Figure 2B**).

3.2.2.2. Orthotopic lung injection with transfected A549 lung adenocarcinoma cells

- Animal species: Four-week-old male nude mice (BALB/cAnN.Cg-Foxnlnu/CrlNARL) was used.

- A total of 2E+6 iRFP-2A-venus A549 cells were directly injected orthotopically into the transpleural cavity on the left lung side of nude mice.
- IVIS imaging recorded lung tumor formation (**Figure 2C**).

3.2.2.3. Histopathologic analysis confirms the tumor formation of orthotopic lung injected nude mice, which had iRFP-2A-venus A549 expression

- By examining the tissues with an H&E stain, we observe abundant tumor cells formation in the orthotopically injected iRFP-2A-venus A549 cells in mice lung tissue (**Figure 2D**, upper panel).
- Using immunohistochemistry (IHC) and staining with antivenus, lung tumor formation was found (**Figure 2D**, lower panel).

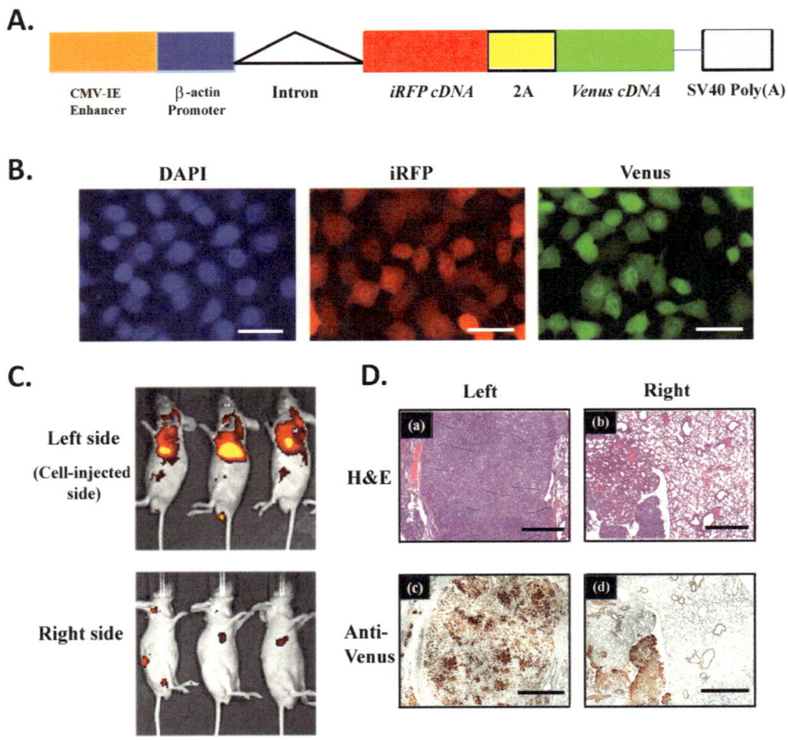

Figure 2. Animal model 2 for dual fluorescence reporting genes expressed by *in vivo* imaging model of orthotopic lung adenocarcinoma in mice. (A) Construction map of dual fluorescence expression vector, pCAG-iRFP-2A-venus transgene. (B) Three different fluorescence signals were used in iRFP-2A-Venus A549 cells expressed under a fluorescent microscope: DAPI (blue), iRFP (red) and venus (green). Scale bar: 50 μm. (C) The IVIS imaging analysis of nude mice that received iRFP-2A-venus A549 cells by orthotopic injection. Color scale: Max: 4.56e+7, Min: 2.02e+7. (D) Histopathologic study of nude mice lung tumors after receiving iRFP-2A-venus A549 cells by orthotopic injection. L and R represent left and right lungs, respectively. The left side column (a) and (c) represent H&E and IHC expression on the longitudinal sections of lung tumors, respectively. The brown color of antivenus expression in column (c) and (d) indicates lung tumor formation. The scale bar in columns (b) and (d) is 100 μm.

http://dx.doi.org/10.5772/67160

4. Conclusion

First, we presented a brief introduction of the antihyperglycemic effect of metformin. More and more studies have involved the repurposing of metformin due to its observed antitumor effects. Observational studies found lung cancer patients with type 2 DM under metformin treatment had better outcomes. Through a literature review, we initially sought to examine the potential antitumorigenic effects of metformin in a preclinical setting. Population-based research revealed the survival benefit of type 2 DM patients with metformin under cancer management. Based on the AMPK-dependent pathway, we attempted to discover an AMPK-independent pathway (such as angiogenesis, inflammation, etc.) related to metformin. Later, we illustrated two animal models of lung cancer utilized in our research group. **Model 1** focused on the angiogenesis pathway. Overexpression of human *VEGF-A*$_{165}$ transgenic mice model provided further clues for tumor formation. **Model 2** emphasizes the *in vivo* image of dual fluorescence reporting gene expression created by orthotopic lung injection. IVIS-aided analysis helped track the lung adenocarcinoma formation in real time. This method could shorten the waiting time for lung tumor formation in animal studies. Furthermore, we aim to integrate these two animal models with metformin in a stepwise manner. We look forward to thoroughly elucidating the antitumor effects of metformin for lung cancer management based on current animal model platforms.

Acknowledgements

We thank Dr. Yu-Tang Tung and Dr. Cheng-Wei Lai for their assistance in performing experiments and data collections. This article was financially supported in part by MOST-104-2313-B-005-043-MY3 from the Ministry of Science and Technology, ATU-105-S0508 from the Ministry of Education, TCVGH-NCHU 1027605 and TCVGH-NCHU 1047610 from Rong-Hsing cooperation project, and TCVGH-1033203B, TCVGH-1043204B from VGHTC research project, Taiwan.

Author details

Chuan-Mu Chen[1,2]*, Jiun-Long Wang[1,3], Yi-Ting Tsai[4], Jie-Hau Jiang[1], and Hsiao-Ling Chen[5]

*Address all correspondence to: chchen1@dragon.nchu.edu.tw

1 Department of Life Sciences, and Agricultural Biotechnology Center, National Chung Hsing University, Taichung, Taiwan

2 Rong-Hsing Translational Medicine Center and iEGG Center, National Chung Hsing University, Taichung, Taiwan

3 Division of Chest Medicine, Department of Internal Medicine, Taichung Veterans General Hospital, Taichung, Taiwan

4 Division of Endocrinology and Metabolism, Department of Internal Medicine, Taichung Veterans General Hospital, Taichung, Taiwan

5 Department of Bioresources, Da-Yeh University, Changhwa, Taiwan

References

[1] Saxena A, Becker D, Preeshagul I, Lee K, Katz E, Levy B. Therapeutic effects of repurposed therapies in non-small cell lung cancer: What is old is new again. Oncologist. 2015 Aug; 20(8):934–45. DOI: 10.1634/theoncologist.2015-0064

[2] Evans JM, Donnelly LA, Emslie-Smith AM, Alessi DR, Morris AD. Metformin and reduced risk of cancer in diabetic patients. BMJ. 2005 Jun 4; 330(7503):1304–5. DOI:10.1136/bmj.38415.708634.F7

[3] Bo S, Ciccone G, Rosato R, Villois P, Appendino G, Ghigo E, et al. Cancer mortality reduction and metformin: A retrospective cohort study in type 2 diabetic patients. Diabetes Obes Metab. 2012 Jan; 14(1):23–9. DOI: 10.1111/j.1463-1326.2011.01480.x

[4] Currie CJ, Poole CD, Jenkins-Jones S, Gale EA, Johnson JA, Morgan CL. Mortality after incident cancer in people with and without type 2 diabetes: Impact of metformin on survival. Diabetes Care. 2012 Feb;35(2):299–304. DOI: 10.2337/dc11-1313

[5] Jiralerspong S, Palla SL, Giordano SH, Meric-Bernstam F, Liedtke C, Barnett CM, et al. Metformin and pathologic complete responses to neoadjuvant chemotherapy in diabetic patients with breast cancer. J Clin Oncol. 2009 Jul 10; 27(20):3297–302. DOI:10.1200/JCO.2009.19.6410

[6] Jiralerspong S, Gonzalez-Angulo AM, Hung MC. Expanding the arsenal: Metformin for the treatment of triple-negative breast cancer? Cell Cycle. 2009 Sep 1; 8(17):2681.DOI: 10.4161/cc.8.17.9502

[7] Algire C, Zakikhani M, Blouin MJ, Shuai JH, Pollak M. Metformin attenuates the stimulatory effect of a high-energy diet on in vivo LLC1 carcinoma growth. Endocr Relat Cancer. 2008 Sep; 15(3):833–9. DOI: 10.1677/ERC-08-0038

[8] Guariguata L, Whiting DR, Hambleton I, Beagley J, Linnenkamp U, Shaw JE. Global estimates of diabetes prevalence for 2013 and projections for 2035. Diabetes Res Clin Pract. 2014 Feb; 103(2):137–49. DOI: 10.1016/j.diabres.2013.11.002

[9] Zakikhani M, Dowling R, Fantus IG, Sonenberg N, Pollak M. Metformin is an AMP kinase-dependent growth inhibitor for breast cancer cells. Cancer Res. 2006 Nov 1; 66(21):10269–73. DOI: 10.1158/0008-5472.CAN-06-1500

[10] Sinnett-Smith J, Kisfalvi K, Kui R, Rozengurt E. Metformin inhibition of mTORC1 activation, DNA synthesis and proliferation in pancreatic cancer cells: Dependence on glucose concentration and role of AMPK. Biochem Biophys Res Commun. 2013 Jan 4; 430(1):352–7. DOI: 10.1016/j.bbrc.2012.11.010

[11] Emami Riedmaier A, Fisel P, Nies AT, Schaeffeler E, Schwab M. Metformin and cancer: From the old medicine cabinet to pharmacological pitfalls and prospects. Trends Pharmacol Sci. 2013 Feb; 34(2):126–35. DOI: 10.1016/j.tips.2012.11.005

[12] El-Mir MY, Nogueira V, Fontaine E, Averet N, Rigoulet M, Leverve X. Dimethylbiguanide inhibits cell respiration via an indirect effect targeted on the respiratory chain complex I. J Biol Chem. 2000 Jan 7; 275(1):223–8.DOI: 10.1074/jbc.275.1.223

[13] Rena G, Pearson ER, Sakamoto K. Molecular mechanism of action of metformin: Old or new insights? Diabetologia. 2013 Sep; 56(9):1898–906. DOI: 10.1007/s00125-013-2991-0

[14] Shaw RJ, Lamia KA, Vasquez D, Koo SH, Bardeesy N, Depinho RA, et al. The kinase LKB1 mediates glucose homeostasis in liver and therapeutic effects of metformin. Science. 2005 Dec 9; 310(5754):1642–6. DOI: 10.1126/science.1120781

[15] Gwinn DM, Shackelford DB, Egan DF, Mihaylova MM, Mery A, Vasquez DS, et al. AMPK phosphorylation of raptor mediates a metabolic checkpoint. Mol Cell. 2008 Apr 25; 30(2):214–26. DOI: 10.1016/j.molcel.2008.03.003

[16] Weis SM, Cheresh DA. Tumor angiogenesis: molecular pathways and therapeutic targets. Nat Med. 2011 Nov 7; 17(11):1359–70. DOI: 10.1038/nm.2537

[17] Arai M, Uchiba M, Komura H, Mizuochi Y, Harada N, Okajima K. Metformin, an antidiabetic agent, suppresses the production of tumor necrosis factor and tissue factor by inhibiting early growth response factor-1 expression in human monocytes in vitro. J Pharmacol Exp Ther. 2010 Jul; 334(1):206–13. DOI: 10.1124/jpet.109.164970

[18] Algire C, Moiseeva O, Deschenes-Simard X, Amrein L, Petruccelli L, Birman E, et al. Metformin reduces endogenous reactive oxygen species and associated DNA damage. Cancer Prev Res (Phila). 2012 Apr; 5(4):536–43. DOI: 10.1158/1940-6207.CAPR-11-0536

[19] Ben Sahra I, Laurent K, Loubat A, Giorgetti-Peraldi S, Colosetti P, Auberger P, et al. The antidiabetic drug metformin exerts an antitumoral effect in vitro and in vivo through a decrease of cyclin D1 level. Oncogene. 2008 Jun 5; 27(25):3576–86. DOI: 10.1038/sj.onc.1211024

[20] Albini A, Tosetti F, Li VW, Noonan DM, Li WW. Cancer prevention by targeting angiogenesis. Nat Rev Clin Oncol. 2012 Sep; 9(9):498–509. DOI: 10.1038/nrclinonc.2012.120

[21] Iliopoulos D, Hirsch HA, Struhl K. Metformin decreases the dose of chemotherapy for prolonging tumor remission in mouse xenografts involving multiple cancer cell types. Cancer Res. 2011 May 1; 71(9):3196–201. DOI: 10.1158/0008-5472.CAN-10-3471

[22] Kato K, Gong J, Iwama H, Kitanaka A, Tani J, Miyoshi H, et al. The antidiabetic drug metformin inhibits gastric cancer cell proliferation in vitro and in vivo. Mol Cancer Ther. 2012 Mar; 11(3):549–60. DOI: 10.1158/1535-7163.MCT-11-0594

[23] Li D. Diabetes and pancreatic cancer. Mol Carcinog. 2012 Jan; 51(1):64–74. DOI: 10.1002/mc.20771

[24] Rattan R, Graham RP, Maguire JL, Giri S, Shridhar V. Metformin suppresses ovarian cancer growth and metastasis with enhancement of cisplatin cytotoxicity in vivo. Neoplasia. 2011 May; 13(5):483–91. DOI 10.1593002Fneo.11148

[25] Li W, Yuan Y, Huang L, Qiao M, Zhang Y. Metformin alters the expression profiles of microRNAs in human pancreatic cancer cells. Diabetes Res Clin Pract. 2012 May; 96(2):187–95. DOI: 10.1016/j.diabres.2011.12.028

[26] Ashinuma H, Takiguchi Y, Kitazono S, Kitazono-Saitoh M, Kitamura A, Chiba T, et al. Antiproliferative action of metformin in human lung cancer cell lines. Oncol Rep. 2012 Jul; 28(1):8–14. DOI: 10.3892/or.2012.1763

[27] Tseng SC, Huang YC, Chen HJ, Chiu HC, Huang YJ, Wo TY, et al. Metformin-mediated downregulation of p38 mitogen-activated protein kinase-dependent excision repair cross-complementing 1 decreases DNA repair capacity and sensitizes human lung cancer cells to paclitaxel. Biochem Pharmacol. 2013 Feb 15; 85(4):583–94. DOI: 10.1016/j.bcp.2012.12.001

[28] Lin CC, Yeh HH, Huang WL, Yan JJ, Lai WW, Su WP, et al. Metformin enhances cisplatin cytotoxicity by suppressing signal transducer and activator of transcription-3 activity independently of the liver kinase B1-AMP-activated protein kinase pathway. Am J Respir Cell Mol Biol. 2013 Aug; 49(2):241–50. DOI: 10.1165/rcmb.2012-0244OC

[29] Morgillo F, Sasso FC, Della Corte CM, Vitagliano D, D'Aiuto E, Troiani T, et al. Synergistic effects of metformin treatment in combination with gefitinib, a selective EGFR tyrosine kinase inhibitor, in LKB1 wild-type NSCLC cell lines. Clin Cancer Res. 2013 Jul 1; 19(13):3508–19. DOI: 10.1158/1078-0432.CCR-12-2777

[30] Li L, Han R, Xiao H, Lin C, Wang Y, Liu H, et al. Metformin sensitizes EGFR-TKI-resistant human lung cancer cells in vitro and in vivo through inhibition of IL-6 signaling and EMT reversal. Clin Cancer Res. 2014 May 15; 20(10):2714–26. DOI: 10.1158/1078-0432.CCR-13-2613

[31] Storozhuk Y, Hopmans SN, Sanli T, Barron C, Tsiani E, Cutz JC, et al. Metformin inhibits growth and enhances radiation response of non-small cell lung cancer (NSCLC) through ATM and AMPK. Br J Cancer. 2013 May 28; 108(10):2021–32. DOI: 10.1038/bjc.2013.187

[32] Lai SW, Liao KF, Chen PC, Tsai PY, Hsieh DP, Chen CC. Antidiabetes drugs correlate with decreased risk of lung cancer: a population-based observation in Taiwan. Clin Lung Cancer. 2012 Mar; 13(2):143–8. DOI: 10.1016/j.cllc.2011.10.002

[33] Tan BX, Yao WX, Ge J, Peng XC, Du XB, Zhang R, et al. Prognostic influence of metformin as first-line chemotherapy for advanced nonsmall cell lung cancer in patients with type 2 diabetes. Cancer. 2011 Nov 15; 117(22):5103–11. DOI: 10.1002/cncr.26151

[34] Lin JJ, Gallagher EJ, Sigel K, Mhango G, Galsky MD, Smith CB, et al. Survival of patients with stage IV lung cancer with diabetes treated with metformin. Am J Respir Crit Care Med. 2015 Feb 15; 191(4):448–54. DOI: 10.1164/rccm.201407-1395OC

[35] Zhu N, Zhang Y, Gong YI, He J, Chen X. Metformin and lung cancer risk of patients with type 2 diabetes mellitus: A meta-analysis. Biomed Rep. 2015 Mar; 3(2):235–41. DOI: 10.3892/br.2015.417

[36] Tosetti F, Ferrari N, De Flora S, Albini A. Angioprevention': Angiogenesis is a common and key target for cancer chemopreventive agents. FASEB J. 2002 Jan; 16(1):2–14. DOI: 10.1096/fj.01-0300rev

[37] Tung YT, Huang PW, Chou YC, Lai CW, Wang HP, Ho HC, et al. Lung tumorigenesis induced by human vascular endothelial growth factor (hVEGF)-A165 overexpression in transgenic mice and amelioration of tumor formation by miR-16. Oncotarget. 2015 Apr 30; 6(12):10222–38. DOI: 10.18632/oncotarget.3390

[38] Shcherbakova DM, Verkhusha VV. Near-infrared fluorescent proteins for multicolor in vivo imaging. Nat Methods. 2013 Aug; 10(8):751–4. DOI: 10.1038/nmeth.2521

[39] Filonov GS, Piatkevich KD, Ting LM, Zhang J, Kim K, Verkhusha VV. Bright and stable near-infrared fluorescent protein for in vivo imaging. Nat Biotechnol. 2011 Aug; 29(8):757–61. DOI: 10.1038/nbt.1918

[40] Lai CW, Chen HL, Yen CC, Wang JL, Yang SH, Chen CM. Using dual fluorescence reporting genes to establish an in vivo imaging model of orthotopic lung adenocarcinoma in mice. Mol Imaging Biol. 2016 Dec; 18(6):849–859. DOI: 10.1007/s11307-016-0967-4

Chapter 10

The Bioenergetic Role of Mitochondria in Lung Cancer

Keely Erin FitzGerald, Purna Chaitanya Konduri,
Chantal Vidal, Hyuntae Yoo and Li Zhang

Additional information is available at the end of the chapter

http://dx.doi.org/10.5772/67238

Abstract

In 1920s, Otto Warburg made the observation that cancer cells utilize significantly more glucose than normal, healthy cells, which led him to believe that cancer cells relied on glycolysis more than healthy cells. However, many subsequent studies have shown that glucose is not only necessary for glycolysis but also for oxidative phosphorylation and production of building blocks for the synthesis of other molecules. There are many challenges associated with studying and treating lung cancer, and there is a diverse set of metabolic factors influencing the tumorigenesis and metastasis of lung cancer. Lung cancer cells rely heavily on mitochondrial respiration, and several studies have shown that inhibiting mitochondrial function is an effective method to combat lung cancer. Several agents have been used to inhibit mitochondrial function, including cyclopamine and metformin. Further, more research has noted increased levels of heme flux and function as critical to intensified oxygen consumption and accompanying amplified pathogenesis and progression of lung cancer. The upregulation of mitochondrial DNA and biogenesis genes are also correlated with lung cancer. In this chapter, we will cover these recent and emerging topics in lung cancer bioenergetics research.

Keywords: heme, mitochondrial respiration, respiration genes, oxidative fuels, glutamine, cyclopamine

1. Introduction

Cells perform a variety of diverse functions and processes, all of which require some form of cellular energy. The general currency of cellular energy exists as adenosine triphosphate, a high energy molecule created by two main bioenergetic pathways: glycolysis and oxidative phosphorylation.

Glycolysis, which translates to "sweet splitting," is the process of breaking down a substrate, usually glucose, through a series of steps to produce two ATP molecules. This process does not require oxygen, and it is sometimes referred to as anaerobic respiration. To begin the process, glucose transporters allow glucose uptake into the cell [1]. Hexokinase then phosphorylates glucose, which becomes glucose-6-phosphate. Glucose-6-phosphate isomerase is an enzyme that catalyzes the reversible isomerization of glucose-6-phosphate and fructose-6-phosphate which follow the pentose phosphate pathway that produces nucleotides and NADPH, or the glycolytic pathway to make lactate. Fructose-6-phosphate undergoes a reaction facilitated by phosphofructokinase-1 to become fructose-1,6 bisphosphate, which then becomes glyceraldehyde-3-phosphate for glycolysis or dihydroxyacetone phosphate to help create lipids. Glyceraldehyde-3-phosphate becomes glycerate-2-phosphate by glyceraldehyde-3-phosphate dehydrogenase. Glycerate-2-phosphate becomes phosphoenol pyruvate via enolase. To produce the two ATP of glycolysis, pyruvate kinase catalyzes the conversion of phosphoenol pyruvate into pyruvate (see **Figure 1**). Finally, pyruvate is converted to lactate, a process which is mediated by the enzyme lactate dehydrogenase-A. This process generates NAD^+ from NADH. The production of NAD^+ allows the process of glycolysis to be cyclical.

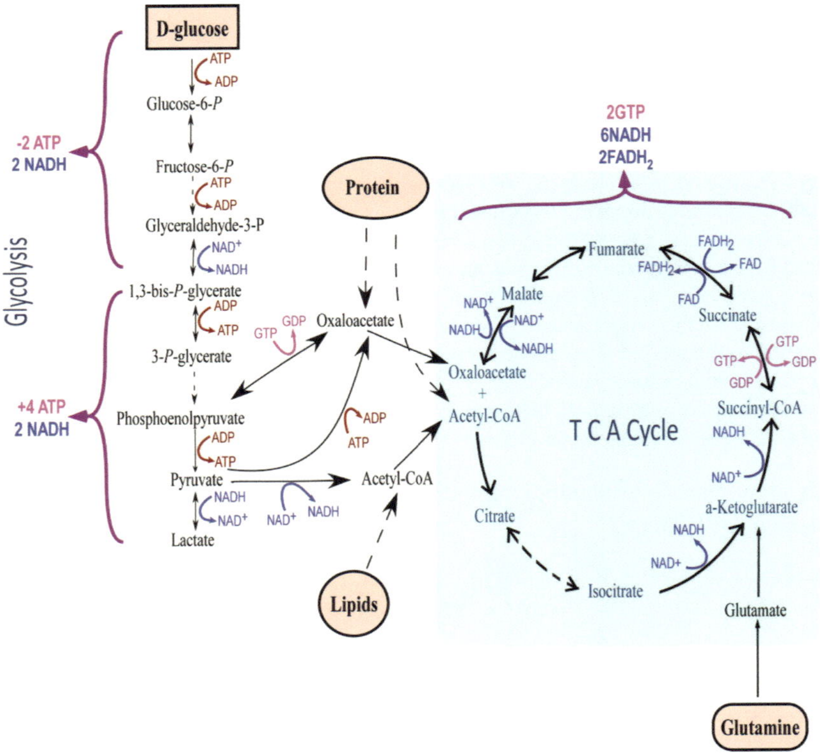

Figure 1. Cells use lipids, glutamine, protein, and glucose in order to gain energy. Many of these substrates, including those produced by glycolysis eventually lead into the tricarboxylic acid (TCA) cycle. The steps involved in ATP synthesis or consumption are marked in red. Those involved in utilization or production of GTP are marked in pink, while NAD^+/NADH and FAD/$FADH_2$ are in blue. The numbers of ATP/GTP and NADH/$FADH_2$ produced by glycolysis and by the tricarboxylic acid cycle are indicated.

Oxidative phosphorylation has many more steps than glycolysis, and it requires oxygen. Oxidative phosphorylation creates significantly more ATP per substrate molecule than does glycolysis. It is a slower process, and it is made possible by mitochondrial respiratory chain complexes.

Mitochondria are the site of oxidative phosphorylation (see **Figure 2**). Mitochondria are present in many diverse types of cells in eukaryotes, and they are capable of producing large quantities of energy. The respiratory chain complexes in mitochondria are responsible for facilitating the reactions associated with oxidative phosphorylation. Consequently, the unique bioenergetics of cancer suggests altered mitochondria. Indeed, some genes have been found to be mutated in mitochondria (see **Figure 2**).

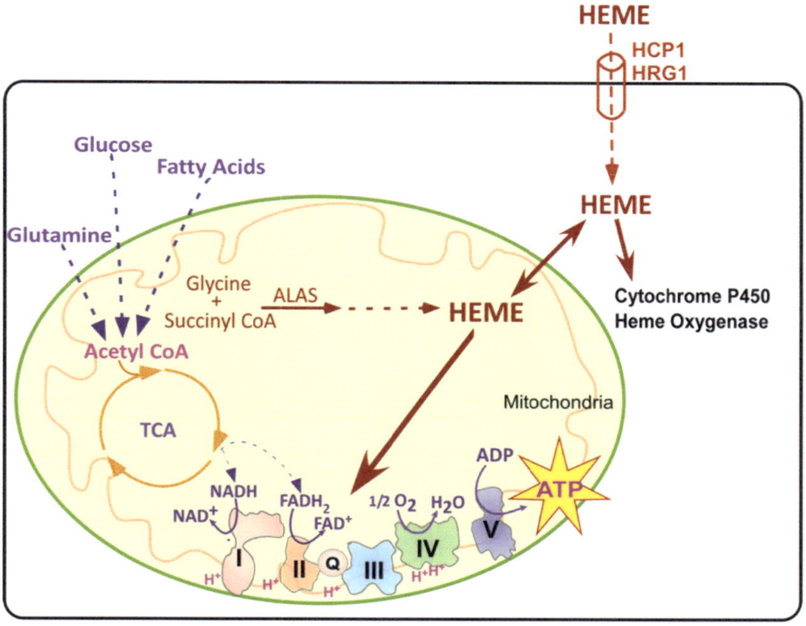

Figure 2. Mitochondrial and heme function in cellular bioenergetics. Bioenergetic fuels, including glucose, glutamine, and fatty acids, can generate metabolites that feed into the tricarboxylic acid (TCA) cycle. Through oxidative phosphorylation, NADH and $FADH_2$ generated from the tricarboxylic acid cycle can be used to generate a large amount of ATP. Heme is a central molecule in mitochondrial function and oxidative phosphorylation. Heme can be taken up from the extracellular space via heme transporters HRG1 and HCP1. Heme is also synthesized in mitochondria in most mammalian cells. Heme serves as a prosthetic group or cofactor for many enzymes in Complexes II–IV. In non-small cell lung cancer cells, it has been shown that heme flux and function are intensified to support enhanced oxidative phosphorylation.

The process of oxidative phosphorylation requires several protein complexes, named Complex I–V, all of which are partly coded by mitochondrial DNA with the exception of Complex II [2]. Within the inner membrane of the mitochondria, there are electron carriers that are critical for mitochondrial respiration. Importantly, up to 2% of electrons cycling through the electron transport chain can escape the process, and this creates reactive oxygen species, or ROS [3]. These ROS can cause significant damage to mitochondrial DNA.

Pyruvate is transported into the mitochondria or transformed into lactate and nicotinamide adenine dinucleotide (NAD) by lactate dehydrogenase (LDH). Direct transport of pyruvate into the mitochondria across the outer mitochondrial membrane, intermembrane space, and inner mitochondrial membrane is facilitated by mitochondrial pyruvate carrier (MPC). Mitochondrial pyruvate carrier also facilitates the removal of hydroxide from the mitochondria. Once within the mitochondrial matrix, pyruvate is converted to acetyl coenzyme A (acetyl CoA) via pyruvate dehydrogenase catalysis. Acetyl CoA enters the tricarboxylic acid cycle, and succinate is formed via organic acid oxidation. NADH contains electrons that go through the electron transport chain (ETC), which consists of mitochondrial Complexes I–IV (see **Figure 2**). Complex I, alternatively called NADH dehydrogenase or NADH ubiquinone oxidoreductase, marks the beginning of the electron transport chain and is also the largest of the five mitochondrial complexes [4]. From Complex I, the electron transport chain brings electrons toward coenzyme Q through the inner mitochondrial membrane. Alternatively, electrons can skip Complex I entirely. The transport of these electrons is mediated by flavin-containing enzyme complexes and they also reach coenzyme Q via this alternative pathway [5]. From coenzyme Q, electrons are transferred to Complex III. Yet another pathway to coenzyme Q is possible via Complex II. Succinate is reduced and the electrons from the reduction of succinate are taken to coenzyme Q and Complex III. Complex III and cytochrome c shift electrons to Complex IV. The movement of electrons over the inner mitochondrial matrix by Complexes I, III, and IV creates a proton gradient. This causes protons to enter the mitochondrial matrix, a process allowed by Complex V, ATP synthase (V), and causes the production of ATP (see **Figure 2**). Taken together, Complexes I–V facilitate oxidative phosphorylation and can create up to 36 mol of ATP per mol glucose. ROS created via oxidative phosphorylation can be used to regenerate NAD^+. It is important to note that many cancer cells prefer glutamine as opposed to glucose [6]. This may be because cancer mimics the effects of starvation on the body. During starvation, the body utilizes amino acids from a pool of amino acids, and then breaks down skeletal muscle to replenish the pool of amino acids. One of the major amino acids consumed in this process is glutamine, the very same amino acid substrate which many cancer cells are remarkably adept at converting for energy. Many glycolytic molecules are considerably upregulated in cancer, including hexokinase II, glucose transporters, pyruvate kinase, and lactate dehydrogenase-A [1]. These molecules serve as targets for chemotherapy drugs. In the same way, many oxidative phosphorylation enzymes and molecules are differentially regulated in cancer.

2. Unique clinical problems of lung cancer

Lung cancer screening with low-dose computer tomography has proven to be effective in significantly reducing mortality of lung cancer patients through detection of nonsymptomatic patients at early stages [7]. These early stage patients are typically treated with surgical or radiological procedures followed by periodical surveillance with radiographic imaging. Although these curative treatments have been successful in saving many of these patients from lung cancer, 30–60% of the patients are predicted to present with local or distant recurrences (mostly within 5 years, but some beyond the first 5 year period) [8]. This is a unique problem for lung cancer that limits overall survival rates in these patients to less than 60% despite early detection, as compared with greater than 95% in the case of early stage prostate or breast cancers [9].

If these patients can be accurately identified at the time of initial treatment, adding appropriate adjuvant therapy to their initial treatment plan may significantly increase their survival rates. However, adjuvant chemotherapy on Stages I–III non-small cell lung cancer (NSCLC) patients showed only marginal 5-year overall survival benefits of less than 6% in meta-analyses of recent clinical trials [10, 11]. Neither epidermal growth factor receptor-targeting therapy nor immunotherapy showed significant benefits in adjuvant settings for early stage NSCLC patients [12, 13]. Thus, no methods are currently available to effectively treat these patients. However, several recent experiments strongly suggest that targeting mitochondria will yield effective strategies to treat lung cancer patients in the future [14–18].

3. Lung cancer cells are extremely susceptible to inhibitors of mitochondria

Several studies have suggested that inhibiting mitochondrial function makes drug-resistant tumors more sensitive to treatment [14–16, 18]. When oxidative phosphorylation was suppressed, cancer became less able to proliferate in an anchorage-independent manner [14]. This drastically limits the tumorigenic capacity of cancer cells. Because mitochondria are crucial for the electron transport chain and therefore oxidative phosphorylation, two processes which are especially prominent in cancer cells, inhibiting mitochondrial function essentially starves the cancer cell of ATP, affecting processes such as growth and metastasis of tumors. However, because healthy cells have drastically lower levels of oxidative phosphorylation and often significantly lower energy requirements, healthy cells are not as strongly impacted as cancer cells and can maintain functionality. Consequently, when the mitochondria of tumor cells are tampered with to inhibit oxidative phosphorylation, these tumor cells become significantly more susceptible to cytotoxic drugs [16, 19]. Agents such as cyclopamine tartrate, a water-soluble derivative of a molecule found in corn lilies [20]; metformin, an antidiabetic drug [18]; BAY 87-2243, a lead structure [15]; and microRNA-126, a microRNA [21] have shown potential to interfere with normal mitochondrial function in cancer cells. These molecules interact with various aspects of mitochondrial function, such as interfering with Hedgehog signaling and inhibiting Complex I. Cyclopamine tartrate functions by inhibiting Hedgehog signaling [20]. Cyclopamine was the first chemical found which effectively inhibited Hedgehog signaling. Cyclopamine tartrate is an analog of cyclopamine, but it is more soluble in water than cyclopamine. The mechanism by which cyclopamine and cyclopamine tartrate work has been studied extensively. Smoothened (SMO) is a G protein-coupled receptor. SMO is responsible for facilitating Hedgehog signaling. Cyclopamine tartrate inhibits SMO, thereby inhibiting Hedgehog signaling. In NSCLC HCC4017 cells, studies have demonstrated intensified oxygen consumption compared to benign HBEC cells from the same patient [20]. Low levels of glucose also contribute to higher oxygen consumption rates, and low levels of glutamine lower oxygen consumption rates. Low levels of glucose also encourage NSCLC cells to utilize glutamine, and low levels of glutamine contribute to increased glucose consumption. Although NSCLC cell lines have varying levels of sensitivity to cyclopamine tartrate, this agent can be used to induce apoptosis by targeting these aerobic respiration pathways. Further, Cyclopamine tartrate helps generate ROS, which disturb the mitochondria in tumor cells. Cyclopamine tartrate can cause mitochondrial fission and fragmentation in several types of NSCLC cells, including H1299, A549, and H460 cells. Consequently, cyclopamine tartrate reduces mitochondrial respiration. Metformin has been used for years to combat Type II diabetes, but as of 2001, scientists were only beginning to take note of the anticancer properties of the drug in mammals [22]. Scientists also noticed that those individuals taking metformin for diabetes had lower overall rates of cancer. Recently, researchers have shed some light onto the mechanism of metformin. Metformin inhibits mitochondrial Complex I by reducing oxygen consumption in the presence of malate and pyruvate, which create NADH as a substrate for Complex I [23]. Metformin has also been reported to interrupt the tricarboxylic acid cycle, the methionine cycle, and the folate cycle, as well as decrease nucleotide synthesis.

4. Enhanced heme function is important for NSCLC cells

Heme, or iron protoporphyrin IX, is notably and inextricably linked with oxygen transport, storage, and utilization. Most mammalian cells can synthesize heme *de novo*. Many cells also uptake heme via heme transporters, such as HRG1 and HCP1. Heme is important for neurogenesis, circadian rhythm, erythroid biogenesis, and pancreatic development and functions as a prosthetic group for hemoglobin, myoglobin, cytochromes, peroxidases, and catalases [24]. Heme directly regulates transcription, cell cycle, cell death, and protein synthesis [25–29]. When heme levels are too low or too high, therefore, many diverse processes are affected. There are several diseases associated with altered heme levels. These include anemia, porphyrias, Alzheimer's disease, Parkinson's disease, Type-2 diabetes, coronary heart disease, and several types of cancer including colorectal, pancreatic, and lung cancers [25, 30].

When levels of heme flux and function are increased, levels of oxygen utilization are also increased. Intensified oxygen consumption allows increased cancer cell proliferation and function [17]. Recent research suggests that non-small cell lung cancer (NSCLC) cells upregulate proteins that stimulate heme synthesis, uptake, and function. When these proteins abound, heme is significantly upregulated, and aids in lung cancer progression. Notably, affected proteins include ALAS, HRG1, HCP1, cytoglobins, and cytochromes [30].

When NSCLC cells were compared to normal cells from the same patient, studies showed that rates of heme biosynthesis were significantly raised in cancerous cells [30]. ALAS1, a rate limiting enzyme in nonerythroid heme synthesis, is higher in NSCLC cells. Succinyl acetone has been used to lower heme levels by inhibiting heme synthesis. Succinyl acetone attacks delta-aminolevulinic acid dehydratase.

5. Mitochondrial respiration and biogenesis genes are upregulated in lung tumor cells

Lung cancer often has a genetic basis. Up to 60% of lung adenocarcinoma tissues have a driver mutation. These genes include Kirsten rat sarcoma viral oncogene (KRAS), epidermal growth factor receptor (EGFR), anaplastic lymphoma kinase (ALK), and proto-oncogene B-Raf (BRAF) [31, 32]. In lung adenocarcinoma, the type of NSCLC most frequently found to plague nonsmokers, smoking causes a very different pathway of tumorigenesis [33]. In nonsmokers, there are four times as many differently expressed genes as in smokers [33]. This is thought to be due to the lung tumor locally evolving in nonsmokers. By contrast, in smokers the lung tumor is thought to evolve from a patch of genetically altered tissue. Furthermore, some of the genes that were found to be upregulated in smokers were upregulated more depending on how frequently the smoker smoked. Malic enzyme (ME) expression is also significantly increased in the lung tissues of smokers compared to nonsmokers [34]. The EGFR pathway is the most common signaling pathway for lung cancer, and the mutation rate of genes of the EGFR pathway reach 70–80% [32]. About 30–35% of lung adenocarcinoma genetic variation is attributable to the KRAS mutation. In NSCLC cells, 97% of KRAS mutations occur in codon 12 or 13, and by testing codon 12 for KRAS mutation in bronchoalveolar lavage, scientists can diagnose lung cancer. Some labs have identified proteins that are overexpressed significantly in lung adenocarcinomas. Particularly, ATP synthase subunit d (ATP5D) is significantly over-expressed in lung adenocarcinomas (tumor: $n = 93$, $1.155 + 0.418$; normal: $n = 10$, $0.663 + 0.210$; p value: <0.0001) [35]. Some common marker genes include neuron-specific enolase, carcinoembryonic antigen, cytokeratin 19 fragments (CYFRA 21-1), squamous cell carcinoma antigen, cancer antigen CA 125, and tissue polypeptide antigen, although no one marker gene is as efficient as multiple marker genes at predicting and diagnosing lung adenocarcinomas. Both ME and ATP-citrase lyase (ACLY) are enzymes related to aerobic glycolysis and fatty acid synthesis. They are both correlated with NSCLC cells, and ACLY tends to be more localized, whereas ME tends to signify mediastinal lymph nodes, a site of metastasis in the human body [34]. Interestingly, in young patients, overexpression of ACLY and/or ME correlated with extended survival compared to patients who did not overexpress ACLY and/or ME. However, in older patients, overexpression of ACLY and/or ME is predictive of shorter period of survival as compared to patients who do not overexpress ACLY and/or ME. It can therefore be inferred that potential rising treatments must take into consideration the age group of the afflicted patient. Mitochondrial respiration genes have also been shown to be upregulated in lung tumor cells. In lung adenocarcinoma, many genes, especially those associated with mitochondrial respiration, have been shown to be differently expressed than in healthy tissue [32]. One study noted 535 upregulated and 465 downregulated differentially expressed genes in lung adenocarcinoma comparing matched tissues of the same patients. One prominent class of upregulated genes is related to mitochondrial oxidative phosphorylation and the electron transport chain. ATP5D, UQCRC2, NDUFA2, NDUFB8, NDUFA7, NDUFA1, NDUFB1, NDUFS7, UQCR11, NDUFV1, NDUFV2, and NDUFS3 are specifically related to bioenergetic pathways including mitochondrial ATP synthesis-coupled electron transport and the electron transport chain [32]. Additionally, genes associated with mitochondrial biogenesis are specifically upregulated in circulating lung cancer cells and have been reported to be essential for their metastatic potential [36]. By studying metastatic cancers, LeBleu et al. investigated the role of peroxisome proliferator-activated receptor gamma, coactivator 1 alpha (PGC-1α) in enhancing metastatic potential by increasing oxygen consumption, mitochondrial biogenesis, and oxidative phosphorylation rates. The effect of PGC-1α on respiration appears to be key to allowing metastasis specifically, and does not appear to strongly affect cancer cell proliferation, epithelial-to-mesenchymal transfer, or primary tumor growth. Activating mutations in Ras guanosine nucleotide-binding proteins result in insensitivity to GTPase-activating proteins [37]. These Ras mutations are common in human cancers [38]. Activated GTP-bound Ras family members increase glucose uptake and flux, which partly promotes the survival and proliferation of lung cancer [37]. This effect is important because it increases the capacity for energy production in lung adenocarcinoma cells. Activated Ras also increases tricarboxylic acid cycle activity and oxygen consumption, which further enables cancerous cells to produce energy and therefore increases carcinogenic and metastatic potential of cancer cells. Cytochrome c oxidase is activated by Ras [39]. Cytochrome c oxidase contains 3 mitochondrial DNA–encoded and 10 genomic DNA–encoded subunits and forms Complex IV of the electron transport chain [40]. In some types of cancer, levels of cytochrome c oxidase are significantly elevated [40, 41]. Without activated cytochrome c oxidase, A549 lung adenocarcinoma is incapable of growth [37]. Still more mutations in nuclear genes affecting mitochondrial form and function have been linked with lung cancer. Succinate dehydrogenase, including SDHB, SDHC, and SDHD genes, and isocitrate dehydrogenase, including IDH1 and IDH2 genes, code for mitochondrial components [42]. By affecting the structure of the mitochondria, these genes affect the function of the mitochondria, and consequently are associated with or considered causal to cancer. Due to the large genetic variation between lung tumor cells, or tumor heterogeneity, chemoresistance is a major problem in lung cancer treatment. Many chemicals which are effective on certain types of lung cancer are not effective on other types of lung cancer. Furthermore, individual tumors possess intratumoral heterogeneity. That is, the tumor has nonidentical cells. Therefore, while some cell types may respond favorably to treatment, other cell types may not. Consequently, over time, these cell types begin to dominate the tumor and the tumor becomes chemoresistant by acquiring genetic and epigenetic changes. This process was first proposed by Nowell as clonal evolution [43]. Understanding tumor heterogeneity and variation among NSCLC categories therefore significantly increases the ability of research to successfully unearth potential treatments and cures for lung cancer.

6. Mitochondrial DNA is correlated with lung cancer

Mitochondrial DNA is especially susceptible to reactive oxygen species because it does not have protective histones and introns [44]. Further, mitochondria lack the capacity to repair damaged mitochondrial DNA. Consequently, mitochondrial DNA mutates more frequently than other genomic DNA [45]. The instability of mitochondrial DNA can have devastating effects on the cell, including mutations and copy number alterations [2]. Both germline and somatic mitochondrial DNA defects are associated with cancer. Mitochondrial DNA is thought to be able to function as a driver or as a complementary gene mutation of carcinogenesis according to the multiple-hit model, thereby allowing increased clonogenic and/or mutagenic capacities in cancer cells [2]. To combat these mutations, mitochondria increase their copy number drastically. Some studies suggest that the number of copies of mitochondrial DNA is strongly correlated with carcinogenesis [44, 46]. This relationship has been supported by several other labs [47, 48]. This relationship has been especially noted in lung adenocarcinoma. It is important to note that some diseases have a causal effect with cancer, and may also increase mitochondrial DNA copy number. To overcome this bias due to a latent disease, mitochondrial DNA was measured in peripheral white blood cells. The results suggested that even in the absence of a causal disease, increased copy number is indicative of an increased risk of lung cancer [44]. Importantly, this connection does not hold true for all types of cancer [47, 48]. Some cancers express lower mitochondrial copy numbers. However, in lung adenocarcinoma, the mitochondrial copy number is increased compared to controls. There is also a strong correlation between mitochondrial DNA copy number and TFAM (Transcriptional Factor A, Mitochondria) expression [48]. TFAM is a factor for transcription and replication and in nucleoids. TFAM binds to mitochondrial DNA. Significantly, the gene set responsible for controlling the tricarboxylic acid cycle and respiratory electron transport is most commonly correlated to copy number. In NSCLC cells, epithelial-to-mesenchymal transition is thought to be the critical moment defining metastatic potential [49]. It is thought that during epithelial-to-mesenchymal transition, the copy number of mitochondrial DNA is altered. In A549 cells, copy number increased from 1700 to 2800 during epithelial-to-mesenchymal transition.

7. Stromal cells in the tumor microenvironment contribute bioenergetic molecules to cancer cells

Despite the deregulation of normal metabolic processes in tumor cells and the many contributors to mitochondrial dysfunction, tumors still have remarkable capacity to perform oxidative phosphorylation. This is in part due to a phenomenon where surrounding tissues contribute fuel sources to tumor tissues [50]. A two-compartment model was proposed in 2012 to explain this process [51–53]. Glycolytic stromal cells produce L-lactate and ketone bodies which are utilized by oxidative epithelial cancer cells. The metabolites produced by these fibroblasts (see **Figure 3**) provide fuel for cancer proliferation via oxidative phosphorylation [54]. This process is thought to be mediated by pyruvate kinase isoforms. Glutamine helps to fuel this process [55–57]. It appears as though the tumor cells take advantage of the stromal cells in a form of micro-level commensalism [52].

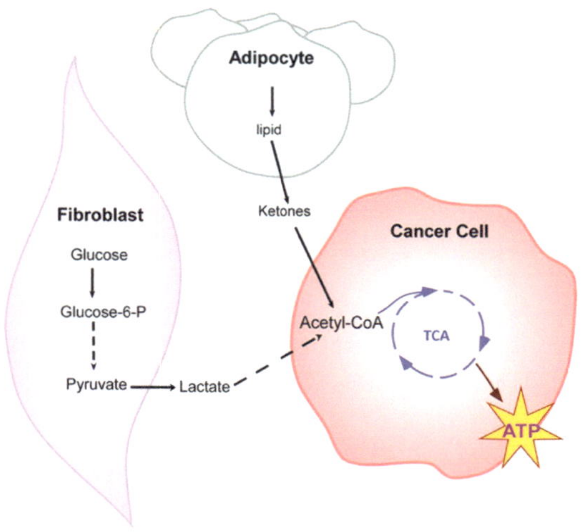

Figure 3. Metabolic fuels for tumor cells. Cancer cells use a variety of bioenergetic substrates including glucose, glutamine, fatty acids, and ketones. Stromal cells in the tumor microenvironment can provide various oxidative fuels depending on their characteristics. Shown here are adipocytes and fibroblasts.

8. Summary

Emerging evidence increasingly shows that mitochondrial respiration is key to cancer bioenergetics. Particularly, heme is a central molecule in mitochondrial respiration. Many lines of evidence from epidemiological studies, gene expression studies of human tumor tissues, and molecular studies of cancer cell lines indicate that functions of heme and oxygen-utilizing hemoproteins are critical for tumorigenesis, particularly lung tumorigenesis. Enhanced heme flux and function is a key feature of non-small cell lung cancer cells. Consistent with these observations, many cancer cells are susceptible to inhibitors of mitochondrial function and heme biosynthesis. A better understanding of the relationships between mitochondrial and heme function with cancer bioenergetics should facilitate the development of effective strategies to treat cancers, particularly lung cancer.

Acknowledgements

Work on lung cancer in Dr. Li Zhang's lab is funded by the CPRIT Grant and the Cecil H and Ida Green Funds from the University of Texas at Dallas.

Author details

Keely Erin FitzGerald, Purna Chaitanya Konduri, Chantal Vidal, Hyuntae Yoo and Li Zhang*

*Address all correspondence to: li.zhang@utdallas.edu

Department of Biological Sciences, Center for Systems Biology, University of Texas at Dallas, Richardson, TX, USA

References

[1] Zhang, Y. and J.M. Yang, Altered energy metabolism in cancer: a unique opportunity for therapeutic intervention. Cancer Biol Ther, 2013. **14**(2): pp. 81–9.

[2] Van Gisbergen, M.W., et al., How do changes in the mtDNA and mitochondrial dysfunction influence cancer and cancer therapy? Challenges, opportunities and models. Mutat Res Rev Mutat Res, 2015. **764**: pp. 16–30.

[3] St-Pierre, J., et al., Topology of superoxide production from different sites in the mitochondrial electron transport chain. J Biol Chem, 2002. **277**(47): pp. 44784–90.

[4] Voets, A.M., et al., Transcriptional changes in OXPHOS complex I deficiency are related to anti-oxidant pathways and could explain the disturbed calcium homeostasis. Biochim Biophys Acta, 2012. **1822**(7): pp. 1161–8.

[5] Smeitin, J., The genetics and pathology of oxidative phosphorylation. Nat Rev, 2001. **2(5): pp. 342–52.**

[6] van den Heuvel, A.P., et al., Analysis of glutamine dependency in non-small cell lung cancer: GLS1 splice variant GAC is essential for cancer cell growth. Cancer Biol Ther, 2012. **13**(12): pp. 1185–94.

[7] National Lung Screening Trial Research Team, et al., Reduced lung-cancer mortality with low-dose computed tomographic screening. N Engl J Med, 2011. **365**(5): pp. 395–409.

[8] Demicheli, R., et al., Recurrence dynamics for non-small-cell lung cancer: effect of surgery on the development of metastases. J Thorac Oncol, 2012. **7**(4): pp. 723–30.

[9] Siegel, R.L., K.D. Miller, and A. Jemal, Cancer statistics, 2015. CA Cancer J Clin, 2015. **65**(1): pp. 5–29.

[10] Burdett, S., et al., Adjuvant chemotherapy for resected early-stage non-small cell lung cancer. Cochrane Database Syst Rev, 2015. **3**: pp. CD011430.

[11] Pignon, J.P., et al., Lung adjuvant cisplatin evaluation: a pooled analysis by the LACE Collaborative Group. J Clin Oncol, 2008. **26**(21): pp. 3552–9.

[12] Kelly, K., et al., Adjuvant erlotinib versus placebo in patients with stage IB-IIIA non-small-cell lung cancer (RADIANT): a randomized, double-blind. Phase III Trial J Clin Oncol, 2015. **33**(34): pp. 4007–14.

[13] Pujol, J.L., et al., Safety and immunogenicity of MAGE-A3 cancer immunotherapeutic with or without adjuvant chemotherapy in patients with resected stage IB to III MAGE-A3-positive non-small-cell lung cancer. J Thorac Oncol, 2015. **10**(10): pp. 1458–67.

[14] Viale, A., D. Corti, and G.F. Draetta, Tumors and mitochondrial respiration: a neglected connection. Cancer Res, 2015. **75**(18): pp. 3685–6.

[15] Ellinghaus, P., et al., BAY 87-2243, a highly potent and selective inhibitor of hypoxia-induced gene activation has antitumor activities by inhibition of mitochondrial complex I. Cancer Med, 2013. **2**(5): pp. 611–24.

[16] Cavelli, L.R., Diminished tumorigenic phenotype after deplition of mitochondrial DNA. Cell Growth Differ, 1997. **8**: pp. 1189–98.

[17] Alam, M.M., et al., A holistic view of cancer bioenergetics: mitochondrial function and respiration play fundamental roles in the development and progression of diverse tumors. Clin Transl Med, 2016. **5**(1): pp. 3.

[18] Luengo, A., Understanding the complex-I-ty of metformin action: limiting mitochondrial respiration to improve cancer therapy. BMC Biol, 2014.

[19] Gao, C., et al., Cancer stem cells in small cell lung cancer cell line H446: higher dependency on oxidative phosphorylation and mitochondrial substrate-level phosphorylation than non-stem cancer cells. PLoS One, 2016. **11**(5): pp. e0154576.

[20] Alam, M.M., et al., Cyclopamine tartrate, an inhibitor of hedgehog signaling, strongly interferes with mitochondrial function and suppresses aerobic respiration in lung cancer cells. BMC Cancer, 2016. **16**: pp. 150.

[21] Tomasetti, M., et al., MicroRNA-126 suppresses mesothelioma malignancy by targeting IRS1 and interfering with the mitochondrial function. Antioxid Redox Signal, 2014. **21**(15): pp. 2109–25.

[22] Jara, J.A. and R. Lopez-Munoz, Metformin and cancer: between the bioenergetic disturbances and the antifolate activity. Pharmacol Res, 2015. **101**: pp. 102–8.

[23] Kuhn, K.S., et al., Glutamine as indispensable nutrient in oncology: experimental and clinical evidence. Eur J Nutr, 2010. **49**(4): pp. 197–210.

[24] Hooda, J., et al., Evaluating the association of heme and heme metabolites with lung cancer bioenergetics and progression. Metabolomics, 2015. **5**(3): pp. 150.

[25] Hooda, J., A. Shah, and L. Zhang, Heme, an essential nutrient from dietary proteins, critically impacts diverse physiological and pathological processes. Nutrients, 2014. **6**(3): pp. 1080–102.

[26] Zhu, Y., T. Hon, and L. Zhang, Heme initiates changes in the expression of a wide array of genes during the early erythroid differentiation stage. Biochem Biophys Res Commun, 1999. **258**(1): pp. 87–93.

[27] Ye, W. and L. Zhang, Heme controls the expression of cell cycle regulators and cell growth in HeLa cells. Biochem Biophys Res Commun, 2004. **315**(3): pp. 546–54.

[28] Yao, X., et al., Heme controls the regulation of protein tyrosine kinases Jak2 and Src. Biochem Biophys Res Commun, 2010. **403**(1): pp. 30–5.

[29] Chen, J.J., Regulation of protein synthesis by the heme-regulated eIF2α kinase: relevance to anemias. Blood, 2007. **109**(7): pp. 2693–9.

[30] Hooda, J., et al., Enhanced heme function and mitochondrial respiration promote the progression of lung cancer cells. PLoS One, 2013. **8**(5): pp. e63402.

[31] Kris, M.G., Identification of driver mutations in tumor specimens from 1000 patients with lung adenocarcinoma: the NCI's Lung Cancer Mutation Consortium (LCMC). J Clin Oncol, 2011. **29(15_suppl): pp. CRA7506.**

[32] Xu, H., et al., Gene expression profiling analysis of lung adenocarcinoma. Braz J Med Biol Res, 2016. **49(3): pp. e4861.**

[33] Powell, C.A., et al., Gene expression in lung adenocarcinomas of smokers and nonsmokers. Am J Respir Cell Mol Biol, 2003. **29**(2): pp. 157–62.

[34] Csanadi, A., et al., Prognostic value of malic enzyme and ATP-citrate lyase in non-small cell lung cancer of the young and the elderly. PLoS One, 2015. **10**(5): pp. e0126357.

[35] Chen, G., Proteomic analysis of lung adenocarcinoma: identification of a highly expressed set of proteins in tumors. Clin Cancer Res, 2002. **8**: pp. 2298–305.

[36] LeBleu, V.S., et al., PGC-1 alpha mediates mitochondrial biogenesis and oxidative phosphorylation in cancer cells to promote metastasis. Nat Cell Biol, 2014. **16**(10): pp. 992–1003, 1–15.

[37] Telang, S, Cytochrome c oxidase is activated by the oncoprotein Ras and is required for A549 lung adenocarcinoma growth. Mol Cancer, 2012.

[38] Minamoto, T., M. Mai, and Z. Ronai, K-ras mutation: early detection in molecular diagnosis and risk assessment of colorectal, pancreas, and lung cancers—a review. Cancer Detect Prev, 2000. **24**(1): pp. 1–12.

[39] Dejean, L., et al., Activation of Ras cascade increases the mitochondrial enzyme content of respiratory competent yeast. Biochem Biophys Res Commun, 2002. **293**(5): pp. 1383–8.

[40] Kadenbach, B., et al., Mitochondrial energy metabolism is regulated via nuclear-coded subunits of cytochrome c oxidase. Free Radic Biol Med, 2000. **29**(3–4): pp. 211–21.

[41] Wang, Z., et al., Cyclin B1/Cdk1 coordinates mitochondrial respiration for cell-cycle G2/M progression. Dev Cell, 2014. **29**(2): pp. 217–32.

[42] Sequist, L.V., et al., Implementing multiplexed genotyping of non-small-cell lung cancers into routine clinical practice. Ann Oncol, 2011. **22**(12): pp. 2616–24.

[43] Nowell, P.C., The clonal evolution of tumor cell populations. Science, 1976. **194**(4260): pp. 23–8.

[44] Hosgood, H.D. et al., Mitochondrial DNA copy number and lung cancer risk in a prospective cohort study. Carcinogenesis, 2010. **31**(5): pp. 847–9.

[45] Wallace, D.C., Mitochondrial DNA sequence variation in human evolution and disease. Proc Natl Acad Sci U S A, 1994. **91**(19): pp. 8739–46.

[46] Akgul, E.O., et al., MtDNA depletions and deletions may also be important in pathogenesis of lung cancer. Respir Med, 2013. **107**(11): pp. 1814.

[47] Mi, J., et al., The relationship between altered mitochondrial DNA copy number and cancer risk: a meta-analysis. Sci Rep, 2015. **5**: pp. 10039.

[48] Reznik, E., et al., Mitochondrial DNA copy number variation across human cancers. Elife, 2016. **5: pp. e10769.**

[49] Xie, M., et al., Activation of notch-1 enhances epithelial-mesenchymal transition in gefitinib-acquired resistant lung cancer cells. J Cell Biochem, 2012. **113**(5): pp. 1501–13.

[50] Galluzzi, L., et al., Metabolic targets for cancer therapy. Nat Rev Drug Discov, 2013. **12**(11): pp. 829–46.

[51] Salem, A.F., et al., Two-compartment tumor metabolism: autophagy in the tumor microenvironment and oxidative mitochondrial metabolism (OXPHOS) in cancer cells. Cell Cycle, 2012. **11**(13): pp. 2545–56.

[52] Icard, P., et al., The metabolic cooperation between cells in solid cancer tumors. Biochim Biophys Acta, 2014. **1846**(1): pp. 216–25.

[53] Martinez-Outschoorn, U.E., M.P. Lisanti, and F. Sotgia, Catabolic cancer-associated fibroblasts transfer energy and biomass to anabolic cancer cells, fueling tumor growth. Semin Cancer Biol, 2014. **25**: pp. 47–60.

[54] Sotgia, F., et al., Mitochondrial metabolism in cancer metastasis: visualizing tumor cell mitochondria and the "reverse Warburg effect" in positive lymph node tissue. Cell Cycle, 2012. **11**(7): pp. 1445–54.

[55] DeBerardinis, R.J. and T. Cheng, Q's next: the diverse functions of glutamine in metabolism, cell biology and cancer. Oncogene, 2010. **29**(3): pp. 313–24.

[56] Fan, J., et al., Glutamine-driven oxidative phosphorylation is a major ATP source in transformed mammalian cells in both normoxia and hypoxia. Mol Syst Biol, 2013. **9**: pp. 712.

[57] Whitaker-Menezes, D., et al., Evidence for a stromal-epithelial "lactate shuttle" in human tumors: MCT4 is a marker of oxidative stress in cancer-associated fibroblasts. Cell Cycle, 2011. **10**(11): pp. 1772–83.

Chapter 11

Long Non-Coding RNA in Non-Small Cell Lung Cancers

Zule Cheng and Hongju Mao

Additional information is available at the end of the chapter

http://dx.doi.org/10.5772/66487

Abstract

Non-small cell lung cancer (NSCLC) accounts for nearly 80% of diagnosed lung cancers. Due to the predominantly late diagnosis of NSCLC and drug resistance in the targeted therapy approaches, the 5-year overall survival rate is still less than 19%. Thus, novel diagnosis and treatment approaches are needed. Many efforts have been made to achieve great progress in understanding the genomic landscape of NSCLC and the molecular mechanisms involved in tumorigenesis. Long non-coding RNAs (lncRNAs) are transcripts longer than 200 nucleotides with little or no protein-coding potential. They are encoded across the genome and are involved in a wide range of cellular and biological processes. Dysregulation of lncRNAs is associated with a number of cancer-related processes, including epigenetic regulation, microRNA silencing, and DNA damage. Furthermore, lncRNAs have been reported to have the potential as biomarker for diagnosis and prognosis, as well as the therapy targets. Here in this chapter, we review some well-characterized lncRNAs associated with NSCLCs and the potential of lncRNAs as biomarkers in the diagnosis and prognosis of NSCLCs.

Keywords: NSCLC, lncRNA, diagnosis, prognosis, epigenetic

1. Introduction

Lung cancer is the leading cause of cancer-related deaths worldwide. According to the estimation of National Cancer Institute, USA, the estimated new cases for lung cancer in 2016 will be 224,390, accounting 13.3% of all new cancer cases, and the estimated deaths of lung cancer in 2016 will be 158,080 accounting 26.5% of all new cancer cases [1]. Non-small cell lung cancer (NSCLC) is the most common type of lung cancer which accounts for nearly 80–85% of diagnosed lung cancers [2]. NSCLC can be further histologically classified into three major subtypes: lung adenocarcinoma (ADC), lung squamous cell carcinoma (SCC), and large cell carcinoma. Much attention has been paid to the clinical diagnosis and treatment of NSCLC, however, the 5-year overall survival rate of NSCLC is still less than 19% in these days [1]. This may attribute to the advanced stage of the disease at the time of diagnosis for many patients. The predominantly late diagnosis of NSCLC has limited the therapy options. The low-dose computed tomography (CT) scan can detect NSCLC early and has become the dominant detection approach. However, the high cost and the risk of false positive has overshadowed the benefits of swift diagnosis [3]. Thus, it is important to develop novel early detection approach with high sensitivity and specificity.

Biomarker is a powerful approach for cancer detection and treatment. It is defined as an indicator of biologic processes, pathogenic processes, or pharmacologic responses to therapeutic interventions. Traditional protein biomarkers such as CEA, SSC, CY211, and CA125 are classic tumour biomarkers commonly used in the diagnoses of NSCLC patients [4]. However, the current lack of diagnostic sensitivity and specificity has limited their usefulness in early detection of NSCLC. The occurrence of NSCLC always comes with the genetic changes. A thorough understanding of the genetic aberrations that contribute to NSCLC would assist in identifying biomarkers that could aid in earlier diagnoses and serve as drug targets, thus increasing treatment efficacy. Considerable efforts have been made to achieve great progress in understanding genomic landscape of NSCLC and the molecular mechanisms involved in tumorigenesis, several cancer-related genes such as TP53, EGFR, and KRAS, have been identified which play a vital role in cancer-related pathways [5–7]. Identification and characterization of specific driver mutations has transformed the diagnosis and treatment of NSCLC.

With the development of sequencing technology and bioinformatics databases, researchers have identified that more than 90% of genome is transcribed; of these transcripts, most are non-coding RNAs with little or no protein-coding potentials [8]. The enormous number and complex kinds of non-coding RNAs have drawn peoples' attention to their roles in biological processes. MicroRNA (miRNA) is a well-studied small non-coding RNA of 18–25 nucleotides [9]. The functions of miRNAs can be summarized as mediating gene silencing by interfering with translational process or inducing mRNA degradation [10, 11]. miRNAs can be classified into oncomiRNAs and tumour suppressor miRNAs in relation to their function in carcinogenic processes; meanwhile, some of them show both oncogenic and suppressive activities under different situations [12]. Another advantage for miRNAs is their high stability and easy detection in tissue and blood [13, 14]. Several studies have reported the deregulation of various miRNAs in NSCLC [13, 15]. Screening studies have uncovered the potential of miRNAs as biomarkers in the diagnosis and prognosis of NSCLC [16, 17]. As the researches for novel biomarkers and therapy targets go further, another class of non-coding RNA molecules, long non-coding RNAs (lncRNAs) with longer length and more complex biological functions have drawn people's attentions and become a new star in the RNA world.

2. Long non-coding RNAs in non-small cell lung cancer

2.1. Long non-coding RNAs

The development of microarray and high-throughput sequencing technologies have enabled us to explore the RNA world. As the understanding of the heterogeneous RNA molecules goes deeper, the functional RNA molecules gain increasing attention again, among these, lncRNAs play a major role in the centre stage. Long non-coding RNAs can be loosely defined as a class of non-coding RNA, which are longer than 200 nucleotides. Different from the small non-coding RNAs, although lncRNAs have little or no protein coding potentials, several common features are still shared with mRNAs. Most of the lncRNAs are transcribed by RNA polymerase II, subsequent post-transcriptional processing including alternative splicing, 5′-capping, and polyadenylation are prevalently found in many lncRNAs [18]. Like mRNAs, the expression of lncRNAs is also under the regulation of transcriptional and epigenetic factors. Active or repressive histone marks that indicate the transcription status can also be found around the transcription start site of the lncRNAs [19]. On the other hand, lncRNAs have their own characters. LncRNAs have shorter median transcript length (2453 nucleotides for mRNAs and 592 nucleotides for lncRNAs) and less median exons number (8 exons for mRNAs and 3 exons for lncRNAs) than mRNAs [18]. Most lncRNAs are located in the nucleus, as most of them are functioned as regulation factors. The expression level of lncRNAs is always lower in cells than mRNAs, but with higher tissue specificities [18]. On the epigenetic level, the transcription start sites of lncRNAs have a higher density of DNA methylation compare with the mRNAs, however, this high methylation density is independent of their expression status [19].

The various features associated with mRNAs imply the complex origin and functions of lncRNAs. Study on the origin of lncRNAs are relatively scant, several hypotheses of the emergence of lncRNAs have been put forward. Some lncRNAs, such as *Xist* lncRNA, are believed to originate by undergoing a metamorphosis from erstwhile protein-coding gene while incorporating transposable sequence [20]. Other studies report the lncRNA can also originate from chromosome's rearrangement, duplication of a non-coding gene by retrotransposition, neighbouring repeat, or transposable elements insertion [21, 22]. Along with the complex originations, lncRNAs also have heterogeneous groups with multiple classifications. The most prevalent classification method is based on the genomic location and context. According to this method, lncRNAs can be defined as: (1) sense lncRNAs; (2) antisense lncRNAs that are transcribed from the sense or antisense strands, respectively, overlapping one or more exons of protein-coding gene on the same or opposite strand; (3) bidirectional lncRNAs, whose transcription and neighbouring coding transcript on the opposite strand is initiated in close genomic proximity; (4) intronic lncRNA that are transcribed entirely from introns of protein-coding genes; (5) intergenic lncRNA that lies within the genomic interval between two genes [20, 23, 24]. Functions of lncRNAs may differ from each category. In general, through molecular mechanisms like signalling, decoying, guiding, and scaffolding [25], lncRNAs are widely involved in gene progresses like chromatin modification, transcriptional regulation, and post-transcriptional regulation [26–29]. As the exploration of lncRNAs goes further, growing evidences demonstrate that lncRNAs play important roles in various cellular processes [25, 30, 31]. Studies have identified the aberrant expression of lncRNAs in various cancers [32, 33] including non-small cell lung cancer [34]. The deregulation of some specific functional lncRNAs is proved to be important drivers implicated in tumour initialization and malignant transformation. Thus, lncRNAs have the potential as cancer biomarkers in the diagnosis and prognosis, as well as the targets for cancer therapy.

2.2. Functional lncRNAs in NSCLC

According to the current version of GENCODE (encyclopaedia of genes and gene variants), 15,767 long non-coding RNA genes encoding 27,692 long non-coding loci RNA have been identified based on manual curation, computational analysis, and experimental validation [35]. Along with it is the plethora of deregulated lncRNAs that are found in plenty of high-throughput lncRNA screen works. However, compared with the numerous screened lncRNAs, only few lncRNAs are well characterized and validated, the roles of most deregulated lncRNAs in diseases still remained unknown, and the data on the mechanism are scarce. In this section, some well characterized lncRNAs with reported deregulation and associated pathophysiological functions in NSCLC are reviewed.

2.2.1. HOX transcript antisense RNA (HOTAIR)

HOX transcript antisense RNA (HOTAIR) is a 2158 bps long antisense lncRNA transcribed from human HOXC locus in chromosome 12q13 [36]. As one of the most well-studied lncRNA implicated in cancer, HOTAIR is mainly involved in the epigenetic regulation as a molecular scaffold. HOTAIR can interact with polycomb repressive complex 2 (PRC2) and lysine-specific demethylase 1 (LSD1) in its 5′- and 3′-domain, respectively, and recruits PCR2 and LSD1 to the HOXD locus located on chromosome 2, inducing H3K27 methylation and H3K4 demethylation, thus silences a gene cluster involved in metastasis suppression.

HOTAIR was first reported to be highly overexpressed in primary breast cancer and metastatic breast cancer tissues. The high expression level of HOTAIR in breast cancer was closely associated with the metastasis [37]. A further study in the breast carcinoma cells showed that the enforced overexpression of HOTAIR led to the methylation of H3K27 [37]. Other researches also reported the up-regulated HORAIR as a negative prognostic predictor in hepatocellular carcinoma [38], colorectal carcinoma [39], pancreatic cancer [40], oesophageal carcinoma [41], lung cancer [42], and gastric cancer [43, 44]. In gastric cancer, HOTAIR was also reported as an endogenous sponge of miR-331-3p, thus abolishing repression of target gene HER2 [44].

In non-small cell lung cancer, Liu et al. analysed the HOTAIR expression level in 42 NSCLC tissues and 4 NSCLC cell lines and reported the high expression of HOTAIR in both NSCLC samples and cell lines compared with corresponding normal counterparts. Results showed that high expression level of HOTAIR was correlated with advanced disease stage, metastasis, and short disease free interval. Furthermore, knockdown of HOTAIR decreased the migration and invasion of NSCLC cells *in vitro* and impeded cell metastasis *in vivo*, without altering cell vitality, which suggests a potential therapeutic role of lncRNA targeted therapies [42]. Nakagawa et al. examined the expression of HOTAIR in 77 NSCLCs and 6 brain metastases. They confirmed the negative prognostic effects of HOTAIR high expression and pointed out the overexpression of HOTAIR enhanced the invasion of NSCLC cells [45]. In lung adenocarcinoma (ADC) cells, the upregulation of HOTAIR contributed to the cisplatin resistance of ADC cells through the regulation of p21 expression, and a silence of HOTAIR resulted in the increase of chemosensitivity, which further led to the inhibition of cell proliferation, induction of G0/G1 cell-cycle arrest and enhancement of apoptosis [46]. Another study of lung ADC found that HOTAIR was an important mediator for the ratio of FOXA1 and FOXA2, which might infect the migration and invasion [47]. A tumour micro-environment study performed in a type I collagen (Col-1) supplemented three-dimensional organotypic culture model found that the expression of HOTAIR could be upregulated by the tumour-promoting Col-1 in lung cancer cells. This finding provided a deeper insight into the mechanism of HOTAIR regulation [48].

In summary, various studies have worked on illuminating the mechanism of HOTAIR deregulation and function in NSCLCs. HOTAIR is widely involved in the chromatin modifications, and can also interact with various molecules like miRNAs and proteins. Although the facts that HOTAIR promotes cancer progress and drug resistance in NSCLC cells have been revealed, there are still many unclarified details in the mechanisms. Hence, more analyses on HOTAIR regulation and modes of action are needed.

2.2.2. Metastasis-associated lung adenocarcinoma transcript 1 (MALAT1)

Metastasis-associated lung adenocarcinoma transcript 1 (MALAT1), also known as nuclear-enriched abundant transcript 2 (NEAT2), is an 8 kbs nuclear lncRNA expressed in chromosome 11q13 [49]. The mature MALAT1 transcript is generated through the procession by RNase P and RNase Z from the primary transcript [50]. MALAT1 is located in the nuclear speckles, and is mainly involved in alternative splicing process [51, 52]. MALAT1 exists widely and conservatively in lung, pancreas, and other healthy organs, the abundant amount of MALAT1 in these organs suggests significant functions for MALAT1 [49].

As one of the earliest identified cancer-associated lncRNAs, MALAT1 was firstly regarded as a high-risk predictor for metastasis in early stage NSCLC patients [49]. Since then, accumulating evidences confirmed the negative prognostic factor of MALAT1 in various cancers. Overexpression of MALAT1 was identified in pancreatic cancers and colorectal cancers, the high expression level was correlated with clinical progression and poor prognosis [53, 54]. Upregulation of MALAT1 was reported to promote the proliferation and metastasis of osteosarcoma and gallbladder cancer via different pathways such as PI3K/AKT and ERK/MAPK pathways [55, 56]. In oesophageal squamous cell carcinoma, silencing the MALAT1 expression resulted in the inhabitation of proliferation, migration, and invasion [57, 58]. Other studies also reported the deregulation of MALAT1 in bladder cancer and renal cancers [59, 60].

High expression of MALAT1 was identified in both early stage lung adenocarcinomas and squamous cell lung cancers [49, 61]. The overexpression of MALAT1 in NSCLC was reported to be associated with poor prognosis, shorter overall survival, and metastasis development. An RNAi-mediated suppression of MALAT1 performed in A549 cells led to the suppression of cell migration and clonogenic growth. Reversely, enforced upregulation of MALAT1 resulted in an increased NSCLC cell growth and colony formation *in vitro* [61]. In a later study, a highly efficient knockdown of MALAT1 in a NSCLC cell line, through zinc finger nuclease-based technique, confirmed the MALAT1 positive influence on the cell metastasis *in vitro* and *in vivo* without affecting cell proliferation. Furthermore, blocking MALAT1 by antisense oligonucleotides (ASO) prevented the tumour metastasis formation in a tumour implanted mouse xenograft module, which provides a potential therapeutic approach to prevent lung cancer metastasis [62].

Numbers of studies have been performed on elucidating the mechanism of MALAT1 regulation. Alternative splicing is one of the major topics in the MALAT1 functions. One example was that MALAT1 could interact with some alternative splicing factors such as Serine/Arginine (SR) proteins, thus affected the gene expression [52]. Another example in human diploid fibroblasts cell lines demonstrated the depletion of MALAT1 might led to the aberrant alternative splicing of the pre-mRNA of oncogenic transcription factor B-MYB, thus reduced the expression of it [63]. Another major topic is the gene expression regulation. MALAT1 displayed a strong association with genes involved in cellular growth, movement, proliferation, signalling, and immune regulation [61]. In lung cancer, MALAT1 could activate the expression of some metastasis-associated genes without affecting the alternative splicing [62]. A study involved in the epigenetic field reported that MALAT1 could interact with demethylated Polycomb 2 protein (Pc2), and controlled the re-localization of growth control genes between polycomb bodies and interchromatin granules [64].

In summary, the poor prognostic role and multiple functions of MALAT1 indicate its potential as predictable biomarker and therapy target. However, detailed studies are still needed as the mechanisms of MALAT1 regulation differ in various situations.

2.2.3. H19

H19 is a paternally imprinted and maternally expressed gene localized on human chromosome 11p15 [65]. Beside the H19 transcripts, the H19 locus also harbours miR-675, an antisense transcript, and an antisense protein-encoding transcript [66]. H19 was first reported as a tumour suppressor gene in mice [65]. However, later studies point out the oncogenic potential of H19.

Loss of imprinting (LOI) in paternal allele and the resulting overexpression of H19 was found in various cancers including lung cancer [67], oesophagus cancer [68], osteosarcoma [69], and bladder cancer [70]. H19 upregulation was found related to a range of risk factors such as smoking, carcinogens exposuring, and hypoxia. Cigarette smoking could induce a LOI-independent upregulation of H19 by activating the H19 maternal allele [71]. This observation was also confirmed in a later *in vitro* study, which reported the increased expression of H19 in human respiratory epithelial cells treated with cigarette smoking condensate [72]. Hypoxia could also induce upregulation of H19 in cell lines with mutated p53, through a critical factor HIF1-alpha [73]. H19 was also directly induced by MYC oncogene in different cell types including fibroblast cells. A study demonstrated that c-Myc selectively increased H19 transcription from the maternally derived allele, and downregulated the reciprocally imprinted gene insulin-like growth factor 2 (IGF2) at the H19/IGF2 locus. This study indicated that c-Myc and H19 expression had strong association in lung carcinomas [74]. The mineral dust-induced gene (MDIG) could conduct the demethylation of H3K9me3 in the promoter region of H19 and activate the H19 expression. High expression of MDIG and H19 were found correlated with poorer survival of the lung cancer patients [75].

In NSCLC, the expression levels of lncRNA H19 in tissues and cells were significantly higher than adjacent tissues and normal cells, overexpression and knockdown of c-Myc could change the H19 expression level significantly. Moreover the higher expression of H19 was positively correlated with advanced tumour-node-metastasis (TNM) stage and tumour size [76].

In summary, the expression level of H19 is related to many risk factors including smoking, which is an important lung cancer factor. Overexpression of H19 may contribute to the cell proliferative in many cancers and is associated with poor prognosis. Since the deregulation of H19 expression may occur from different mechanism, future studies should focus on the different functions of H19 in physiological and pathological processes and evaluate the potential of H19 as biomarkers and therapy targets under different situations.

2.2.4. Cancer-associated region long non-coding RNA 5 (CARLo-5)

LncRNAs cancer-associated region long non-coding RNA 5 (CARLo-5) is transcribed from the (−) strand of the 8q24.21 genomic region, where two other transcripts, sharing significant overlap in their sequences, colon cancer-associated transcript 1 (CCAT1) and CCAT1 long isoform (CCAT1-L) are also transcribed [66].

CARLo-5 was originally reported to be overexpressed in colorectal cancer patient tissues [77]. Later study revealed the overexpression of CARLo-5 in NSCLC and in some other cancers such as gastric cancer [78, 79]. In NSCLC patients, high CARLo-5 expression level was associated with advanced pathological stage and lymph node metastasis and was a significant predictor of shorter overall survival. An *in vitro* knockdown experiment showed a significant inhibition of proliferation in tumour cells, mainly due to the induction of the G0/G1 arrest [77, 78]. Furthermore, silencing CARLo-5 could result in the inhibitory effects in the cell invasion and migration, possibly by modulating the EMT process [78].

The regulatory mechanism of CARLo-5 may be related to the adjacent region of the cancer-associated variant rs6983267, as the region including rs6983267 has enhancer activity and can interact with the proto-oncogene MYC [80]. Evidences were provided in a colon cancer study that demonstrated a strong connection between the cancer-associated variant rs6983267 and the expression of CARLo-5. The chromosome conformation capture method revealed the MYC enhancer region could physically interact with the active regulatory region of the CARLo-5 promoter and enhanced the expression of CARLo-5, this finding suggested there was a long-range interaction of MYC enhancer with the CARLo-5 promoter [77]. Since CARLo-5 is proved to have an oncogenic function, further studies focus on elucidating the mechanism of CARLo-5 regulation may provide potential therapy target for cancer treatment.

2.2.5. Other functional lncRNAs in NSCLC

LncRNA colon cancer-associated transcript 2 (CCAT2) is expressed from a highly conserved MYC enhancer region within chromosome 8q24.21. It was initially reported to be involved in metastatic progress and chromosome instability in colorectal cancer [81]. Further studies reported its association with poor prognosis in various cancers including NSCLC [82]. CCAT2 was significantly overexpressed in NSCLC tissues, in particular, the overexpression of CCAT2 was associated with adenocarcinomas specifically but not with squamous cell carcinoma.

Silencing CCAT2 by siRNA led to the inhibition of proliferation and invasion in NSCLC cell lines *in vitro*, supporting the role of CCAT2 in the metastatic progression. Further analysis found that CCAT2 combined with CEA could predict lymph node metastasis. These findings implied the potential of CCAT2 as a specific ADC biomarker for lymph node metastasis.

Growth arrest-specific transcript 5 (GAS5) is expressed from human chromosome 1q25 [83]. GAS5 was found significantly downregulated in NSCLC tissues, which was correlated with advanced TNM stage and increased tumour size [84]. GAS5 could compete with the glucocorticoid response elements (GRE) on DNA by directly interacting with the DNA-binding domain of glucocorticoid receptor (GR), thus prevented the activation of glucocorticoid-responsive genes. This competition resulted in the reduction of cell growth and metabolism, while sensitizing cells to apoptosis [85]. Recent study demonstrated that downregulation of GAS5 was associated with cisplatin resistance in NSCLC. GAS5 could inhibit autophagy and therefore enhance cisplatin sensitivity in NSCLC cells [86]. Another study found that GAS5 overexpression was inversely correlated with EGFR pathway and the expression of IGF-1R proteins in human ADC cell line, indicating its role in reversing EGFR-TKIs resistance [87]. These findings indicate the tumour suppressor lncRNA GAS5 may represent a potential biomarker for diagnosis and therapy target for NSCLC intervention.

SRY-box containing gene 2 overlapping transcript (SOX2OT) locates in the chromosome region 3q26.33, and is transcribed form the same orientation of gene SOX2 [88]. SOX2OT was reported upregulated in NSCLC, along with the upregulation of SOX2, meanwhile, the expression level was significantly higher in lung SCCs than ADCs [89]. Further study found high SOX2OT expression predicted poor survival in lung cancer patients. In lung cancer cell lines, knocking down SOX2OT inhibited the cell proliferation. These finding suggest the oncogenic SOX2OT may be prognostic indicator for NSCLC [89].

BRAF-activated non-coding RNA (BANCR) is a 693 bps lncRNA located on (−) strand of chromosome 9q21, which is initially found as a tumour suppressor factor involved in melanoma cell migration [90]. BANCR expression level was reported to be significantly decreased in NSCLC tumour tissues samples, the reduction of BANCR was related to the larger tumour size, advanced TNM stage, metastasis development, and shorter overall survival. BANCR was also an independent poor prognostic predictor of poor survival for NSCLC. An investigation on the mechanisms of tissue-specific expression revealed that histone deacetylase might be involved in the repression of BANCR. Furthermore, upregulation of BANCR inhibited NSCLC cell viability, migration, and invasion, while promoting the apoptosis process. Reversely, knockdown of BANCR promoted migration and invasion of NSCLC cells *in vitro*. These inhibitory effects were reported to be associated with EMT [91]. Interestingly, although BANCR was downregulated in NSCLC, some studies reported the significant upregulation of BANCR in other cancers, which suggested a tissue-dependent regulation mechanism of BANCR [66].

Maternally expressed gene 3 (MEG3) is expressed in chromosome 14q32.3 with a full length of 1.6 kb nucleotides [92]. Alternative splicing process was found associated with the gene MEG3, which consisted of 10 exons and could generate multiple transcripts [93]. It was reported that the expression level of MEG3 in NSCLC tissues was significantly lowered than normal tissues, which might due to the higher methylation rate of MEG3-DMR in NSCLC cells. Downregulation of MEG3 in NSCLC patients was associated with poor prognosis. In addition, overexpression of MEG3 by transfecting exogenous pCDNA-MEG3 into NSCLC cells inhibited cell proliferation and induced cell apoptosis *in vitro*, partially through activating the p53 signalling pathway [94].

3. Long noncoding RNA as novel NSCLC biomarkers

The high mortal rate of NSCLC may be mainly attributed to the late diagnosis and tumour metastasis. In addition, the heterogeneity of disease also increases the difficulty in the diagnosis and treatment, the molecular characters are different from each subtypes. Early detection, precise diagnosis, and treatment may increases the survival rate of NSCLC. To meet these ends, it is of great importance to identify novel NSCLC biomarkers.

As a new class of functional RNA molecules, lncRNAs are involved in a wide range of cellular and biological processes. Dysregulation of lncRNAs is associated with many cancer-related processes. In addition, the expression of lncRNA can be very tissue specific. These advantageous features imply a potential role of lncRNAs in cancer detection and treatment. Reduced BANCR expression was found to be an independent prognostic factor for NSCLC [91]. Huang et al. found small amount of lncRNAs (3.36%) in circulating vesicles [95]. Later research detected lncRNA HOTAIR, MALAT1, and H19 in the plasma of patients with gastric cancer and identified the expression level of plasma H19 was significantly higher than normal samples, furthermore, plasma H19 level was reduced in postoperative samples, which suggested H19 might be a biomarkers for gastric cancer [96]. Ren et al. identified fragments of lncRNA MALAT1 in plasma of prostate cancer (Pca) and named one of them as MALAT1-derived miniRNA (MD-miniRNA). Researchers then evaluated the diagnostic performance of MD-miniRNA in plasma samples of 192 patients. The results showed a sensitivity of 58.6% and specificity of 84.8% for discriminating PCa from non-PCa [97]. Although the functional lncRNAs mentioned above have been well-characterized, only few of them have been evaluated as biomarkers for diagnosis and prognosis in NSCLC, further validations is still need.

With the development of high-throughput technology, an increasing number of previously unidentified lncRNAs have been found. More and more researchers started to explore novel biomarkers from these unidentified lncRNAs. MiTranscriptome is a database, which derived from computational analysis of high-throughput RNA sequencing (RNA-Seq) data comprising 6500 samples spanning diverse cancer and tissue types. In database, 1128 ADC-related lncRNAs and 1309 lung SCC-related lncRNAs are identified, among these, 4 lncRNAs in ADC and 11 lncRNAs in lung SCC are predicted to be tissue specific, indicating that lncRNAs can discriminate not only between tumour and normal samples, but also between different subtypes [98]. Although most of these lncRNAs remain to be annotated and validated, the large number of cancer-related lncRNAs provides great hope for further screening of biomarkers and therapy targets. Some groups have investigated the potential of lncRNAs as biomarkers in early detection of NSCLCs. Wang et al. examined the expression of lncRNAs in three pairs of early stage ADC samples by high-throughput microarray technology and identified

LncRNA	Regulation	Region	p-Value	AUC	Sensitivity (%)	Specificity (%)	Type of sample	Reference
BC034684	Up	Chr1:203,148,063–203,148,611	1.486E−06	0.719	79.4	60.3	Tissue	Wang et al. [99]
RP11-1008C21.2	Down	Chr15:38,363,827–38,364,884	1.193E−07	0.843	81	79.4		
AK094413	Down	Chr9:104,235,441–104,237,132	6.634E−08	0.821	85.2	62.4		
RP11-598F7.5	Down	Chr12:273,829–275,487	4.108E−11	0.882	79.4	84.1		
VNN2	Down	Chr6:133,065,008–133,079,022	1.063E−05	0.835	77.8	79.4		
Combination				0.987	92	98		
SPRY4-IT1	Up	Chr5:142,317,620–142,318,322	<0.01	0.603	/	/	Plasma	Hu et al. [102]
ANRIL	Up	Chr9:21,994,791–22,120,646	<0.001	0.798	/	/		
NEAT1	Up	Chr11:65,422,800–65,423,368	<0.001	0.693	/	/		
Combination				0.876	88	81		
MALAT1	Up	Chr11:65,497,762–65,506,469	<0.0001	0.79	56	96	Peripheral blood	Weber et al. [101]

Table 1. List of NSCLC-associated lncRNA biomarkers identified in different researches.

1170 differentially expressed lncRNAs (DE-lncRNAs) between early stage ADC tissues and their adjacent normal tissues. Further analysis identified 20 candidates of lncRNAs from 1170 DE-lncRNAs through a screening pipeline, the pipeline could be summarized briefly as follows: if an lncRNA's average inter-group difference between tumour group and normal group was 10 times bigger than the inner group difference, it would be selected as a candidate. These 20 candidates were then validated by real-time quantitative PCR (qPCR) on a total of 102 pairs of early stage ADC samples. A panel of five lncRNAs (**Table 1**) was finally identified which can distinguish early stage adenocarcinoma samples from normal samples with high sensitivity (97%) and specificity (92%) [99]. Another study, which integrated two NSCLC microarray datasets comprising 165 and 90 patients, reported a list of 64 significantly deregulated lncRNAs in NSCLC tumours compared with normal lung tissues and a panel of 181 lncRNAs that were specific to histological subtypes of NSCLC [100].

An ideal biomarker should be of high sensitivity and specificity, and it should be easy to detect, better with non-invasive methods from body liquids. Weber et al. detected the expression level of MALAT1 in the cellular fraction of blood of a small NSCLC patients group (**Table 1**), they found that MALAT1 was detectable in peripheral human blood and the expression level between cancer patients and cancer-free controls was different, the sensitivity and specificity for discrimination was 56% and 96%, respectively [101]. Another study reported circulating SPRY4-IT1, ANRIL, and NEAT1 were significantly increased in plasma samples of NSCLC patients (**Table 1**). Combination with the three factors indicated a high power of discrimination (AUC, 0.876; sensitivity, 82.8%; and specificity, 92.3%) [102].

4. Conclusion

Since the researchers have identified that most of the genome is actively transcribed, while only small part of the human genome has the coding potential as protein-coding genes, the roles of non-coding RNAs have been transferred from transcriptional noises to the important functional molecules. This finding has led the classical view of the central dogma, which considers that the RNA functions mainly as an intermediate bridge between DNA sequences and protein synthesis, into a deeper understanding.

The roles of lncRNAs in the upstream of whole cellular signal system indicate that lncRNAs are closely associated with cellular differentiation, mitosis, and apoptosis. In the view of epigenetics, the functions of lncRNAs are mainly involved in three levels, including chromatin remodelling, transcriptional control, and post-transcriptional processes. LncRNA can act as transcriptional regulators and modulate the expression of protein-coding genes in *cis* or *trans* manner through directly or indirectly binding to DNA or protein molecules. Thus, the occurrences of diseases including cancers are always along with the dysregulation of lncRNAs. In this chapter, we have discussed several lncRNAs that have been reported to be associated with NSCLCs. Some of them are well-characterized and also identified in other cancers, while some still remain to be studied. Most of these lncRNAs have the potential as biomarkers in diagnosis and prognosis of NSCLCs. However, these lncRNAs lack NSCLC tissue specificity, thus great efforts are still needed to identify NSCLC tissue-specific lncRNAs.

Despite the high performance of these lncRNA panels in diagnosis, most of them are identified from statistical analysis, which means the biological meanings of lncRNAs have not been taken into consideration. In addition, the candidate screening methods are mainly based on p-value, fold change, absolute expression level, and PAM method, outcomes of the candidates may differs for different methods [103]. Thus, a better candidate screening method combining the biological meaning of lncRNAs and robust statistical pipeline is need for future studies. Also, up to now, most of the samples in these studies are collected from patient tissues through invasive methods, more works are still needed to explore circulating lncRNA expressions in blood plasma, urine, or sputum, which can meet the non-invasive demands.

Considering the sophisticated functions and large number of lncRNAs, we have now identified just the tip of the lncRNA iceberg. Lots of questions are waiting to be clarified, for example, what does the classification of lncRNAs looks like, and what the mechanistic basis of their functions is. Huge gaps are still in front of us in understanding the big picture of the lncRNA world. Fortunately, new technology such as the third generation sequencing, which allows the longer read length, are now providing more reliable and accurate information of lncRNAs. In future, we believe that understanding the lncRNA world will bring us new answers to old questions in evolution, development, and the understanding of NSCLCs. There may be a long way before the clinical application of lncRNAs in NSCLC, however, fast progressing in the lncRNA filed opens up numerous opportunities for diagnosis and therapeutic intervention against NSCLC.

Author details

Zule Cheng[1, 2] and Hongju Mao[1*]

*Address all correspondence to: hjmao@mail.sim.ac.cn

1 State Key Laboratory of Transducer Technology, Shanghai Institute of Microsystem and Information Technology, Chinese Academy of Science, Shanghai, China

2 University of Chinese Academy of Sciences, Beijing, China

References

[1] National Cancer Institute. SEER Stat fact sheets: lung and bronchus cancer [Internet]. 2016 [Updated: 2016]. Available from: http://seer.cancer.gov/statfacts/html/lungb.html

[2] Davidson MR, Gazdar AF, Clarke BE. The pivotal role of pathology in the management of lung cancer. Journal of Thoracic Disease. 2013; **5**(4):S463–S478. DOI: 10.3978/j.issn.2072-1439.2013.08.43

[3] Hasan N, Kumar R, Kavuru MS. Lung cancer screening beyond low-dose computed tomography: the role of novel biomarkers. Lung. 2014; **192**(5):639–648. DOI: 10.1007/s00408-014-9636-z

[4] Molina R, Filella X, Augé JM, Fuentes R, Bover I, Rifa J, et al. Tumor markers (CEA, CA 125, CYFRA 21-1, SCC and NSE) in patients with non-small cell lung cancer as an aid in histological diagnosis and prognosis. Comparison with the main clinical and pathological prognostic factors. Tumour Biology. 2003; **24**(4):209–218. DOI: 74432

[5] Mogi A, Kuwano H. TP53 mutations in nonsmall cell lung cancer. BioMed Research International. 2011; **2011**(1):50–56. DOI: 10.1155/2011/583929

[6] Paez JG, Jänne PA, Lee JC, Tracy S, Greulich H, Gabriel S, et al. EGFR mutations in lung cancer: correlation with clinical. Science. 2004; **304** (5676):1497–1500. DOI: 10.1126/science.1099314

[7] Tam IY, Chung LP, Suen WS, Wang E, Wong MC, Ho KK, et al. Distinct epidermal growth factor receptor and KRAS mutation patterns in non-small cell lung cancer patients with different tobacco exposure and clinicopathologic features. Clinical Cancer Research. 2006; **12**(5): 1647–1653. DOI: 10.1158/1078-0432.CCR-05-1981

[8] Ponting CP, Belgard TG. Transcribed dark matter: meaning or myth? Human Molecular Genetics. 2010; **15**(19):162–168. DOI: 10.1093/hmg/ddq362

[9] Bartel DP. MicroRNAs: target recognition and regulatory. Cell. 2009; **136**(2):215–233. DOI: 10.1016/j.cell.2009.01.002

[10] Chen X, Ba Y, Ma L, Cai X, Yin Y, Wang K, Guo J, et al. Characterization of microRNAs in serum: a novel class of biomarkers for diagnosis of cancer and other diseases. Cell Research. 2008; **18**(10):997–1006. DOI: 10.1038/cr.2008.282

[11] Russell RB, Cohen SM. Principles of microRNA-target recognition. PLoS Biology. 2005; **3**(3):e85. DOI: 10.1371/journal.pbio.0030085

[12] O'Carroll D, Mecklenbrauker I, Das PP, Santana A, Koenig U, Enright AJ, et al. Slicer-independent role for Argonaute 2 in hematopoiesis and the microRNA pathway. Genes & Development. 2007; **21**(16):1999–2004. DOI: 10.1101 /gad. 1565607

[13] Ji Q, David M. MicroRNAs and lung cancers: from pathogenesis to clinical implications. Frontiers of Medicine. 2012; **6**(2):134–155. DOI: 10.1007/s11684-012-0188-4

[14] Mattia B, Carla V, Davide C, Luca R, Piergiorgio M, Federica F, et al. MicroRNA signatures in tissues and plasma predict development and prognosis of computed tomography detected lung cancer. PNAS. 2010; **108**(9):3713–3718. DOI: 10.1073/pnas.1100048108

[15] Nozomu Y, Natasha C, Elise B, Masahiro S, Kensuke K, Ming Y, et al. Unique microRNA molecular profiles in lung cancer diagnosis and prognosis. Cancer Cell. 2006; **9**(3):189–198. DOI: 10.1016/j.ccr.2006.01.025

[16] Wang P, Yang D, Zhang H, Wei X, Ma T, Cheng Z, et al. Early detection of lung cancer in serum by a panel of microRNA biomarkers. Clinical Lung Cancer. 2015; **16**(4):313–319. DOI: 10.1016/j.cllc.2014.12.006

[17] Li X, Shi Y, Yin Z, Xue X, Zhou B. An eight-miRNA signature as a potential biomarker for predicting survival in lung adenocarcinoma. Journal of Translational Medicine. 2014; **4**(12):159. DOI: 10.1186/1479-5876-12-159

[18] Derrien T, Johnson R, Bussotti G, Tanzer A, Djebali S, Tilgner H, et al. The GENCODE v7 catalog of human long noncoding RNAs: analysis of their gene structure, evolution, and expression. Genome Research. 2012; **22**(9):1775–1789. DOI: 10.1101/ gr.132159.111

[19] Sati S, Ghosh S, Jain V, Scaria V, Sengupta S. Genome-wide analysis reveals distinct patterns of epigenetic features in long non-coding RNA loci. Nucleic Acids Research. 2012; **40**(20):10018–10031. DOI: 10.1093/nar/gks776

[20] Elisaphenko EA, Kolesnikov NN, Shevchenko AI, Rogozin IB, Nesterova TB, Brockdorff N, et al. A dual origin of the Xist gene from a protein-coding gene and a set of transposable elements. PLoS One. 2008; **3**(6):e2521. DOI: 10.1371/journal.pone.0002521

[21] Chris PP, Peter LO, Wolf R. Evolution and functions of long noncoding RNAs. Cell. 2009; **136**(4):629–641. DOI: 10.1016/j.cell.2009.02.006

[22] Conley AB, Miller WJ, Jordan IK. Human cis natural antisense transcripts initiated by transposable elements. Trends in Genetics 2008; **24**(2):53–56. DOI: 10.1016/j.tig.2007. 11. 008

[23] St Laurent G, Wahlestedt C, Kapranov P. The landscape of long noncoding RNA classification. Trends in Genetics. 2015; **31**(5):239–251. DOI: 10.1016/j.tig.2015.03.007

[24] Ma L, Bajic VB, Zhang Z. On the classification of long non-coding RNAs. RNA Biology. 2013; **10**(6):925–933. DOI: 10.4161/rna.24604

[25] Wang KC, Chang HY. Molecular mechanisms of long noncoding RNAs. Molecular Cell. 2011;**43**(6):904–914. DOI: 10.1016/j.molce2011.08.018

[26] John LR, Michael K, Jordon KW, Sharon LS, Xiao X, Samantha A, et al. Functional demarcation of active and silent chromatin domains in human HOX loci by non-coding RNAs. Cell. 2007; **129**(7):1311–1323. DOI: 10.1016/j.cell.2007.05.022

[27] Ogawa Y, Sun BK, Lee JT. Intersection of the RNA interference and X-inactivation pathways. Science. 2008; **320**(5881):1336–1341. DOI: 10.1126/science.1157676

[28] Wang X, Arai S, Song X, Reichart D, Du K, Pascual G, et al. Induced ncRNAs allosterically modify RNA-binding proteins in cis to inhibit transcription. Nature. 2008; **454**(7200):126–130. DOI: 10.1038/nature06992

[29] Manuel B, Isabel P, Cristina P, José MG, Ana BÁ, Raúl P, et al. A natural antisense transcript regulates Zeb2/Sip1 gene expression during Snail1-induced epithelial–mesenchymal transition. Genes & Development. 2008; **22**(6):756–769.DOI: 10.1101/gad. 455708

[30] Batista PJ, Chang HY. Long noncoding RNAs: cellular address codes in development and disease. Cell. 2013; **152**(6):1298–1307. DOI: 10.1016/j.cell.2013.02.012

[31] Tim RM, Marcel ED, John SM. Long non-coding RNAs: insights into functions. Nature Reviews Genetics. 2009; **10**(3):155–159. DOI: 10.1038/nrg2521

[32] Tsai MC, Spitale RC, Chang HY. Long intergenic non-coding RNAs—new links in cancer progression. Cancer Research. 2011; **71**(1):3–7. DOI: 10.1158/0008-5472.CAN-10-2483

[33] Yang G, Lu X, Yuan L. LncRNA: a link between RNA and cancer. Biochimica et Biophysica Acta. 2014; **1839**(11):1097–1109. DOI: 10.1016/j.bbagrm.2014.08.012

[34] Yang Y, Li H, Hou S, Hu B, Liu J, Wang J. The noncoding RNA expression profile and the effect of lncRNA AK126698 on cisplatin resistance in non-small-cell lung cancer cell. PLoS One. 2013; **8**(5):e65309. DOI: 10.1371/journal.pone.0065309

[35] The GENCODE Project. Encyclopaedia of genes and gene variants. Statistics about the current human GENCODE release (version 25) [Internet]. 2016 freeze, GRCh38. Available from: http://www.gencodegenes.org/stats/current.html

[36] Rinn JL, Kertesz M, Wang JK, Squazzo SL, Xu X, Brugmann SA, et al. Functional demarcation of active and silent chromatin domains in human HOX loci by noncoding RNAs. Cell. 2007; **129**(7):1311–1323. DOI: 10.1016/j.cell.2007.05.022

[37] Gupta RA, Shah N, Wang KC, Kim J, Horlings HM, Wong DJ, et al. Long noncoding RNA HOTAIR reprograms chromatin state to promote cancer metastasis. Nature. 2010; **464**(7291):1071–1076. DOI: 10.1038/nature08975

[38] Yang Z, Zhou L, Wu LM, Lai MC, Xie HY, Zhang F, et al. Overexpression of long non-coding RNA HOTAIR predicts tumor recurrence in hepatocellular carcinoma patients following liver transplantation. Annals of Surgical Oncology. 2011; **18**(5):1243–1250. DOI: 10.1245/s10434-011-1581-y

[39] Svoboda M, Slyskova J, Schneiderova M, Makovicky P, Bielik L, Levy M, et al. HOTAIR long non-coding RNA is a negative prognostic factor not only in primary tumors, but also in the blood of colorectal cancer patients. Carcinogenesis. 2014; **35**(7): 1510–1515. DOI: 10.1093/carcin/bgu055

[40] Kim K, Jutooru I, Chadalapaka G, Johnson G, Frank J, Burghardt R, et al. HOTAIR is a negative prognostic factor and exhibits pro-oncogenic activity in pancreatic cancer. Oncogene. 2013; **32**(13):1616–1625. DOI: 10.1038/onc.2012.193

[41] Li X, Wu Z, Mei Q, Guo M, Fu X, Han W, et al. Long non-coding RNA HOTAIR, a driver of malignancy, predicts negative prognosis and exhibits oncogenic activity in oesophageal squamous cell carcinoma. British Journal of Cancer. 2013; **109**(109):2266–2278. DOI: 10.1038/bjc.2013.548

[42] Liu XH, Liu ZL, Sun M, Liu J, Wang ZX, De W. The long non-coding RNA HOTAIR indicates a poor prognosis and promotes metastasis in non-small cell lung cancer. BMC Cancer. 2013; **13**(1):1–10. DOI: 10.1186/1471-2407-13-464

[43] Hiroyuki E, Takeharu S, Takayuki N, Misa Y, Keiichi T, Hideaki Y, et al. Enhanced expression of long non-coding RNA HOTAIR is associated with the development of gastric cancer. PLoS One. 2013; **8**(10):e77070. DOI: 10.1371/journal.pone.0077070

[44] Liu XH, Sun M, Nie FQ, Ge YB, Zhang EB, Yin DD, et al. Lnc RNA HOTAIR functions as a competing endogenous RNA to regulate HER2 expression by sponging miR-331-3p in gastric cancer. Molecular Cancer. 2014; **13**(1):2739–2748. DOI: 10.1186/1476-4598-13-92

[45] Nakagawa T, Endo H, Yokoyama M, Abe J, Tamai K, Tanaka N, et al. Large noncoding RNA HOTAIR enhances aggressive biological behavior and is associated with short disease-free survival in human non-small cell lung cancer. Biochemical and Biophysical Research Communications. 2013; **436**(2):319–324. DOI: 10.1016/ j.bbrc.2013. 05.101

[46] Liu Z, Sun M, Lu K, Liu J, Zhang M, Wu W, et al. The long noncoding RNA HOTAIR contributes to cisplatin resistance of human lung adenocarcinoma cells via downregualtion of p21 (WAF1/CIP1) expression. PLoS One. 2013; **8**(10):e77293. DOI: 10.1371/journal.pone.0077293

[47] Wang R, Shi Y, Chen L, Jiang Y, Mao C, Yan B, et al. The ratio of FoxA1 to FoxA2 in lung adenocarcinoma is regulated by LncRNA HOTAIR and chromatin remodeling factor LSH. Scientific Reports. 2015; **5**(17):826. DOI: 10.1038/srep17826

[48] Zhuang Y, Wang X, Nguyen HT, Zhuo Y, Cui X, Fewell C, et al. Induction of long intergenic non-coding RNA HOTAIR in lung cancer cells by type I collagen. Journal of Hematology & Oncology. 2013; **6**(35). DOI: 10.1186/1756-8722-6-35

[49] Ji P, Diederichs S, Wang W, Böing S, Metzger R, Schneider PM, et al. MALAT-1, a novel noncoding RNA, and thymosin beta4 predict metastasis and survival in early-stage non-small cell lung cancer. Oncogene. 2003; **22**(39): 8031–8041. DOI: 10.1038 /sj. onc.1206 928

[50] Wilusz JE, Freier SM, Spector DL. 3′ end processing of a long nuclear-retained noncoding RNA yields a tRNA-like cytoplasmic RNA. Cell. 2008; **135**(5):919–932. DOI: 10.1016/j.cell.2008.10.012

[51] Hutchinson JN, Ensminger AW, Clemson CM, Lynch CR, Lawrence JB, Chess A. A screen for nuclear transcripts identifies two linked noncoding RNAs associated with SC35 splicing domains. BMC Genomics. 2007; **8**(39):1–16. DOI: 10.1186/1471-2164-8-39

[52] Tripathi V, Ellis JD, Shen Z, Song DY, Pan Q, Watt AT, et al. The nuclear-retained noncoding RNA MALAT1 regulates alternative splicing by modulating SR splicing factor phosphorylation. Molecular Cell. 2010; **39**(6):925–938. DOI: 10.1016/j.molcel.2010. 08.011

[53] Pang EJ, Yang R, Fu XB, Liu YF. Overexpression of long non-coding RNA MALAT1 is correlated with clinical progression and unfavorable prognosis in pancreatic cancer. Tumour Biol: J Int Soc Oncodevelopmental Biol Med. 2014; **36**(4):2403–2407. DOI: 10.10 07/s13277-014-2850-8

[54] Zheng HT, Shi DB, Wang YW, Li XX, Xu Y, Tripathi P, et al. High expression of lncrna malat1 suggests a biomarker of poor prognosis in colorectal cancer. International Journal of Clinical and Experimental Pathology. 2014; **7**(6):3174–3181.

[55] Dong Y, Liang G, Yuan B, Yang C, Gao R, Zhou X. Malat1 promotes the proliferation and metastasis of osteosarcoma cells by activating the PI3K/AKT pathway. Tumour Biology: The Journal of the International Society for Oncodevelopmental Biology & Medicine. 2014; **36**(3):1477–1486. DOI: 10.1007/s13277-014-2631-4.

[56] Wu XS, Wang XA, Wu WG, Hu YP, Li ML, Ding Q, et al. Malat1 promotes the proliferation and metastasis of gallbladder cancer cells by activating the ERK/MAPK pathway. Cancer Biology & Therapy, 2014; **15**(6): 806–814. DOI: 10.4161/cbt.28584

[57] Hu L, Wu Y, Tan D, Meng H, Wang K, Bai Y, et al. Up-regulation of long noncoding RNA MALAT1 contributes to proliferation and metastasis in esophageal squamous cell carcinoma. Journal of Experimental & Clinical Cancer Research. 2015; **34**(7). DOI: 10.1186/s13046-015-0123-z.

[58] Wang X, Li M, Wang Z, Han S, Tang X, Ge Y, et al. Silencing of long noncoding RNA malat1 by mir-101 and mir-217 inhibits proliferation, migration, and invasion of esophageal squamous cell carcinoma cells. Journal of Biological Chemistry. 2015; **290**(7): 3925–3935. DOI: 10.1074/jbc.M114.596866

[59] Fan Y, Shen B, Tan M, Mu X, Qin Y, Zhang F, Liu Y. TGF-β-induced upregulation of malat1 promotes bladder cancer metastasis by associating with suz12. Clinical Cancer Research. 2014; **20**(6):1531–1541. DOI: 10.1158/1078-0432.CCR-13-1455

[60] Hirata H, Hinoda Y, Shahryari V, Deng G, Nakajima K, Tabatabai ZL, et al. Long noncoding RNA MALAT1 promotes aggressive renal cell carcinoma through Ezh2 and interacts with miR-205. Cancer Research. 2015; **75**(7):1322–1331. DOI: 10.1158/0008-5472.CAN-14-2931

[61] Schmidt LH, Spieker T, Koschmieder S, Humberg J, Jungen D, Bulk E, et al. The long noncoding MALAT-1 RNA indicates a poor prognosis in non-small cell lung cancer and induces migration and tumor growth. Journal of Thoracic Oncology. 2011; **6**(12):1984–1992. DOI: 10.1097/JTO.0b013e3182307eac

[62] Gutschner T, Hämmerle M, Eissmann M, Hsu J, Kim Y, Hung G, et al. The non-coding RNA MALAT1 is a critical regulator of the metastasis phenotype of lung cancer cells. Cancer Research. 2013; **73**(3):1180–1189. DOI: 10.1158/0008-5472.CAN-12-2850

[63] Tripathi V, Shen Z, Chakraborty A, Giri S, Freier SM, Wu X, et al. Long noncoding RNA MALAT1 controls cell cycle progression by regulating the expression of oncogenic transcription factor B-MYB. PLoS Genetics. 2013; **9**(3):e1003368. DOI: 10.1371/journal.pgen.1003368

[64] Yang L, Lin C, Liu W, Zhang J, Ohgi K, Grinstein J, et al. NcRNA- and Pc2 methylation-dependent gene relocation between nuclear structures mediates gene activation programs. Cell. 2011; **147**(4):773–788. DOI: 10.1016/j.cell.2011.08.054

[65] Gabory A, Jammes H, Dandolo L. The H19 locus: role of an imprinted non-coding RNA in growth and development. Bioessays: News & Reviews in Molecular Cellular & Developmental Biology. 2010; **32**(6):473–480. DOI: 10.1002/bies.200900170

[66] Roth A, Diederichs S. Long noncoding RNAs in lung cancer. Curent Topics in Microbiology & Immunolog. 2016; **394**:57–110. DOI: 10.1007/82_2015_444

[67] Kondo M, Suzuki H, Ueda R, Osada H, Takagi K, Takahashi T, et al. Frequent loss of imprinting of the H19 gene is often associated with its overexpression in human lung cancers. Oncogene. 1995; **10**(6):1193–1198.

[68] Gao T, He B, Pan Y, Gu L, Chen L, Nie Z, et al. H19 dmr methylation correlates to the progression of esophageal squamous cell carcinoma through igf2 imprinting pathway. Clinical and Translational Oncology. 2014; **16**(4):410–417. DOI: 10.1007/s12094-013-1098-x

[69] Ulaner GA, Vu TH, Li T, Hu JF, Yao XM, Yang Y, et al. Loss of imprinting of IGF2 and H19 in osteosarcoma is accompanied by reciprocal methylation changes of a CTCF-binding site. Human Molecular Genetics. 2003; **12**(5):535–549. DOI: 10.1093/hmg/ddg034

[70] Byun HM, Wong HL, Birnstein EA, Wolff EM, Liang G, Yang AS. Examination of IGF2 and H19 loss of imprinting in bladder cancer. Cancer Research. 2007; **67**(22):10753–10758. DOI: 10.1158/0008-5472.CAN-07-0329

[71] Kaplan R, Luettich K, Heguy A, Hackett NR, Harvey BG, Crystal RG. Monoallelic up-regulation of the imprinted H19 gene in airway epithelium of phenotypically normal cigarette smokers. Cancer Research. 2003; **63**(7):1475–1482.

[72] Liu F, Killian JK, Yang M, Walker RL, Hong JA, Zhang M, et al. Epigenomic alterations and gene expression profiles in respiratory epithelia exposed to cigarette smoke condensate. Oncogene. 2010; **29**(25):3650–3664. DOI: 10.1038/onc.2010.129

[73] Matouk IJ, Mezan S, Mizrahi A, Ohana P, Abu-Lail R, Fellig Y, et al. The oncofetal h19 rna connection: hypoxia, p53 and cancer. Biochimica et Biophysica Acta, Molecular Cell Research. 2010; **1803**(4):443–451. DOI: 10.1016/j.bbamcr.2010.01.010

[74] Barsyte-Lovejoy D, Lau SK, Boutros PC, Khosravi F, Jurisica I, Andrulis IL, et al. The c-Myc oncogene directly induces the H19 noncoding RNA by allele-specific binding to potentiate tumorigenesis. Cancer Research. 2006; **66**(10):5330–5337. DOI: 10.1158/0008-5472.CAN-06-0037

[75] Chen B, Yu M, Chang Q, Lu Y, Thakur C, Ma D, et al. Mdig de-represses h19 large intergenic non-coding rna (lincrna) by down-regulating h3k9me3 and heterochromatin. Oncotarget. 2013; **4**(9):1427-1437. DOI: 10.18632/oncotarget.1155

[76] Cui J, Mo J, Luo M, Yu Q, Zhou S, Li T, et al. c-Myc-activated long non-coding RNA H19 downregulates miR-107 and promotes cell cycle progression of non-small cell lung cancer. International Journal of Clinical and Experimental Pathology. 2015; **8**(10):12400–12409.

[77] Kim T, Cui R, Jeon YJ, Lee JH, Sim H, Park JK, et al. Long-range interaction and correlation between MYC enhancer and oncogenic long noncoding RNA CARLo-5. PNAS. 2014; **111**(11):4173–4178. DOI: 10.1073/pnas.1400350111

[78] Luo J, Tang L, Zhang J, Ni J, Zhang HP, Zhang L, et al. Long non-coding RNA CARLo-5 is a negative prognostic factor and exhibits tumor pro-oncogenic activity in non-small cell lung cancer. Tumour Biology. 2014; **35**(11):11541–11549. DOI: 10.1007/ s13277-014-2442-7

[79] Zhang Y, Ma M, Liu W, Ding W, Yu H. Enhanced expression of long noncoding RNA CARLo-5 is associated with the development of gastric cancer. International Journal of Clinical and Experimental Pathology. 2014; **7**(12):8471–8479.

[80] Pomerantz MM, Ahmadiyeh N, Jia L, Herman P, Verzi MP, Doddapaneni H, et al. The 8q24 cancer risk variant rs6983267 shows long-range interaction with MYC in colorectal cancer. Nature Genetics. 2009; **41**(8):882–884. DOI: 10.1038/ng.403

[81] Ling H, Spizzo R, Atlasi Y, Nicoloso M, Shimizu M, Redis RS, et al. CCAT2, a novel noncoding RNA mapping to 8q24, underlies metastatic progression and chromosomal instability in colon cancer. Genome Research. 2013; **23**(9):1446–1461. DOI: 10.1101/gr. 152942.112

[82] Qiu M, Xu Y, Yang X, Wang J, Hu J, Xu L, et al. CCAT2 is a lung adenocarcinoma-specific long non-coding RNA and promotes invasion of non-small cell lung cancer. Tumour Biology: The Journal of the International Society for Oncodevelopmental Biology & Medicine. 2014;**35**(6):5375–5380. DOI: 10.1007/s13277-014-1700-z

[83] Coccia EM, Cicala C, Charlesworth A, Ciccarelli C, Rossi GB, Philipson L, et al. Regulation and expression of a growth arrest-specific gene (gas5) during growth, differentiation, and development. Molecular and Cellular Biology. 1992; **12**(8):3514–3521.

[84] Shi X, Sun M, Liu H, Yao Y, Kong R, Chen F. et al. A critical role for the long non-coding RNA GAS5 in proliferation and apoptosis in non-small-cell lung cancer. Molecular Carcinogenesis. 2013; **54**(S1):E1–E12. DOI: 10.1002/mc.22120

[85] Kino T, Hurt DE, Ichijo T, Nader N, Chrousos GP. Noncoding RNA gas5 is a growth arrest- and starvation-associated repressor of the glucocorticoid receptor. Science Signaling. 2010; **3**(107):692–702. DOI: 10.1126/scisignal.2000568

[86] Zhang N, Yang GQ, Shao XM, Wei L. GAS5 modulated autophagy is a mechanism modulating cisplatin sensitivity in NSCLC cells. European Review for Medical and Pharmacological Sciences. 2016; **20**(11):2271–2277.

[87] Dong S, Qu X, Li W, Zhong X, Li P, Yang S, et al. The long non-coding RNA GAS5 enhances gefitinib-induced cell death in innate EGFR tyrosine kinase inhibitor-resistant lung adenocarcinoma cells with wide-type EGFR via downregulation of the IGF-1R expression. Journal of Hematology & Oncology. 2015; **8**(1):1–13. DOI: 10.1186/ s13045-015-0140-6

[88] Amaral PP, Neyt C, Wilkins SJ, Askarian-Amiri ME, Sunkin SM, Perkins A, et al. Complex architecture and regulated expression of the SOX2OT locus during vertebrate development. RNA. 2009; **15**(11):2013–2027. DOI: 10.1261/rna.1705309

[89] Hou Z, Zhao W, Zhou J, Shen L, Zhan P, Xu C. et al. A long noncoding RNA Sox2ot regulates lung cancer cell proliferation and is a prognostic indicator of poor survival. The International Journal of Biochemistry & Cell Biology. 2014; **53**(8):380–388. DOI: 10.1016/j.biocel.2014.06.004

[90] Flockhart RJ, Webster DE, Qu K, Mascarenhas N, Kovalski J, Kretz M, et al. $BRAF^{V600E}$ remodels the melanocyte transcriptome and induces BANCR to regulate melanoma cell migration. Genome Research. 2012; **22**(6):1006–1014. DOI: 10.1101/gr. 140061.112

[91] Sun M, Liu XH, Wang KM, Nie FQ, Kong R, Yang JS, et al. Downregulation of braf activated non-coding rna is associated with poor prognosis for non-small cell lung cancer and promotes metastasis by affecting epithelial-mesenchymal transition. Molecular Cancer. 2014; **13**(1):1–12. DOI: 10.1186/1476-4598-13-68

[92] Miyoshi N, Wagatsuma H, Wakana S, Shiroishi T, Nomura M, Aisaka K, et al. Identification of an imprinted gene, Meg3/Gtl2 and its human homologue MEG3, first mapped on mouse distal chromosome 12 and human chromosome 14q. Genes to Cells. 2000; **5**(3):211–220.

[93] Zhou Y, Zhong Y, Wang Y, Zhang X, Batista DL, Gejman R, et al. Activation of p53 by meg3 non-coding RNA. Journal of Biological Chemistry. 2007; **282**(34):24731–24742. DOI: 10.1074/jbc.M702029200

[94] Lu KH, Li W, Liu XH, Sun M, Zhang ML, Wu WQ, et al. Long non-coding RNA MEG3 inhibits NSCLC cells proliferation and induces apoptosis by affecting p53 expression. BMC Cancer. 2013; **13**(1):1–11. DOI: 10.1186/1471-2407-13-461

[95] Huang X, Yuan T, Tschannen M, Sun Z, Jacob H, Du M, et al. Characterization of human plasma-derived exosomal RNAs by deep sequencing. BMC Genomics. 2013; **14**(319):1–14. DOI: 10.1186/1471-2164-14-319

[96] Arita T, Ichikawa D, Konishi H, Komatsu S, Shiozak, A, Shoda, K, et al. Circulating long non-coding RNAs in plasma of patients with gastric cancer. Anticancer Research. 2013; **33**(8):3185–3193.

[97] Ren S, Wang F, Shen J, Sun Y, Xu W, Lu J, et al. Long non-coding RNA metastasis associated in lung adenocarcinoma transcript 1 derived miniRNA as a novel plasma-based biomarker for diagnosing prostate cancer. European Journal of Cancer. 2013; **49** (13):2949–2959. DOI: 10.1016/j.ejca.2013.04.026

[98] Iyer MK, Niknafs YS, Malik R, Singhal U, Sahu A, Hosono Y, et al. The landscape of long noncoding RNAs in the human transcriptome. Nature Genetics. 2015; **47**(3):199–208. DOI: 10.1038/ng.3192

[99] Wang P, Lu SH, Mao HH, Bai YN, Ma TL, Cheng ZL, et al. Identification of biomarkers for the detection of early stage lung adenocarcinoma by microarray profiling of long noncoding RNAs. Lung Cancer. 2015; **88**(2):147–153. DOI: 10.1016/j.lungcan.2015.02.009

[100] Yu H, Xu Q, Liu F, Ye X, Wang J, Meng X. Identification and validation of long noncoding RNA biomarkers in human non-small-cell lung carcinomas. Journal of Thoracic Oncology. 2015; **10**(4):645–654. DOI: 10.1097/JTO.0000000000000470.

[101] Weber DG, Johnen G, Casjens S, Bryk O, Pesch B, Jöckel KH, et al. Evaluation of long noncoding RNA MALAT1 as a candidate blood-based biomarker for the diagnosis of non-small cell lung cancer. BMC Research Notes. 2013; **6**(518):1–9. DOI: 10.1186/1756-0500-6-518.

[102] Hu X, Bao J, Wang Z, Zhang Z, Gu P, Tao F, et al. The plasma lncRNA acting as fingerprint in non-small-cell lung cancer. Tumour Biology. 2016; **37**(3):3497–3504. DOI: 10.1007/s13277-015-4023-9

[103] Tibshirani R, Hastie T, Narasimhan B, Chu G. Diagnosis of multiple cancer types by shrunken centroids of gene expression. Proceedings of the National Academy of Sciences of the United States of America. 2002; **99**(10):6567–6572. DOI: 10.1073/pnas.082099299

Chapter 12

Antitumor Effect of Natural Product Molecules against Lung Cancer

Wei-long Zhong, Yuan Qin, Shuang Chen and Tao Sun

Additional information is available at the end of the chapter

http://dx.doi.org/10.5772/67241

Abstract

Lung cancer treatment remains difficult because of multidrug resistance and adverse effects, and natural product molecules show powerful activity in lung cancer with few side effects. The molecular targets and efficacy of natural product molecules remain unclear. We described the molecular regulation of natural product molecules with antitumor activities, the antilung cancer activities and the clinical trials for lung cancer treatment of natural product molecules. The results support the updated systemic information on the use of natural product molecules to prevent cancer progression and their constituents for lung cancer treatment.

Keywords: lung cancer, natural product molecules, antitumor activity

1. Introduction

Lung cancer treatment remains difficult because of multidrug resistance and adverse effects. Natural product molecules represent an attractive approach for lung cancer therapy with few side effects but high treatment outcome. Various natural product molecules have proven to be useful and effective in sensitizing conventional agents. Several natural product molecules can prevent the side effects of chemotherapy. Moreover, natural product molecules can improve the quality of life (QoL) and prolong the survival time of lung cancer patients. In this chapter, we summarize the molecular regulation mechanisms of natural product molecules and their antitumor effects on lung cancer *in vitro* and *in vivo*.

In lung cancer treatment, the molecular targets and efficacy of natural product molecules remain unclear. Thus, we reviewed the antitumor activities of natural product molecules in lung cancer therapy. This chapter is mainly divided into three parts: the molecular regulation of natural product molecules with antitumor activities, the antilung cancer activities of natural product molecules *in vivo*, and the clinical trials on natural product molecules for lung cancer treatment.

On the basis of our critical analyses, we suggest the potential of natural product molecules that have been traditionally used for lung diseases, including cancer, and the discussion of data from *in vitro* or *in vivo* laboratory experimental models and clinical trials. We suggest that natural product molecules can be potent anticancer agents for lung cancer treatment and prevention by regulating multimolecular targets. The effects of natural product molecules are involved in angiogenesis, metastasis, and severe side effects.

Lung cancer is the leading cause of cancer death worldwide. Small-cell lung cancer (SCLC) and non–small-cell lung cancer (NSCLC) are the two main types of lung cancer. Smoking can induce most kinds of lung cancer. In addition, vinyl chloride, arsenic, cadmium, beryllium, chloride, and nickel chromates contribute to the occurrence of lung cancer. For lung cancer patients who are nonsmokers, their cancer is usually caused by a combination of genetic factors, as well as exposure to radon gas and air pollution [1, 2]. For lung cancer, early diagnosis is very important for patients to improve their survival rate. The cause of lung cancer did not show any obvious symptoms until the cancer began to metastasize to other organs.

Chemotherapy, radiotherapy, and surgery are the most widely used strategies in lung cancer treatment. However, standard chemotherapies present severe toxicity for patients and may result in limited survival benefit. Given that phytochemicals and antitumor herbs are less toxic, these agents are used to treat lung cancer, and the outcome has attracted recent reports and investigations [3]. To date, antilung cancer herbs have included 130 Chinese herbal medicines with effective treatment effects. These herbs are classified on the basis of their actions: (1) clearing heat and toxin, (2) resolving dampness and phlegm, (3) regulating blood and Qi, (4) reinforcing Qi, and (5) nourishing Yin through their ethnopharmacological efficacies.

In this chapter, we discuss the ethnopharmacological effects of natural product molecules focusing on metastasis, angiogenesis, apoptosis, and clinical trial efficacy. In these reviews, the results support the updated systemic information on the use of natural product molecules to prevent cancer progression and their constituents for lung cancer treatment.

2. Molecular regulation of natural product molecules with antitumor activities

To develop useful agents for cancer therapy, the unique activity mechanisms of natural product molecules should be studied. The molecular mechanisms of natural product molecules with anticancer activities are important for the development of many drug-targeted therapies for cancer treatment [4]. Molecular biology methods for high-risk individuals during early diagnosis, screening, and identification can help determine the prognosis of innovative treatment and provide a novel point of view [5]. Significantly, target molecules should be considered for lung cancer treatment.

2.1. Apoptosis and natural product molecules

Apoptosis involves a series of morphological alterations, such as plasma and nuclear membrane blebbing, cell shrinkage, dissolution of nuclear lamina, and biochemical processes, which are responsible for the activation of apoptosis [6]. In Chinese medicine, the fruit and roots of *Toona sinensis* (Meliaceae) have been used for cancer therapy. Toona displayed glucose uptake in 3T3-L1 adipocyte differentiation of fat and enhanced the antidiabetic activity [7]. *T. sinensis* leaf extract (TSL-1) inhibition of lung adenocarcinoma cell proliferation after 24 hours can mediate apoptosis at 0.5 or 1 mg/mL. *Ocimum gratissimum* (OG) (Lamiaceae) is a perennial aromatic herb with antibacterial and antidiabetic activity in Taiwan and is traditionally used to treat gastrointestinal diseases. OG can activate apoptotic signaling molecules, such as caspase-3 and caspase-9, in A549 cells at a concentration of 0.5 or 0.8 mg/mL; thus, OG is a potentially useful candidate [8]. In lung cancer cell apoptosis, medicinal plants from many biologically active compounds are also known as potent inducers. Acacetin flavonoid polyphenol compound (5,7-dihydroxy-4′-methoxy-flavonoids) from *Robinia pseudoacacia* (legumes) can inhibit A549 cell proliferation (IC50 = 9.46 μm). By upregulating p53 and p21/WAF1 proteins, acacia-induced apoptosis and cell cycle at the concentrations of 5 or 10 μM in A549 cells [9]. Dihydroartemisinin (DHA) is a derivative of artemisinin from *Artemisia annua* Altai Michael (Asteraceae) and is used to treat malaria; DHA can also induce apoptosis in human lung cancer cells. PG490 (triptolide), a diterpene triepoxide from *Tripterygium wilfordii* (Celastraceae), was significantly sensitized to Apo2L/TRAIL-induced apoptosis, but it did not significantly induce cell death in A549 cells. Acutiaporberine is a bisalkaloid from the pointed leaves of Thalictrum (Ranunculaceae); ritterazine B is one of the ritterazine analogues from *Ritterella tokioka* (Polyclinidae), and ursolic acid is a pentacyclic triterpene from *Hedyotis diffusa* (Rubiaceae); these agents were all reported to induce apoptosis *in vitro*. Ginseng extract (EAG) (Panax ginseng C.A. Meyer) exerts anticancer effects on Lewis lung carcinoma cells (LLC) and demonstrates weak activity in breast cancer and liver cancer cells; the results showed that lung cancer cells may be more likely to prompt treatment by EAG.

By modulation of ERK-p53 and NF-κB signaling, EAG revealed inhibition *in vitro* and *in vivo* of mouse LLC. Traditional Chinese herbal medicine significantly inhibited the proliferation of A549 cells, partly because of the inhibition of NF-κB activation induced by tumor necrosis factor alpha (TNF-α) [10]. H460 cell viability was reduced by plumbagin from *Plumbago indica*, and the A549 cell survival rate decreased to 17.6% at 15 μM [11]. By inhibiting the survival proteins Akt, NF-κB, Bcl-2, and survivin in H460 cells, plumbagin can induce apoptosis. In addition, many traditional herbs have induced apoptosis in lung cancer cells; other biologically active substances have also induced apoptosis: glossogin from *Glossogyne tenuifolia* (Asteraceae), a novel ginsenoside 25-OCH(3)-PPD from *Panax notoginseng* (Araliaceae), deguelin from *Lonchocarpus utilis* or *Lonchocarpus urucu* (Fabaceae), and elemene from *Curcuma kwangsiensis* (Zingiberaceae) [12].

2.2. Inhibitory effects of natural product molecules on angiogenesis and metastasis

Among the contributing factors to the spread and growth of lung cancer, angiogenesis is the most important process because it involves the growth of new blood vessels from preexisting vessels. Angiogenesis is associated with the development and spread of lung cancer because it influences the growth of novel blood vessels [13]. Thus, blockage of angiogenesis is considered an important therapeutic target for lung cancer. In the past decade, clinical trials have been conducted on angiostatin, endostatin, solimastat, bevacizumab, and angiozyme-targeting vascular endothelial growth factor (VEGF) as a key factor of angiogenesis. Selected VEGF targets have shown survival benefits in patient therapy [14]. VEGF is also related to other indirect angiogenic factors, such as basic fibroblast growth factor (bFGF), platelet-derived growth factor (PDGF), and tumor growth factor alpha (TGF-α) [15].

As a medicinal herb, *Ganoderma lucidum* (Ganodermataceae) is a basidiomycete white rot fungus, which is helpful to the treatment of various diseases such as cancer, HIV infection, diabetes, asthma, and ulcers, as demonstrated in Korea, China, and Japan [16]. Thus, many experts suggest the use of *G. lucidum* for prostate, skin, ovarian, and colon cancer therapy [17–19].

The growth of PG cells in Balb/c nude mice significantly inhibited *G. lucidum* polysaccharides. For human umbilical vein endothelial cells (HUVECs), *G. lucidum* polysaccharides also inhibited cell proliferation. Under hypoxic condition, *G. lucidum* polysaccharides inhibited the secretion of VEGF in lung cancer cells. By using chick chorioallantoic membrane (CAM) assay, *G. lucidum* polysaccharides were proven to exert an antiangiogenic effect on Balb/c mice. Overall, these results suggest that *G. lucidum* polysaccharides inhibited vascular cell proliferation in HUVECs. In human lung carcinoma PG cells, *G. lucidum* polysaccharides also reduced the secretion of VEGF. Generally, clinical researchers unexpectedly found that *G. lucidum* polysaccharides might positively influence chemo/radiotherapy by combining these compounds with the subgroups of advanced lung cancer patients, resulting in reversed immunosuppressive effects on traditional cancer therapy [20]. Although the antitumor activity against lung cancer has been recognized, we need to study its efficacy, safety, optimal concentration, and molecular targets for further research. The effect of VEGF alone or in combination with current therapies for lung cancer is also very important to be investigated through future pharmacokinetic research on animals and humans.

The most characteristic aspect of malignant neoplasm is metastasis, which is the leading cause of death in cancer patients [21]. Tumor cell dissociation, intravasation, invasion, and distribution to distant organs arrest cells in small vessels, resulting in adhesion to endothelial cells, extravasation, invasion of the target organ, and proliferation, which are all related to tumor metastasis. matrix metalloproteinases (MMPs) are related to metastasis and cancer invasion and are proteolytic enzymes in the extracellular matrix (ECM). MMP-2 and MMP-9 significantly influence the metastatic processes among the MMP family [22, 23].

2.3. Reversion of multidrug resistance

The largest difficulty of chemotherapy against cancers is multidrug resistance (MDR) [24]. Cellular overproduction of p-glycoprotein (p-gp) is one of the influencing factors leading to MDR because it can transport various anticancer drugs outward the cell. To date, a series of compounds to reverse MDR by interfering with the p-gp function have been determined [25–27]. However, some MDR reversal agents may lead to the change of pharmacokinetics and even cause serious side effects. Many anticancer drugs such as docetaxel, gemcitabine, and vinorelbine can overexpress MDR-associated proteins (MRPs), including pgp. Although this effect is helpful for inducing MDR in the treatment of NSCLC, new MDR reversal agents should be developed to avoid MDR and improve the effects of lung cancer therapy.

Stephania tetrandra (Menispermaceae) comprises a herbal formula, which is also called "Supplement energy and nourish lung" (SENL) in herbal medicines. Both *S. tetrandra* and *G. lucidum* (Ganodermataceae) demonstrate a MDR-reversal potential in SW1573/2R 120, adriamycin (ADM)-resistant lung cancer cells, and valproic acid (VPA) MDR SCLC. Solamargine (SM) suppressed MRPs in lung cancer cells, although SM is traditionally used to treat chest pains, pleurisy, pneumonia, toothache, and sore throat in India because of the major steroidal glycoalkaloid from *Solanum incanum* (Solanaceae). SM enhanced the sensitivity of apoptosis induction in tumor necrosis factor (TNF) and cisplatin-resistant lung cancer cells. After combining the treatment of SM and epirubicin, we observed that the apoptosis effect of chemotherapy was improved in A549 cells [28, 29]. Hence, we believe that SM is a potential MDR-reversal agent [30]. A test also showed that additional bioactive phytochemicals might be potential MDR-reversal agents, which include a novel monoketone curcumin analog, EF24 from *Curcuma longa* (Zingiberaceae), emodin (1,3,8-trihydroxy-6-methyl-anthraquinone) from *Rheum palmatum* (Polygonaceae), and elemene from *C. kwangsiensis* (Zingiberaceae) [31].

2.4. Reactive oxygen species (ROS) and lung cancer therapy

Recently, ROS signaling became the focus of research on lung cancer as well as other cancer therapies [32]. In recent lung cancer therapies, targeting ROS signaling was thought to be a striking method [33]. Notably, smoke-oxidative stress results in DNA damage and restrains survival signaling, which make proliferation out of control during the transfer of lung epithelial cells [34–36]. Few studies have shown that some herbal extracts and their components can eliminate active oxygen in lung cancer cells.

In Korea, people maintain oral health by using *Polygonum cuspidatum* (Polygonaceae) because of its effect in reducing oral microorganisms; Koreans also use *P. cuspidatum* in the treatment of arthritis and urinary diseases [37]. *P. cuspidatum* extract contains alkaloids, phenolics, and sterol/terpenes and induces biological activities such as anti-inflammation, antioxidation, and anticancer effects [38]. In A549 and H1650 cells, the ethanol and ethyl acetate extracts of *P. cuspidatum* can eliminate 1,1-diphenyl-2-hydrazyl (DPPH) and hydroxyl radicals. The ethyl acetate fraction (EAF) of wampee peel [*Clausena lansium* Skeels (Rutaceae)] is obtained from a species of strongly scented evergreen trees in Southeast Asia. Similarly, in comparison with cisplatin, the EAF of wampee peel exerted increased antioxidant and anticancer effects on A549 lung cancer cells, SGC-7901 gastric cancer cells, and HepG2 liver cancer cells. Thus, wampee peel should be studied to develop a natural antioxidant and pharmaceutical supplement because of the DPPH radical scavenging activity, reducing power, and superoxide scavenging activity.

Recently, Lawless et al. advised in their review paper that histone deacetylase (HDAC) can significantly regulate the oxidative stress pathways in the development of cancer in NSCLC [39–41]. The authors advised that HDAC can be consumed in several common foods such as sulforaphane from *Brassica oleracea* (Brassicaceae), curcumin from *C. longa* L. (Zingiberaceae), and epigallocatechin 3-gallate (EGCG) from *Camellia sinensis* (Theaceae) to combat NSCLC and chronic obstructive pulmonary disease (COPD). Nevertheless, further research on HDAC inhibition is necessary to develop more efficient antitumor drugs from herbal medicine. The mechanism and molecular targets of natural product molecules against lung cancer were shown in **Figures 1** and **2**.

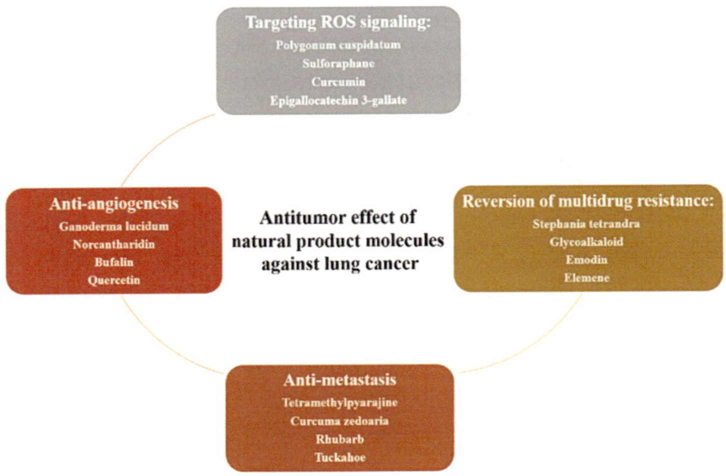

Figure 1. Mechanism of natural product molecules against lung cancer.

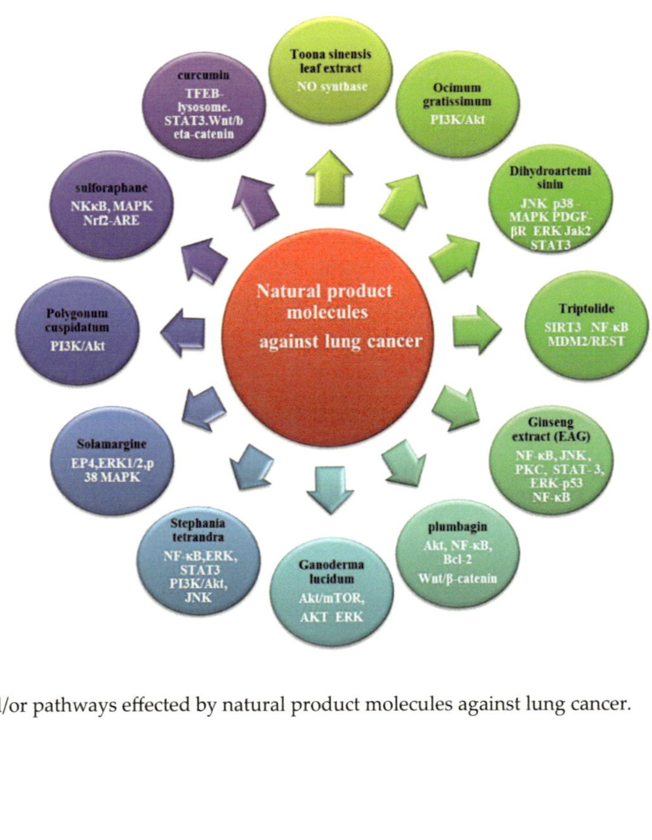

Figure 2. Targets and/or pathways effected by natural product molecules against lung cancer.

3. Antilung cancer natural product molecules in the body

The allogeneic graft model or mice xenograft is a valuable tool in cancer biology evaluation of novel anticancer activity of drug(s). Antitumor activity test is employed to measure the inhibition of the tumor growth and survival time. In vivo mouse models and some active natural product molecules also showed influence on antilung cancer.

3.1. Green tea polyphenols and lung cancer

Tea extract from the plant *C. sinensis* is the most common beverage for consumption worldwide. Important data from different studies provide evidence that drinking tea can prevent carcinogenic effects [42, 43]. All activities related to a major component of green tea exert the effects of (−)-epigallocatechin gallate (EGCG). Some mechanisms showed that EGCG-induced apoptosis and cell-cycle arrest modulation in carcinogen-metabolizing enzymes and regulate cellular signaling pathways and inhibit transcription factors in cancer cells, resulting in the inhibition of cancer development, which facilitated the prevention and treatment by green tea and its composition, particularly EGCG.

Green tea can help prevent and treat lung cancer, especially EGCG and guanosine triphosphate (GTP). Dietary supplementation of EGCG (0.1, 0.3, and 0.5%) inhibited tumor growth in nude mice implanted with thymus H1299 cells. EGCG treatment increased phosphorylated histone 2A variants X and tumor cell apoptosis, as well as oxidative DNA damage assessment of the formation of 8-hydroxy-2′-deoxyguanosine (8-OHdG). This finding presents the first evidence of EGCG induction of ROS generation, leading to tumor cell DNA oxidative damage. EGCG is commonly referred to as a powerful antioxidant, but the current results showed that EGCG can also act as an antioxidant in some cases [44]. In different stages of an experimental lung cancer, EGCG and theaflavins have been proven to reduce the proliferation index in a benzo(a)pyrene[B(a)P]-induced lung carcinogenesis mouse model. When used theaflavins in 0.02 mg/mouse/day and EGCG dose of 0.01 mg/mouse/day, results show that both of them reduced the obvious carcinoma and dysplasia in situ at 8th, 17th, and 26th weeks. In Swiss albino rats, GTP treatment and black tea polyphenols (BTP) at dosage of 0.1 and 0.2% resulted in low incidence of diethylnitrosamine-induced alveologenic tumors, which resulted in the inhibition of the expression of lung cancer caused by Akt, cyclooxygenase (COX)-2, and nuclear factor kappa-B (NF-κB) [45]. The combination of liquid Polyphenon E (0.25 or 0.25%) and atorvastatin-inhibited lung cancer induced by 4-(methylnitrosamino)-1-(3-pyridyl)-1-butanone (NNK) in mice. Low-dose combination of Polyphenon E and atorvastatin significantly reduced the lung tumor diversity and enhanced cell apoptosis but inhibited tumor burden at myelogenous leukemia 1 (Mcl-1) level. Results show that lung tumors were effectively inhibited by atorvastatin and Polyphenon E, and *in vitro* and *in vivo*, the action between the two agents was synergistic. The inhibition activity of atomized difluoromethylornithine (DFMO) and Polyphenon E (1% wt/wt diet) administration was investigated in A/J mice injected with B(a)P. Polyphenon E did not suppress tumor treatment on average diversity but decreased the animal tumor load and significantly reduced the largest carcinoma [46].

3.2. Isothiocyanates and lung cancer

Isothiocyanates (ITCs) existed in cruciferous vegetables, which are converted into glucose and ITC by the enzyme myrosinase. Benzyl isothiocyanate (BITC), phenethyl isothiocyanate (PEITC), and sulforaphane are widely studied for their chemopreventive and anticancer effects [47]. Recently, BITC-inhibited gefitinib-resistant human NSCLC growth, induction of apoptosis, caspase-3 activation, cell-cycle arrest in G2/M phase, ROS generation, glutathione depletion, inhibition of protein kinase activity, NF-κB transcription activation, and activation of mitogen-activated protein kinase (MAPK) and activating protein (AP)-1. PEITC declined the first phase of enzymes involved in the activation of several carcinogenic substances. PEITC also activated the second phase of enzyme activity, which is responsible for many carcinogenic metabolism and oxidative stresses. Isothiocyanates are proven to demonstrate anticancer behavior by inducing apoptosis and inhibition of the cell-cycle stage.

Some reports showed that several mechanisms have been postulated to determine the ITC against the mechanism of lung cancer. Importantly, researchers thought that tubulin is one of the targets in the body for ITC binding and covalent binding of BITC, PEITC, sulforaphane tubulin. Binding with cell apoptosis induced the cell ability and mitosis arrest [48]. The effect of oral sulforaphane (9 μmol/mouse/day) in reducing the oxidative damage caused by B(a)P (100 mg/kg body weight, i.p.) in Swiss albino rats was determined. Oral sulforaphane reduced hydrogen peroxide production, increased the release of mitochondrial cytochrome c, and reduced the expression of Bcl2, Bax, and caspase-3. Newborn mice were exposed to cigarette smoke for 120 consecutive days, beginning at birth, as well as to budesonide in diet (2.4 mg/kg in diet) and PEITC (1000 mg/kg in diet) and N-acetylcysteine in drinking water (1000 mg/kg) of oral drugs, until 210 days. High incidence of benign lung tumor multiplicity and an increase in pulmonary malignant tumor exposure to cigarette smoke and budesonide were observed in the carcinogenicity of PEITC and NAC treatment of mice lung exposed to cigarette smoke. Budesonide, PEITC, and NAC treatments reduced the yield of cigarette mainstream smoke, which induced lung benign or malignant tumor, showing mirror smokers' intervention in the experimental situation. As compared with the NNK-treated control group, Conaway et al. investigated the influence of sulforaphane, PEITC, and NAC yoke compound progress/J mice lung adenoma and adenocarcinoma [49] by reducing the incidence of adenocarcinoma PEITC in treated group of 3 and 1.5 mmol/kg each diet and PEITC-NAC, which used in 8 and 4 mmol/kg each diet in treatment group. Low incidence of lung cancer was showed in the treatment of sulforaphane-NAC (8 and 4 mmol/kg diet) in the diet. The results show that sulforaphane, and NAC yoke, and PEITC compound reducing cell proliferation and inducing apoptosis in tobacco carcinogen-treated A/J mice and resulting in inhibited the progress of adenocarcinoma in lung adenoma [27]. The influence of PEITC diet (3 μmol/g diet) and BITC (1 μmol/g diet) and a mixture of BITC + PEITC (1 and 3 μmol/g diet) on hemoglobin (Hb) adducts of B(a)P and DNA and NNK and two urinary metabolites are worthy of investigation. In urine, NNAL-Gluc and 4-(Methylnitrosamino)-1-(3-pyridyl)-1-butanol (NNAL) were measured. After 2 and 4 months, a significant reduction in the level of 4-hydroxy-1-(3-pyridyl)-1-butanone releasing DNA adducts of the NNK lung was caused by BITC + PEITC or PEITC, whereas no effect was demonstrated by BITC. From 2 weeks to 12 weeks, BITC + PEITC or PEITC also inhibited the Hb adduct of NNK and showed no effect on B(a)P adduct. A significant increase in the NNK level was also observed in rats after treatment with NNAL and NNAL-Gluc PEITC, as well as with PEITC or BITC + PEITC [50]. These findings suggest that PEITC or BITC + PEITC Hb released the DNA adduct formation in the lungs of mice that received B(a)P + nitrosamines. However, the BITC adduct was not influenced by B(a)P or nitrosamines. Before each of the three carcinogenic polycyclic aromatic hydrocarbons (PAHs) were found in cigarettes, treatment with BITC (6.7 and 13.4 μmol) was performed: B(a)P, 5-methylchrysene (5-MeC), and dibenz[a,h] anthracene [DBahA]; Compared with beta hydroxyl acid (BHA) and sulforaphane, these PAHs more effectively inhibited lung tumor multiplicity [51].

3.3. Indole-3-carbinol and lung cancer

An autolysis product of glucosinolate has been reported to exert anticancer effects; this product is indole-3-carbinol (I3C), which is present in Brassica plants like cabbage, cauliflower kale, broccoli, and Brussels sprouts [52].

After the postinitiation or progression protocol in A/J mice, we assessed how I3C inhibited tobacco carcinogen–induced lung adenocarcinoma. After treatment with I3C during the postinitiation period, reduction was observed in the tumor multiplicity, hyperplastic foci, adenoma, adenoma with dysplasia, and adenocarcinoma. When I3C was given during tumor progression, an increase was observed in the multiplicities of smaller tumors and decrease in larger tumors. I3C was found to efficiently inhibit the development of pulmonary adenocarcinoma. Moreover, via modulation of the phosphatidylinositol-3-kinase (PI3K)/Akt signaling pathway, the anticancer effects of I3C were mediated [53]. Silibinin used in 7 μmol/g/diet and I3C used in 10 μmol/g each diet reduced the multiplicities of tumors on the adenocarcinoma and surface of the lung in NNK-treated mice. Additionally, as compared with I3C or silibinin alone, I3C and silibinin were strongly affect cyclin D1 and poly (ADP-ribose) polymerase (PARP), p-Akt, p-ERK cleavage expression levels. Thus, against the development of lung cancer in A/J mice, this study proved that the findings of the combined treatment of silibinin and I3C afforded more protection and can be used to prevent cancer in current and former smokers [54]. Investigation of this effect showed that I3C (100 or 150 μM) on vinyl carbamate (VC) induced deregulation of microRNA (miRNA) levels in lung tissues of female A/J mice. Compared with mice treated with VC alone, the miR-21, mir-31, miR-130a, miR-146b, and miR-377 expression levels decreased in mice treated with VC and I3C in their diet. The development of lung cancer showed a significant relationship with abnormal miRNA expression. In lung tumors, compared with normal lungs, the results explained distinctive changes in the expression of several miRNAs. I3C exerted effects on most of the miRNAs. Myo-inositol (MI; 56 μmol/g/diet) and I3C (30 or 70 μmol/g/diet) against VC-induced lung cancer were applied. With higher dose on the lung surface, incidence of cancer, multiplicity, size, and adenoma with cellular pleomorphism, the lower dose of I3C showed fewer effects, whereas the higher dose of I3C decreased the multiplicities of tumors on treatment of mice. IκBα degradation, NF-κB activation, COX-2, p-Akt, and activation of caspase-3 and PARP cleavage were inhibited by treatment with higher dose of I3C [55].

3.4. Genistein and lung cancer

The most abundant isoflavone in soybean, genistein (4,5,7-trihydroxyisoflavone), has been widely reported for its chemotherapeutic and chemopreventive effects. Recently, lung tumor growth was suppressed *in vivo* in a dose-dependent manner and apparently showed no toxicity on a derivative of genistein, 7-difluoromethyl-5,4′-dimethoxygenistein [56]. A significant decrease in tumor growth was found in a xenograft model for treatment of mice with a combination of gefitinib and genistein [57]. During the phase of pneumonitis, in rats receiving genistein (750 mg/kg body weight), the increase of breathing rate was inhibited after irradiation with 18 Gy at approximately 0.5 Gy/min and a delay of 50–80 days in Sprague-Dawley rats. After irradiation for 28 weeks and treatment with genistein, TNF-α, IL-1β, TGF-β, and collagen also decreased. The levels of 8-OHdG content also decreased, and the protection against DNA damage was measured in surviving rats. Treatment with genistein after irradiation indicated that DNA damage is caused by the production of ROS, which also reduced DNA damage in the form of micronuclear formation [57].

For lung metastasis induced by B16F-10 melanoma cells in C57BL/6 mice, the inhibition effects of dietary soybean isoflavones, genistein, and daidzein were investigated. Compared with untreated tumor-bearing animals, treatment with genistein (200 μmol/kg body weight) caused lung tumor nodule formation inhibition, and the lung collagen hydroxyproline content and serum sialic acid level were inhibited. The life span of the tumor-bearing animals was also increased by treatment with genistein [58].

3.5. Curcumin and lung cancer

Curcumin (diferuloylmethane) is derived from the plant *C. longa*. The antiangiogenic, analgesic, antioxidant, anti-inflammatory, and antiseptic properties of curcumin have been widely studied [59].

Experiments showed that curcumin (0.6%) can decrease the expression of COX2 in subcutaneous tumor *in vivo* and the weight of intralung tumors but can increase the survival rate. Curcumin also increased the survival of athymic nude mice and inhibited the tumor growth of orthotopic human NSCLC xenografts [60]. Curcumin and erlotinib significantly inhibited tumor growth of erlotinib-resistant NSCLC cells *in vivo* compared with the control, and this finding suggested that during treatment with erlotinib, curcumin might be a prospective adjuvant for NSCLC patients. The growth of human lung cancer xenografts in nude mice was inhibited by oral intake of curcumin (500 mg/kg/body/day) and phosphosulindac (200 mg/kg/day); curcumin may improve the phosphosulindac bioavailability and inhibition of efflux transporters [61]. Curcumin (50-mg/kg body weight) was found to increase cell survival, which contributed to T-cell–mediated adaptive immune response and decrease in tumor growth. Low-dose curcumin increased T cells derived from 3LL-tumor-bearing mice, particularly $CD8^+$ T cells, but high-dose curcumin (100-mg/kg body weight) decreased T cells which exhibited the enhancement of cytotoxicity and interferon-γ (IFN-γ) secretion and proliferation against 3LL tumor cells. In lung-tumor-bearing models, the results pointed out that curcumin may support the immune system and induce antitumor immune response via the T-cell-mediated effect. Cancer treatment by curcumin can prove it as an immunologically safe drug. These data provide further evidence that curcumin can play a role in lung cancer therapy [62].

3.6. Fisetin and lung cancer

Fisetin (3,3′,4′,7-tetrahydroxyflavone) is found in strawberry, persimmon, grape, apple, cucumber, and onion. It is a naturally occurring flavonoid with apoptotic and antiangiogenic properties, as well as antiproliferative effects in cancer cells [63].

A previously published study showed that treatment with fisetin (25-mg/kg body weight) decreased histological lesions and lipid peroxidation levels and modulated the enzymatic and nonenzymatic antioxidants in B(a)P-treated Swiss albino mice [64]. In LLC-bearing mice, Matrigel plug assay showed that when fisetin was treated with dose of 223 mg/kg inhibited angiogenesis. Tumor growth was also inhibited by fisetin, which is similar to the effect of low-dose cyclophosphamide (30-mg/kg body weight). Combination of fisetin and cyclophosphamide led to the striking improvement in antitumor activity and decrease in microvessel density and low systemic toxicity. Fisetin exhibited anticancer activities and antiangiogenic properties in LLC-bearing mice.

3.7. Pomegranate polyphenols and lung cancer

Pomegranate (*Punica granatum*, Punicaceae) was cultivated in Afghanistan, India, China, Japan, Russia, and the United States. It is an edible fruit widely comprising about 80% juice and 20% seed.

Pomegranate can provide oral administration of pomegranate fruit extract (PFE), which caused tumor growth inhibition in athymic nude mice implanted with human lung cancer A549 cells. Pomegranate can induce the appearance of small solid tumors, which prolonged survival time in animal models [65]. B(a)P and N-nitroso-tris-chloroethylurea (NTCU) in A/J mice were investigated, caused of effects of oral consumption of a human-achievable dose of PFE dose of 0.2%, w/v effect on progression, angiogenesis, growth, and signaling pathways in two models of lung cancer. For treatment with PFE and B(a)P or NTCU, we found little lung tumor multiplicities of tumor incidence in mice. Oral administration of PFE caused inhibition of NF-κB, MAPK, and PI3K, as well as phosphorylation of Akt, mammalian target of rapamycin (mTOR), c-met, and lung markers that inhibited B(a)P- and NTCU-treated mice; cell proliferation and angiogenesis were also inhibited. By targeting multiple signaling pathways and associated events, PFE demonstrated activity against lung cancer, and these events are critical for the development and progression of lung carcinoma [66]. Molecular targets of antilung cancer natural product molecules in the body were shown in **Table 1**.

Active natural products for antilung cancer	**Molecular targets**					
Green tea	MAPK	mTOR	EGFR	p53	PKC	TGF-β
Isothiocyanates	MAPK	AP-1	NF-κB	Akt	Nrf2	Keap1
Genistein	EGFR	PGE2	Akt	NF-κB	Cox-2	TNF-α
Pomegranate	PI3K	Akt	mTOR	MAPK	c-met	NF-κB
Fisetin	Akt	mTOR	PI3K	AMPKα	AP-1	NF-κB
Curcumin	Wnt/β-catenin	Cox-2	NF-κB	EGFR	STAT-3	Survivin
Indole-3-carbinol	IL-6	IL-1β	p53	PI3K	Akt	Cox-2

Table 1. Antilung cancer natural product molecules in the body and molecular targets.

4. Natural product molecules for the treatment of lung cancer in clinical trials

Complementary and alternative medicine (CAM), including natural product molecules, increased survival in cancer patients [67]. Recently, 453 cancer patients in a cohort study showed that 77% of patients use herbal medicines combined with conventional treatment to reduce the therapy-associated toxicity and cancer-related symptoms, improve the immune system, and even eliminate cancer directly [68].

Conventional chemotherapy is combined with natural product molecules to increase the therapeutic effect and QoL. Sixty-three in-patients diagnosed with IV NSCLC and stage IIIb were treated as randomized-controlled trial, Gujin granules (Jiangyin Tianjiang Pharmaceutical Co., China) and Shengmai injection (Ya'an Sanjiu Pharmaceutical Co., China) were administered intravenously and orally. Navelbine and cisplatin (NP) chemotherapy were treated in all the groups. This combination therapy enhanced median survival time (P = 0.014) and response rate to 48.5% (16/33) compared to untreated control (32.2% = 9/28) in the control group (P = 0.0373). However, herbal medicine did not affect the bone marrow inhibition occurrence, median time to progression, 1-year survival rate, and mean cycles of chemotherapy applied. Among 232 NSCLC patients, by using the QoL scale of the European Organization for Research on Treatment of Cancer (QLQ-C30) (Lin and Li, 2007), treated with Shenqi-fuzheng injection (Lizhu Co., China), improved QoL and the response rate. In another trail, Yiqi Yangyin Jiedu Decoction significantly increased the immunological parameters and Karnofsky (KPS) score, including $CD4^+$, $CD4^+/CD8^+$, $CD3^+$, and $CD8^+/CD28^+$, and all the patients were treated with NP or gemcitabine and cisplatin (GP) compared with the untreated control [69].

Natural product molecules can improve the QoL of patients with lung cancer. Recently, QoL is improved in NSCLC patients with long-term prognostic factors of survival. In a RCT and herbal Feiji recipe, Feiji was found to improve the clinical therapeutic effect, reduce the side effects of chemotherapy before this research by adding higher scores in the role, as well as the social and economic status ($P < 0.05$ or $P < 0.01$) based on the QLQ C30 questionnaire. Similarly, in a clinical trial of 294 patients with advanced NSCLC and treated with Shenfu injection of traditional Chinese medicine, on the basis of the functional assessment of cancer therapy-lung (FACT-L), Chinese medicine positively affected health when used alone, as well as with emotional, functional, and additional care when performing traditional chemotherapy ($P < 0.05$) [70].

The negative influence of natural product molecules is shown by traditional intervention. One of the main risks of conventional treatment is pneumonia in patients with lung cancer, and this complication may be caused by radiation therapy intervention and symptoms of severe dyspnea, cough, fever, respiratory failure and/or verticillium wilt in severe cases. With Dixiong soup in clinical trials of 46 NSCLC patients who underwent radiotherapy, based on the incidence of pneumonia after radiotherapy and QoL using continued to shrink the clinical imaging physical difficulty breathing (CRP) score, tumor radiotherapy group (RTOG) rating scores, and KPS score, Dixiong Shang Xianzhu reduced the incidence of radioactive pneumonia (treatment, 10.0%; control, 26.3%; $P = 0.0032$) and improved the continued decline of CRP dyspnea score, RTOG classification score ($P < 0.05$), and KPS score ($P < 0.01$). Similarly, substantial evidence demonstrated good effect of herbal Liangxue jiedu huoxue soup, Qingjin runfei decoction, and Shenqi fuzheng injection. Hydrochloric acid, stand for kang, topoisomerase inhibitors, and Chinese tree *Camptotheca acuminata* (Cornaceae) are used for lung cancer treatment combined with other conventional drugs, in spite of the side effects including leukopenia and diarrhea. With Hangeshash into RCTs, 44 irinotecan-treated NSCLC patients showed that TJ-14 can significantly improve the grade ($P = 0.044$) and frequency of diarrhea to grades 3 and 4 ($P = 0.018$). A list of therapeutic approaches and outcome assessment and the quality of herbal medication were listed in **Table 2** [71].

CHM formula	No. of participants/ dropout or withdrawal	TNM stage	Control group intervention	Assessment of outcome	Duration (week)	Jadad scale
Shengmai injection Gujin grand decoction	106/6 dropout patients	IIIB–IV	NP	Tumor response, survival rate, chemotoxicity	12	3
Feiji recipe	77/0	IIIB–IV	NP/TP	Tumor response, survival rate, CD62P	8	3
Yinqi Yangyin decoction	60/3 withdrawals	IIIB–IV	GP	Tumor response, survival rate, chemotoxicity, KPS	8	3
Fuzheng Kangai decoction	129/drop out: 5 patients in CTC and 4 patients in CT; withdraw: 2 patients in CTC and 3 patients in CT	IIIB–IV	MVP combined with radiotherapy	Tumor response, chemotoxicity, KPS	12	3
Shengmai injection	60/0	IIB–IV	DP	Tumor response, chemotoxicity	8	3

Table 2. Therapeutic approaches and outcome assessment of herbal medication.

5. Constraints and current clinical trials and the challenges of natural product molecules

The traditional Chinese medicine (TCM) clinical research also presents some limitations and difficulties. As mentioned in a recent review, TCM, including herbal medicine, establishes its unique features, such as holism and personalization. According to the theory of traditional Chinese medicine, a patient is diagnosed with symptoms rather than the disease itself and prescribed with a personalized herbal formula to treat the symptoms. Although RCT is a powerful tool to verify the clinical curative effect of health care, a RCT on the application of personalized herbs remains a challenge because of heterogeneous batch management. Likewise, Chinese medicine intervention heterogeneity leads to some difficulties for high-performance analysis of natural product molecules. Therefore, for cancer research in the future, particularly on herbs and plant chemicals, we suggest that the quality control should be performed consistently with batch and pharmacokinetic studies on TCM and its components, which perform antitumor activities in lung cancer.

There still exist some problems to standardize in the use of natural products in prevention or treatment lung cancer. First, the purity of traditional Chinese medicine is not high, most of the traditional Chinese medicine preparations from to the original drug, powder, or crude extract, so it works slowly. Second, inconvenient to use, taking traditional Chinese medicine generally to a large package of herbs, and not easy to drink because of bitterness. Third, the dose of natural products is difficult to grasp, and the available activity contents are different due to the different plants.

As a result, the problems should be specified to herbs in the QoL in a sense, and the therapeutic effect may vary among different batches. Furthermore, the lack of rigorous methods, risk of possible bias, and a relatively small number of patients involved were repeatedly pointed out in the previous literature on herbal application in lung cancer patients.

However, the most recent basic and clinical research showed a growing body of evidence to support the notion indicating that herbs may be beneficial and effective in the treatment and improvement of the QoL of patients with lung cancer, as well as prevent the side effects of conventional therapy and improve the immune parameters. However, researchers must develop novel specific methods to completely solve the challenges of the present study and verify the credibility of possible herbs.

Despite the great progress of lung cancer treatment, lung cancer remains a leading cause of cancer death worldwide. Molecule-targeted therapy has recently attracted research attention; for example, the treatment of tyrosine kinase inhibitors and erlotinib for epidermal growth factor receptor (EGFR) and its downstream mTOR signaling factors and bevacizumab, as well as humanized monoclonal antibody, can bind to VEGF to increase the response rate and progression-free survival (PFS) of patients on treatment with carboplatin, paclitaxel, cisplatin, and gemcitabine in phase II trials. Plenty of evidence from a previous study showed that the eastern medicine herbal therapy is effective in lung cancer treatment by regulating cell proliferation, apoptosis, angiogenesis, and metastasis in multidrug-resistant tuberculosis patients. These activities can participate in a biological process of target molecule toxicity to normalize lung epithelial cells in lung cancer. Although various herbal formulas and plants are traditionally used to treat lung diseases since the ancient times, the folk prescription of lung cancer guidelines and standards is the first published by the American College of Chest Physicians including complementary and alternative medicine in 2007, as well as the systematic review of the potential of herbs and its active compounds in lung cancer treatment without execution. In the current review, we recommend the potential of herbs and plant chemicals, which are commonly used for the treatment of lung diseases, including cancer, for folk prescription of critical data analysis and discussion *in vitro* or *in vivo* laboratory experimental models and clinical trials. Overall, we conclude that herbs and plant chemicals are potentially effective anticancer drugs for the treatment and prevention of lung cancer by adjusting the multimolecular targets involved in angiogenesis, metastasis, and serious side effects, thereby providing only quality control and reproducibility of problem solving.

Author details

Wei-long Zhong[1], Yuan Qin[1], Shuang Chen[2] and Tao Sun[1]*

*Address all correspondence to: sunrockmia@hotmail.com

1 State Key Laboratory of Medicinal Chemical Biology and College of Pharmacy, Nankai University, Tianjin, People's Republic of China

2 Tianjin Key Laboratory of Molecular Drug Research, Tianjin International Joint Academy of Biomedicine, Tianjin, People's Republic of China

References

[1] Gorlova, O.Y., et al., Aggregation of cancer among relatives of never-smoking lung cancer patients. Int J Cancer, 2007. 121(1): pp. 111–8.

[2] Catelinois, O., et al., Lung cancer attributable to indoor radon exposure in France: impact of the risk models and uncertainty analysis. Environ Health Perspect, 2006. 114(9): pp. 1361–6.

[3] Broker, L.E. and G. Giaccone, The role of new agents in the treatment of non-small cell lung cancer. Eur J Cancer, 2002. 38(18): pp. 2347–61.

[4] Kukunoor, R., J. Shah, and T. Mekhail, Targeted therapy for lung cancer. Curr Oncol Rep, 2003. 5(4): pp. 326–33.

[5] Hirsch, F.R., et al., Epidermal growth factor family of receptors in preneoplasia and lung cancer: perspectives for targeted therapies. Lung Cancer, 2003. 41(Suppl 1): pp. S29–42.

[6] Jacobson, M.D., J.F. Burne, and M.C. Raff, Mechanisms of programmed cell death and Bcl-2 protection. Biochem Soc Trans, 1994. 22(3): pp. 600–2.

[7] Yang, Y.C., et al., Enhancement of glucose uptake in 3 T3-L1 adipocytes by *Toona sinensis* leaf extract. Kaohsiung J Med Sci, 2003. 19(7): pp. 327–33.

[8] Li, M., X. Li, and J.C. Li, Possible mechanisms of trichosanthin-induced apoptosis of tumor cells. Anat Rec (Hoboken), 2010. 293(6): pp. 986–92

[9] Hsu, Y.L., et al., Acacetin-induced cell cycle arrest and apoptosis in human non-small cell lung cancer A549 cells. Cancer Lett, 2004. 212(1): pp. 53–60.

[10] Wang, J.Y., et al., Effects of Feiyanning Decoction on gene expression of nuclear factor-kappaB activated by tumor necrosis factor-alpha in lung adenocarcinoma cell line. Zhong Xi Yi Jie He Xue Bao, 2009. 7(3): pp. 249–54.

[11] Gomathinayagam, R., et al., Anticancer mechanism of plumbagin, a natural compound, on non-small cell lung cancer cells. Anticancer Res, 2008. 28(2A): pp. 785–92.

[12] Hsu, H.F., et al., Glossogin, a novel phenylpropanoid from *Glossogyne tenuifolia*, induced apoptosis in A549 lung cancer cells. Food Chem Toxicol, 2008. 46(12): pp. 3785–91.

[13] Kilarski, W.W., et al., An *in vivo* neovascularization assay for screening regulators of angiogenesis and assessing their effects on pre-existing vessels. Angiogenesis, 2012. 15(4): pp. 643–55.

[14] Revannasiddaiah, S. and S.P. Susheela, Chemically enhanced radiotherapy: visions for the future. Ann Transl Med, 2016. 4(3): p. 52.

[15] Cao, Y., Future options of anti-angiogenic cancer therapy. Chin J Cancer, 2016. 35: p. 21.

[16] Hsu, C.L. and G.C. Yen, Ganoderic acid and lucidenic acid (triterpenoid). Enzymes, 2014. 36: pp. 33–56.

[17] Dan, X., et al., A ribonuclease isolated from wild *Ganoderma lucidum* suppressed autophagy and triggered apoptosis in colorectal cancer cells. Front Pharmacol, 2016. 7: p. 217.

[18] Saylam Kurtipek, G., et al., Resolution of cutaneous sarcoidosis following topical application of *Ganoderma lucidum* (reishi mushroom). Dermatol Ther (Heidelb), 2016. 6(1): pp. 105–9.

[19] Kim, T.H., et al., Induction of apoptosis in MCF7 human breast cancer cells by Khz (fusion of *Ganoderma lucidum* and *Polyporus umbellatus* mycelium). Mol Med Rep, 2016. 13(2): pp. 1243–9.

[20] Gao, Y., et al., Effects of water-soluble *Ganoderma lucidum* polysaccharides on the immune functions of patients with advanced lung cancer. J Med Food, 2005. 8(2): pp. 159–68.

[21] Lee, J.M., et al., Inflammation in lung carcinogenesis: new targets for lung cancer chemoprevention and treatment. Crit Rev Oncol Hematol, 2008. 66(3): pp. 208–17.

[22] Han, M., Y. Song, and X. Zhang, Quercetin suppresses the migration and invasion in human colon cancer Caco-2 cells through regulating toll-like receptor 4/nuclear factor-kappa B pathway. Pharmacogn Mag, 2016. 12(Suppl 2): pp. S237–44.

[23] Jiang, Q., et al., Lunasin suppresses the migration and invasion of breast cancer cells by inhibiting matrix metalloproteinase-2/-9 via the FAK/Akt/ERK and NF-kappaB signaling pathways. Oncol Rep, 2016. 36(1): pp. 253–62.

[24] Hipfner, D.R., et al., Monoclonal antibodies that inhibit the transport function of the 190-kDa multidrug resistance protein, MRP. Localization of their epitopes to the nucleotide-binding domains of the protein. J Biol Chem, 1999. 274(22): pp. 15420–6.

[25] Lima, J.P., et al., Optimal duration of first-line chemotherapy for advanced non-small cell lung cancer: a systematic review with meta-analysis. Eur J Cancer, 2009. 45(4): pp. 601–7.

[26] Einhorn, L.H., First-line chemotherapy for non-small-cell lung cancer: is there a superior regimen based on histology? J Clin Oncol, 2008. 26(21): pp. 3485–6.

[27] Abou-Mourad, Y., et al., Docetaxel and irinotecan as first-line chemotherapy in patients with advanced non-small-cell lung cancer: a pilot study. J Med Liban, 2008. 56(1): pp. 16–21.

[28] Sadava, D., et al., Effect of Ganoderma on drug-sensitive and multidrug-resistant small-cell lung carcinoma cells. Cancer Lett, 2009. 277(2): pp. 182–9.

[29] Sadava, D., et al., Effects of four Chinese herbal extracts on drug-sensitive and multidrug-resistant small-cell lung carcinoma cells. Cancer Chemother Pharmacol, 2002. 49(4): pp. 261–6.

[30] Thomas, S.L., et al., Activation of the p38 pathway by a novel monoketone curcumin analog, EF24, suggests a potential combination strategy. Biochem Pharmacol, 2010. 80(9): pp. 1309–16.

[31] Xu, M., et al., Reversal effect of *Stephania tetrandra*-containing Chinese herb formula SENL on multidrug resistance in lung cancer cell line SW1573/2R120. Am J Chin Med, 2010. 38(2): pp. 401–13.

[32] Trachootham, D., J. Alexandre, and P. Huang, Targeting cancer cells by ROS-mediated mechanisms: a radical therapeutic approach?. Nat Rev Drug Discov, 2009. 8(7): pp. 579–91.

[33] Faux, S.P., et al., The role of oxidative stress in the biological responses of lung epithelial cells to cigarette smoke. Biomarkers, 2009. 14(Suppl 1): pp. 90–6.

[34] Dandona, P., et al., Angiotensin II receptor blocker valsartan suppresses reactive oxygen species generation in leukocytes, nuclear factor-kappa B, in mononuclear cells of normal subjects: evidence of an antiinflammatory action. J Clin Endocrinol Metab, 2003. 88(9): pp. 4496–501.

[35] Binda, M.M., et al., Effect of reactive oxygen species scavengers, antiinflammatory drugs, and calcium-channel blockers on carbon dioxide pneumoperitoneum-enhanced adhesions in a laparoscopic mouse model. Surg Endosc, 2007. 21(10): pp. 1826–34.

[36] Ghanim, H., et al., An antiinflammatory and reactive oxygen species suppressive effects of an extract of *Polygonum cuspidatum* containing resveratrol. J Clin Endocrinol Metab, 2010. 95(9): pp. E1–8.

[37] Li, Y.B., et al., Protective, antioxidative and antiapoptotic effects of 2-methoxy-6-acetyl-7-methyljuglone from *Polygonum cuspidatum* in PC12 cells. Planta Med, 2011. 77(4): pp. 354–61.

[38] Shin, J.A., et al., Apoptotic effect of *Polygonum cuspidatum* in oral cancer cells through the regulation of specificity protein 1. Oral Dis, 2011. 17(2): pp. 162–70.

[39] Lawless, M.W., K.J. O'Byrne, and S.G. Gray, Oxidative stress induced lung cancer and COPD: opportunities for epigenetic therapy. J Cell Mol Med, 2009. 13(9A): pp. 2800–21.

[40] Kachadourian, R., et al., Casiopeina IIgly-induced oxidative stress and mitochondrial dysfunction in human lung cancer A549 and H157 cells. Toxicology, 2010. 268(3): pp. 176–83.

[41] Lee, Y.M., et al., Inhibition of glutamine utilization sensitizes lung cancer cells to apigenin-induced apoptosis resulting from metabolic and oxidative stress. Int J Oncol, 2016. 48(1): pp. 399–408.

[42] Jin, L., et al., Epigallocatechin gallate promotes p53 accumulation and activity via the inhibition of MDM2-mediated p53 ubiquitination in human lung cancer cells. Oncol Rep, 2013. 29(5): pp. 1983–90.

[43] Liu, L.C., et al., EGCG inhibits transforming growth factor-beta-mediated epithelial-to-mesenchymal transition via the inhibition of Smad2 and Erk1/2 signaling pathways in nonsmall cell lung cancer cells. J Agric Food Chem, 2012. 60(39): pp. 9863–73.

[44] Li, G.X., et al., Pro-oxidative activities and dose-response relationship of (-)-epigallocatechin-3-gallate in the inhibition of lung cancer cell growth: a comparative study *in vivo* and *in vitro*. Carcinogenesis, 2010. 31(5): pp. 902–10.

[45] Roy, P., et al., Tea polyphenols inhibit cyclooxygenase-2 expression and block activation of nuclear factor-kappa B and Akt in diethylnitrosoamine induced lung tumors in Swiss mice. Invest New Drugs, 2010. 28(4): pp. 466–71.

[46] Katiyar, S.K., R. Agarwal, and H. Mukhtar, Protective effects of green tea polyphenols administered by oral intubation against chemical carcinogen-induced forestomach and pulmonary neoplasia in A/J mice. Cancer Lett, 1993. 73(2–3): pp. 167–72.

[47] Shapiro, T.A., et al., Chemoprotective glucosinolates and isothiocyanates of broccoli sprouts: metabolism and excretion in humans. Cancer Epidemiol Biomarkers Prev, 2001. 10(5): pp. 501–8.

[48] Mi, L., et al., Covalent binding to tubulin by isothiocyanates. A mechanism of cell growth arrest and apoptosis. J Biol Chem, 2008. 283(32): pp. 22136–46.

[49] Balansky, R., et al., Prevention of cigarette smoke-induced lung tumors in mice by budesonide, phenethyl isothiocyanate, and N-acetylcysteine. Int J Cancer, 2010. 126(5): pp. 1047–54.

[50] Boysen, G., et al., Effects of benzyl isothiocyanate and 2-phenethyl isothiocyanate on benzo[a]pyrene and 4-(methylnitrosamino)-1-(3-pyridyl)-1-butanone metabolism in F-344 rats. Carcinogenesis, 2003. 24(3): pp. 517–25.

[51] Hecht, S.S., et al., Benzyl isothiocyanate: an effective inhibitor of polycyclic aromatic hydrocarbon tumorigenesis in A/J mouse lung. Cancer Lett, 2002. 187(1–2): pp. 87–94.

[52] Steinmetz, K.A. and J.D. Potter, Vegetables, fruit, and cancer prevention: a review. J Am Diet Assoc, 1996. 96(10): pp. 1027–39.

[53] Qian, X., et al., Indole-3-carbinol inhibited tobacco smoke carcinogen-induced lung adenocarcinoma in A/J mice when administered during the post-initiation or progression phase of lung tumorigenesis. Cancer Lett, 2011. 311(1): pp. 57–65.

[54] Dagne, A., et al., Enhanced inhibition of lung adenocarcinoma by combinatorial treatment with indole-3-carbinol and silibinin in A/J mice. Carcinogenesis, 2011. 32(4): pp. 561–7.

[55] Kassie, F., et al., Inhibition of vinyl carbamate-induced pulmonary adenocarcinoma by indole-3-carbinol and myo-inositol in A/J mice. Carcinogenesis, 2010. 31(2): pp. 239–45.

[56] Peng, B., et al., Inhibition of proliferation and induction of G1-phase cell-cycle arrest by dFMGEN, a novel genistein derivative, in lung carcinoma A549 cells. Drug Chem Toxicol, 2013. 36(2): pp. 196–204.

[57] Zhu, H., et al., Synergistic inhibitory effects by the combination of gefitinib and genistein on NSCLC with acquired drug-resistance *in vitro* and *in vivo*. Mol Biol Rep, 2012. 39(4): pp. 4971–9.

[58] Menon, L.G., et al., Effect of isoflavones genistein and daidzein in the inhibition of lung metastasis in mice induced by B16F-10 melanoma cells. Nutr Cancer, 1998. 30(1): pp. 74–7.

[59] Ye, M.X., et al., Curcumin: updated molecular mechanisms and intervention targets in human lung cancer. Int J Mol Sci, 2012. 13(3): pp. 3959–78.

[60] Lev-Ari, S., et al., Curcumin induces apoptosis and inhibits growth of orthotopic human non-small cell lung cancer xenografts. J Nutr Biochem, 2014. 25(8): pp. 843–50.

[61] Cheng, K.W., et al., Curcumin enhances the lung cancer chemopreventive efficacy of phospho-sulindac by improving its pharmacokinetics. Int J Oncol, 2013. 43(3): pp. 895–902.

[62] Moghaddam, S.J., et al., Curcumin inhibits COPD-like airway inflammation and lung cancer progression in mice. Carcinogenesis, 2009. 30(11): pp. 1949–56.

[63] Arai, Y., et al., Dietary intakes of flavonols, flavones and isoflavones by Japanese women and the inverse correlation between quercetin intake and plasma LDL cholesterol concentration. J Nutr, 2000. 130(9): pp. 2243–50.

[64] Ravichandran, N., et al., Fisetin, a novel flavonol attenuates benzo(a)pyrene-induced lung carcinogenesis in Swiss albino mice. Food Chem Toxicol, 2011. 49(5): pp. 1141–7.

[65] Khan, N., et al., Pomegranate fruit extract inhibits prosurvival pathways in human A549 lung carcinoma cells and tumor growth in athymic nude mice. Carcinogenesis, 2007. 28(1): pp. 163–73.

[66] Khan, N., et al., Oral consumption of pomegranate fruit extract inhibits growth and progression of primary lung tumors in mice. Cancer Res, 2007. 67(7): pp. 3475–82.

[67] Boon, H.S., F. Olatunde, and S.M. Zick, Trends in complementary/alternative medicine use by breast cancer survivors: comparing survey data from 1998 and 2005. BMC Women's Health, 2007. 7: p. 4.

[68] Richardson, M.A., et al., Complementary/alternative medicine use in a comprehensive cancer center and the implications for oncology. J Clin Oncol, 2000. 18(13): pp. 2505–14.

[69] Liu, L.S., J.X. Liu, and C.J. Li, Clinical effect of yiqi yangyin jiedu decoction in treating patients with advanced non-small cell lung cancer. Zhongguo Zhong Xi Yi Jie He Za Zhi, 2008. 28(4): pp. 352–5.

[70] Lin, L.Z., D.H. Zhou, and X.T. Zheng, Effect of traditional Chinese medicine in improving quality of life of patients with non-small cell lung cancer in late stage. Zhongguo Zhong Xi Yi Jie He Za Zhi, 2006. 26(5): pp. 389–93.

[71] Li, S.G., H.Y. Chen, C.S. Ou-Yang, et al., The efficacy of Chinese herbal medicine as an adjunctive therapy for advanced non-small cell lung cancer: a systematic review and meta-analysis. PLoS One, 2013. 8(2): p. e57604.